P9-CQY-328

1996
YEAR BOOK OF
SPORTS MEDICINE®

Statement of Purpose

The YEAR BOOK Service

The YEAR BOOK series was devised in 1901 by practicing health professionals who observed that the literature of medicine and related disciplines had become so voluminous that no one individual could read and place in perspective every potential advance in a major specialty. In the final decade of the 20th century, this recognition is more acutely true than it was in 1901.

More than merely a series of books, YEAR BOOK volumes are the tangible results of a unique service designed to accomplish the following:

- to *survey* a wide range of journals of proven value
- to *select* from those journals papers representing significant advances and statements of important clinical principles
- to provide *abstracts* of those articles that are readable, convenient summaries of their key points
- to provide *commentary* about those articles to place them in perspective

These publications grow out of a unique process that calls on the talents of outstanding authorities in clinical and fundamental disciplines, trained literature specialists, and professional writers, all supported by the resources of Mosby, the world's preeminent publisher for the health professions.

The Literature Base

Mosby and its editors survey more than 1,000 journals published worldwide, covering the full range of the health professions. On an annual basis, the publisher examines usage patterns and polls its expert authorities to add new journals to the literature base and to delete journals that are no longer useful as potential YEAR BOOK sources.

The Literature Survey

The publisher's team of literature specialists, all of whom are trained and experienced health professionals, examines every original, peer-reviewed article in each journal issue. More than 250,000 articles per year are scanned systematically, including title, text, illustrations, tables, and references. Each scan is compared, article by article, to the search strategies that the publisher has developed in consultation with the 270 outside experts who form the pool of YEAR BOOK editors. A given article may be reviewed by any number of editors, from one to a dozen or more, regardless of the discipline for which the paper was originally published. In turn, each editor who receives the article reviews it to determine whether or not the article should be included in the YEAR BOOK. This decision is based on the article's inherent quality, its probable usefulness to readers of that YEAR BOOK, and the editor's goal to represent a balanced picture of a given field in each volume of the YEAR BOOK. In addition, the editor indicates when to include figures and tables from the article to help the YEAR BOOK reader better understand the information.

Of the quarter million articles scanned each year, only 5% are selected for detailed analysis within the YEAR BOOK series, thereby assuring readers of the high value of every selection.

The Abstract

The publisher's abstracting staff is headed by a seasoned medical professional and includes individuals with training in the life sciences, medicine, and other areas, plus extensive experience in writing for the health professions and related industries. Each selected article is assigned to a specific writer on this abstracting staff. The abstracter, guided in many cases by notations supplied by the expert editor, writes a structured, condensed summary designed so that the reader can rapidly acquire the essential information contained in the article.

The Commentary

The YEAR BOOK editorial boards, sometimes assisted by guest commentators, write comments that place each article in perspective for the reader. This provides the reader with the equivalent of a personal consultation with a leading international authority—an opportunity to better understand the value of the article and to benefit from the authority's thought processes in assessing the article.

Additional Editorial Features

The editorial boards of each YEAR BOOK organize the abstracts and comments to provide a logical and satisfying sequence of information. To enhance the organization, editors also provide introductions to sections or individual chapters, comments linking a number of abstracts, citations to additional literature, and other features.

The published YEAR BOOK contains enhanced bibliographic citations for each selected article, including extended listings of multiple authors and identification of author affiliations. Each YEAR BOOK contains a Table of Contents specific to that year's volume. From year to year, the Table of Contents for a given YEAR BOOK will vary depending on developments within the field.

Every YEAR BOOK contains a list of the journals from which papers have been selected. This list represents a subset of the more than 1,000 journals surveyed by the publisher and occasionally reflects a particularly pertinent article from a journal that is not surveyed on a routine basis.

Finally, each volume contains a comprehensive subject index and an index to authors of each selected paper.

The 1996 Year Book Series

Year Book of Allergy, Asthma, and Clinical Immunology: Drs. Rosenwasser, Borish, Gelfand, Leung, Nelson, and Szefler

Year Book of Anesthesiology and Pain Management: Drs. Tinker, Abram, Chestnut, Roizen, Rothenberg, and Wood

Year Book of Cardiology®: Drs. Schlant, Collins, Engle, Gersh, Kaplan, and Waldo

Year Book of Chiropractic®: Dr. Lawrence

Year Book of Critical Care Medicine®: Drs. Parrillo, Balk, Calvin, Franklin, and Shapiro

Year Book of Dentistry®: Drs. Meskin, Berry, Kennedy, Leinfelder, Roser, Summitt, and Zakariasen

Year Book of Dermatologic Surgery®: Drs. Swanson, Glogau, and Salasche

Year Book of Dermatology®: Drs. Sober and Fitzpatrick

Year Book of Diagnostic Radiology®: Drs. Federle, Clark, Gross, Latchaw, Madewell, Maynard, and Young

Year Book of Digestive Diseases®: Drs. Greenberger and Moody

Year Book of Drug Therapy®: Drs. Lasagna and Weintraub

Year Book of Emergency Medicine®: Drs. Wagner, Dronen, Davidson, King, Niemann, and Roberts

Year Book of Endocrinology®: Drs. Bagdade, Braverman, Horton, Kannan, Landsberg, Molitch, Morley, Nathan, Odell, Poehlman, Rogol, and Ryan

Year Book of Family Practice®: Drs. Berg, Bowman, Davidson, Dexter, and Scherger

Year Book of Geriatrics and Gerontology®: Drs. Beck, Burton, Rabins, Reuben, Roth, Shapiro, and Whitehouse

Year Book of Hand Surgery®: Drs. Amadio and Hentz

Year Book of Hematology®: Drs. Spivak, Bell, Ness, Quesenberry, Wiernik, and Blume

Year Book of Infectious Diseases®: Drs. Keusch, Barza, Bennish, Klempner, Skolnik, and Snydman

Year Book of Infertility and Reproductive Endocrinology: Drs. Mishell, Lobo, and Sokol

Year Book of Medicine®: Drs. Bone, Cline, Epstein, Greenberger, Malawista, Mandell, O'Rourke, and Utiger

Year Book of Neonatal and Perinatal Medicine®: Drs. Fanaroff and Klaus

Year Book of Nephrology, Hypertension, and Mineral Metabolism: Drs. Coe, Curtis, Favus, Henderson, Kashgarian, Luke, and Myers

Year Book of Neurology and Neurosurgery®: Drs. Bradley and Wilkins

Year Book of Neuroradiology: Drs. Osborn, Eskridge, Grossman, Hudgins, and Ross

Year Book of Nuclear Medicine®: Drs. Gottschalk, Blaufox, McAfee, Wackers, and Zubal

Year Book of Obstetrics and Gynecology®: Drs. Mishell, Herbst, and Kirschbaum

Year Book of Occupational and Environmental Medicine®: Drs. Emmett, Frank, Gochfeld, and Hessl

Year Book of Oncology®: Drs. Simone, Bosl, Cohen, Glatstein, Ozols, and Tallman

Year Book of Ophthalmology®: Drs. Cohen, Augsburger, Eagle, Flanagan, Grossman, Laibson, Maguire, Nelson, Rapuano, Sergott, Tasman, Tipperman, and Wilson

Year Book of Orthopedics®: Drs. Sledge, Cofield, Dobyns, Griffin, Poss, Springfield, Swiontkowski, Wiesel, and Wilson

Year Book of Otolaryngology–Head and Neck Surgery®: Drs. Paparella and Holt

Year Book of Pain: Drs. Gebhart, Haddox, Jacox, Janjan, Marcus, Rudy, and Shapiro

Year Book of Pathology and Laboratory Medicine: Drs. Mills, Bruns, Gaffey, and Stoler

Year Book of Pediatrics®: Dr. Stockman

Year Book of Plastic, Reconstructive, and Aesthetic Surgery®: Drs. Miller, Cohen, McKinney, Robson, Ruberg, and Whitaker

Year Book of Podiatric Medicine and Surgery®: Dr. Kominsky

Year Book of Psychiatry and Applied Mental Health®: Drs. Talbott, Ballenger, Breier, Frances, Meltzer, Schowalter, and Tasman

Year Book of Pulmonary Disease®: Drs. Bone and Petty

Year Book of Rheumatology®: Drs. Sergent, LeRoy, Meenan, Panush, and Reichlin

Year Book of Sports Medicine®: Drs. Shephard, Drinkwater, Eichner, Torg, Col. Anderson, and Mr. George

Year Book of Surgery®: Drs. Copeland, Bland, Deitch, Eberlein, Howard, Luce, Seeger, Souba, and Sugarbaker

Year Book of Thoracic and Cardiovascular Surgery®: Drs. Ginsberg, Wechsler, and Williams

Year Book of Ultrasound®: Drs. Merritt, Carroll, and Fleischer

Year Book of Urology®: Drs. DeKernion and Howards

Year Book of Vascular Surgery®: Dr. Porter

1996
The Year Book of SPORTS MEDICINE®

Editor-in-Chief

Roy J. Shephard, M.D., Ph.D., D.P.E.

School of Physical and Health Education and Professor Emeritus of Applied Physiology, Department of Preventive Medicine and Biostatistics, University of Toronto; and CTAL Resident Scholar in Health Studies, Brock University, St. Catharine's, Ontario

Editors

Col. James L. Anderson, PE.D.

Director of Physical Education, United States Military Academy, West Point

Barbara L. Drinkwater, Ph.D.

Research Physiologist, Department of Medicine, Pacific Medical Center, Seattle

Edward R. Eichner, M.D.

Professor of Medicine, University of Oklahoma Health Sciences Center, Oklahoma City

Francis J. George, A.T.C., P.T.

Head Athletic Trainer, Brown University, Providence

Joseph S. Torg, M.D.

Professor of Orthopedic Surgery, and Director, Sports Medicine Center, Hahnemann University, Philadelphia

American College of Sports Medicine Liaison Representative

Kent B. Pandolf, Ph.D.

Director, Environmental Physiology and Medicine Directorate, U.S. Army Research Institute of Environmental Medicine, Natick, Massachusetts

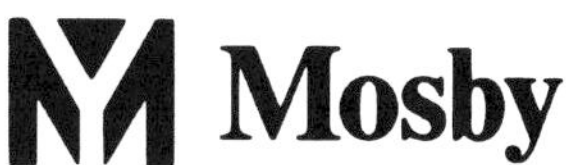

St. Louis Baltimore Boston Carlsbad Chicago Naples New York Philadelphia Portland London Madrid Mexico City Singapore Sydney Tokyo Toronto Wiesbaden

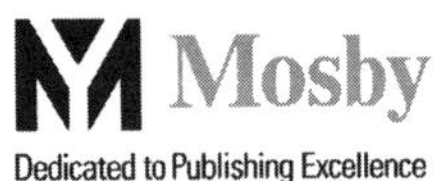

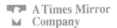

Vice President and Publisher, Continuity Publishing: Kenneth H. Killion
Director, Editorial Development: Gretchen C. Murphy
Acquisitions Editor: Linda Sheehan
Illustrations and Permissions Coordinator: Steven J. Ramay
Manager, Continuity–EDP: Maria Nevinger
Project Supervisor, Editing: Rebecca Nordbrock
Freelance Staff Supervisor: Barbara M. Kelly
Director, Editorial Services: Edith M. Podrazik, B.S.N., R.N.
Information Specialist: Kathleen Moss, R.N.
Circulation Manager: Lynn D. Stevenson

1996 EDITION

Printed in the United States of America
Composition by Reed Technology and Information Services, Inc.
Printing/binding by Maple-Vail

Mosby–Year Book, Inc.
11830 Westline Industrial Drive
St. Louis, MO 63146

Editorial Office:
Mosby–Year Book, Inc.
161 North Clark Street
Chicago, IL 60601

International Standard Serial Number: 0162-0908
International Standard Book Number: 0-8151-7701-1

Table of Contents

Journals Represented

Mosby and its editors survey more than 1,000 journals for its abstract and commentary publications. From these journals, the editors select the articles to be abstracted. Journals represented in this YEAR BOOK are listed below.

Acta Dermato-Venereologica
Acta Ophthalmologica Scandinavica
Acta Oto-Laryngologica
American Heart Journal
American Journal of Cardiology
American Journal of Epidemiology
American Journal of Obstetrics and Gynecology
American Journal of Orthopedics
American Journal of Perinatology
American Journal of Physiology
American Journal of Public Health
American Journal of Respiratory and Critical Care Medicine
American Journal of Roentgenology
American Journal of Sports Medicine
American Journal of the Medical Sciences
Annals of Emergency Medicine
Annals of Epidemiology
Annals of Internal Medicine
Annals of Otology, Rhinology and Laryngology
Annals of Plastic Surgery
Archives of Ophthalmology
Archives of Physical Medicine and Rehabilitation
Arthroscopy
Australian Journal of Science and Medicine in Sport
Biological Psychiatry
Bone
British Heart Journal
British Journal of Radiology
British Journal of Sports Medicine
British Medical Journal
Chest
Chiropractic Technique
Circulation
Clinical Biomechanics
Clinical Orthopaedics and Related Research
Clinical and Experimental Optometry
European Heart Journal
European Respiratory Journal
Foot & Ankle International
Gerontologist
Injury
International Journal of Eating Disorders
Journal of Adolescent Health
Journal of Applied Physiology: Respiratory, Environmental and Exercise Physiology
Journal of Athletic Training
Journal of Biomechanics

Journal of Bone and Joint Surgery (American Volume)
Journal of Bone and Joint Surgery (British Volume)
Journal of Bone and Mineral Research
Journal of Cardiopulmonary Rehabilitation
Journal of Clinical Endocrinology and Metabolism
Journal of Clinical Rheumatology
Journal of Epidemiology and Community Health
Journal of Gerontology
Journal of Orthopaedic Trauma
Journal of Orthopaedic and Sports Physical Therapy
Journal of Pediatric Surgery
Journal of Shoulder and Elbow Surgery
Journal of Sports Medicine and Physical Fitness
Journal of Sports Sciences
Journal of Trauma: Injury, Infection, and Critical Care
Journal of Vascular Surgery
Journal of the American Academy of Orthopaedic Surgeons
Journal of the American College of Cardiology
Journal of the American Geriatrics Society
Journal of the American Medical Association
Journal of the American Society of Nephrology
Lancet
Maturitas
Mayo Clinic Proceedings
Medical Journal of Australia
Medicine and Science in Sports and Exercise
New England Journal of Medicine
Ophthalmology
Orthopedics
Paraplegia
Pediatrics
Physical Therapy
Physician and Sportsmedicine
Postgraduate Medicine
Radiology
Skeletal Radiology
Southern Medical Journal
Spine
Sports Medicine
Sports Medicine and Arthroscopy Review
Thorax
Western Journal of Medicine

Standard Abbreviations

The following terms are abbreviated in this edition: acquired immunodeficiency syndrome (AIDS), cardiopulmonary resuscitation (CPR), central nervous system (CNS), cerebrospinal fluid (CSF), computed tomography (CT), deoxyribonucleic acid (DNA), electrocardiography (ECG), health maintenance organization (HMO), human immunodeficiency virus (HIV), intensive care unit (ICU), intramuscular (IM), intravenous (IV), magnetic resonance (MR) imaging (MRI), and ribonucleic acid (RNA).

Note

The Year Book of Sports Medicine is a literature survey service providing abstracts of articles published in the professional literature. Every effort is made to assure the accuracy of the information presented in these pages. Neither the editors nor the publisher of the Year Book of Sports Medicine can be responsible for errors in the original materials. The editors' comments are their own opinions. Mention of specific products within this publication does not constitute endorsement.

To facilitate the use of the Year Book of Sports Medicine as a reference tool, all illustrations and tables included in this publication are now identified as they appear in the original article. This change is meant to help the reader recognize that any illustration or table appearing in the Year Book of Sports Medicine may be only one of many in the original article. For this reason, figure and table numbers will often appear to be out of sequence within the Year Book of Sports Medicine.

Publisher's Preface

Mosby–Year Book, Inc. would like to extend its sincerest congratulations and warmest goodbyes to Col. James L. Anderson, PE.D. This will be Col. Anderson's final year on the editorial board of the YEAR BOOK OF SPORTS MEDICINE, as he will be retiring from his professional duties in 1997. Col. Anderson has been a devoted editor on the YEAR BOOK OF SPORTS MEDICINE board since the book's inception, and he will be sorely missed.

Introduction

One of the attractions of sports medicine for physicians and scientists is the enormous breadth of the topic. A good understanding of sports medicine provides a worthy challenge, even to the Renaissance man or woman, as he or she explores not only the traditional areas of infection, injury, and rehabilitation, but also the limiting performance of every biological system, both in normal environments and under conditions that are severely challenging to the nonacclimated individual. The YEAR BOOK OF SPORTS MEDICINE provides an invaluable service to the busy practitioner by offering a rapid overview of new developments in this vast field. The 1996 edition is no exception to this rule.

As always, a major section of this volume is devoted to insightful selections that survey recent developments in the prevention and treatment of sports injuries. In terms of prevention, ambient temperature is shown to influence the adhesion of shoes to a playing surface and thus to modify injury rates. The vertigo induced by rapid turns during downhill skiing may be another source of injuries, and at least in adolescents, risks of injury are higher for left- than for right-handed individuals. Uitenbroek discusses the need for Poisson statistics in the analysis of injuries and suggests the need to identify other categories of injury-prone individuals. Several long-term follow-ups of middle-aged and older runners emphasize that the benefits of regular exercise outweigh injuries and possible arthritic sequelae.

Changes in the design of skiing equipment seem to have shifted the main site of injury from the ankle to the knee joint. The trampoline is identified as a frequent source of severe injury, and in-line skating is also shown to be responsible for a number of serious head injuries. Concern is expressed that musculoskeletal allografts have sometimes served as vehicles for the transmission of HIV infection. Knowledge of the inflammatory process is growing; distance running in the heat does not seem to cause endotoxemia, but Mishra et al. query whether it is a good idea to suppress early inflammatory changes.

Four papers examine the catastrophe of eye injuries in basketball, golf, football, and other sports, raising important questions of policy—Do open eye-guards merely funnel dangerous objects into the eyes, and does the wearing of eye protection increase the risk of incurring other types of injury? One of my panel of distinguished co-editors, Dr. Joseph S. Torg, was awarded the Nicholas Andry Award of the Association of Bone and Joint Surgeons for a study that looks at the treatment of spinal cord injuries in terms of cellular events (membrane permeability failure and increases of cytosolic calcium).

In the shoulder, the diagnosis and treatment of rotator cuff injuries and glenoid labral lesions continue to be prominent concerns of the orthopedist. Promising results are reported from the use of titanium anchors in the rotator cuff and bioabsorbable stabilizing devices for the glenoid labrum. One paper describes six cases of suprascapular nerve entrapment by ganglion cysts, a sometimes overlooked differential diagnosis. A discussion of partial medial collateral ligament tears stresses the importance of guarding against ulnar injuries when carrying out arthroscopic procedures in the posterior medial gutter. Two papers consider painful nonunion of olecranon physeal fractures, pointing out that bone grafting or internal fixation may be required for satisfactory resolution. Tennis elbow continues to attract attention, and one of four papers on this topic explores tennis elbow from a kinematic perspective. Play on artificial turf seems to be associated with a preponderance of distal wrist fractures incurred by soccer players.

Back injuries continue to be a major concern, and Col. James L. Anderson provides a substantial section of recent research in this area. A review of 12 cases of osteitis pubis reports impressive results from local injection of 4 mg of dexamethasone. Stiell et al. describe the use of decision rules to increase the cost-effectiveness of injury treatment and avoid unnecessary radiography. In a similar vein, a number of authors critique the overuse of MRI. Increased reliance on outpatient treatment is reflected by a discussion of femoral nerve block in pain control after anterior cruciate ligament reconstruction, and the costs and benefits of local anesthesia are evaluated for arthroscopy of the knee. The diagnosis of peroneal entrapment is apparently facilitated by prior exercise, because this increases local tissue pressures and compression of the nerve. The high incidence of osteoarthritis after menisectomy points to the need for a prolonged follow-up when evaluating the surgical treatment of knee injuries. Concern is raised regarding the potential for a laser beam of inappropriate wavelength characteristics to cause osteonecrosis, and a late follow-up of tendon grafts has shown a disturbing continued abnormality of collagen fibrils.

The viewpoint that modest amounts of physical activity can improve the health and quality of life of the older individual gains credence, and a major paper from *JAMA* presents new recommendations on the minimum dose of physical activity required for population health. A meta-analysis suggests that moderate home-based exercise is the most effective treatment in terms of patient compliance. Despite the fears that are sometimes expressed, older people seem to tolerate exercise at moderate altitudes quite well. Programs to develop back endurance are shown to decrease the likelihood of future lower back pain.

Those determining body composition by dual-energy x-ray absorptiometry are cautioned against errors that can be introduced by a change of software package during the course of an investigation. The use of inaccurate body fat prediction equations as a basis of employment decisions is vigorously attacked. The interpretation of osteoporosis data is clouded by site-specificity of changes and the influence of associated menstrual irregularities. Surprisingly, ordinary physical work seems to provide sufficient mechanical stimulation to reduce the likelihood of osteoporosis in older North American women. Cross-sectional studies suggest that the high peak forces developed in activities such as aerobic dance and speed skating are particularly effective in increasing bone density. Osteoporosis is noted as a potential complication of anorexia nervosa, and if energy intake is poor, there is little response to estrogens. Older patients continue to show large increases in muscle strength in response to resistance training; it leads to a substantial enhancement of function, and CT confirms that it reflects more than a simple learning of technique.

Patients receiving β-blocker treatment continue to complain of muscular fatigue, and a recent paper demonstrates that (at least in prolonged exercise) the reduction of performance is not caused by an inadequate rate of glycolysis. Pregnant women are advised that walking can induce a higher metabolic rate than aerobic dance, with less influence on fetal heart rates. New attempts are made to define the sick sinus syndrome, but it remains elusive and there seems to be an excessive prescription of pacemakers. In some patients with dilated cardiomyopathy, a part of the problem may arise from a downregulation of β-receptors in the region of the sinoatrial pacemaker. The possibility of reducing angina by means of a warm-up exercise continues to attract attention. Even five to six hours of exercise per week fail to stimulate ventricular collateral vessel formation, although if such activity is coupled with a low-fat diet, it may lead to some regression of coronary vascular disease. The ECG is shown to be a less cost-effective method of diagnosis than echocardiography in women (once account is taken of the costs associated with false positive diagnoses), and continuous monitoring of the ECG during rehabilitation also has a poor cost-effectiveness.

A welcome review of gastroesophageal reflux points out that the condition is by no means unknown in athletes, and it may easily be confounded with myocardial ischemia. Gas tonometry has been used to examine gastric blood flow during vigorous rowing; the data suggest that there may be almost complete occlusion of the mesenteric vessels during such exercise. Both ultrafiltration and exercise programs are providing their worth in the treatment of congestive heart failure. Improvements in treadmill data do not always seem to match functional gains, and one interesting technique of estimating functional capacity in this class of patient is to examine the magnitude of the recovery oxygen consumption after a standard bout of exercise. A paper from *BMJ* notes that when people travel to a hot climate, individuals with undetected cystic fibrosis may experience hyponatremic heat exhaustion.

Investigators continue to emphasize differences of psychosocial and physiologic characteristics between patients with chronic obstructive lung disease and "postcoronary" patients, pointing to the need for separate rehabilitation programs; however, much of the loss of cardiorespiratory fitness in the continuing smoker appears to result from cardiac rather than respiratory problems. Debate continues on the contribution of respiratory muscle fatigue to the symptoms experienced in chronic obstructive lung disease and on the merits of adding respiratory muscle training to other forms of rehabilitation; much of any benefit from exercise programs in chronic obstructive lung disease is still thought to be a placebo effect.

The value of low back programs in controlling back pain continues to provoke vigorous debate. Intra-arterial pressure measurements demonstrate both the enormous pressures that can be reached during weight lifting and the ability to limit pressure increases by careful control of breathing patterns. Studies continue to attest to the value of regular physical activity in protection against some forms of cancer, although it remains unclear whether benefit is mediated through the control of obesity or through some other mechanism.

Divers are warned against various pulmonary and periocular manifestations of exposure to high ambient pressures and of the risks associated with flying home from remote diving locations in unpressurized aircraft! Issues are also raised about the rules of synchronized swimming and the danger that such rules may encourage participants to develop a dangerous hypoxia. Those interested in high altitudes continue to explore the value of Doppler measurements in the diagnosis of pulmonary vascular hypersensitivity to hypoxia.

Horror stories continue to emerge about the extent of self-medication among abusers of anabolic steroids, with strong linkages between steroid abuse and other adverse health habits. A study of patients with acromegaly provides a useful warning regarding the negative effects of long-term human growth hormone administration. A new test has been developed that can detect erythropoietin for up to 48 hours after it has been administered. There is growing evidence that selective β_2-agonists can act synergistically with resistance training to enhance the growth of skeletal muscle, and there may thus be a need to review the long-term use of such agents by athletes with asthma. A case history warns that ibuprofen can precipitate renal failure in marathon runners. A paper on electromyostimulation demonstrates that the price of any gain in strength realized by this technique is an increased risk of muscle damage.

In all, our editorial panel has once again succeeded in bringing together and critiquing a fascinating collection of current reports. This material should not only provide stimulating reading but should also enhance the practice of sports medicine in the year ahead.

Roy J. Shephard, M.D., Ph.D., D.P.E.

Exercise Testing by Nonphysician Health Care Providers: Competency, Safety, and Legal Considerations

ROY J. SHEPHARD, M.D., Ph.D., D.P.E.
School of Physical and Health Education and Professor Emeritus of Applied Physiology, Department of Preventive Medicine and Biostatistics, University of Toronto; CTAL Resident Scholar in Health Studies, Brock University, St. Catharine's, Ontario

Canada introduced comprehensive prepaid health care in 1967, and (contrary to much rhetoric in the U.S. media) this scheme has worked well, offering to all Canadian citizens, irrespective of their income, first-class medical service at a much lower fraction of the gross national product than in the United States. However, to achieve universal health coverage, it has been necessary to look critically at certain areas of traditional medical practice that could be offered more economically—and sometimes more effectively—by well-trained paramedical specialists. One such area has been the screening and testing of subjects before they begin an exercise program.

From the early 1970s, Canadians recognized that health promotion held the key to containing the costs of universal medical coverage.[1] An increase of habitual physical activity was a key component of a healthy lifestyle, and, if 10 million Canadian adults were to begin exercising, the question immediately arose concerning what type of preliminary screening such individuals would require. It was decided that a full, medically supervised stress test of an apparently healthy individual could not be an insured service. The American dictum of the period was that everyone over the age of 30 years who wished to enter an exercise program needed a medical examination with ECG, and those over the age of 35 years also needed an exercise ECG.[2] The American College of Sports Medicine[3] was heavily influenced by this restrictive philosophy. It recommended a resting ECG for well individuals younger than 35 years of age who were contemplating a change in the type, intensity, or duration of physical activity; a field stress test or a laboratory stress test for asymptomatic physically inactive people younger than age 35 years; and for those over the age of 35 years, there was to be a complete medical evaluation plus a graded exercise test with a physician in the testing area, even if the person was without risk factors for coronary heart disease!

In Canada, both government and practitioners quickly acknowledged the negative motivational impact that such a policy would have on potential exercisers. Clear evidence was presented that despite the high cost of such examinations, they had very limited diagnostic value[4, 5]: when confronted with a typical adult population, the exercise exclusion rates of different physicians ranged from 1% to 15%, and there was no evidence that physicians with a high exclusion rate were any more successful than their peers in avoiding the cardiac complications of exercise. Indeed, because of the Bayesian constraints imposed by the testing of a healthy, normal population with a low prevalence of abnormalities, a warning based on exercise-induced ECG abnormalities was likely to be wrong two times out of three, and a more accurate verdict would have been obtained had the patient simply tossed a coin. At a time when U.S. equipment companies were advising doctors that if they performed graded exercise tests on all of their patients, they could recoup the costs of a treadmill and ECG setup within six months, the Public Health Committee of the Ontario Medical Association[6] unequivocally advised medical practitioners that (Table 1) "Exercise testing is not only expensive and time consuming, it is medically unnecessary for most persons who plan to exercise." Six years later, a joint committee of the American College of Cardiology and the American Heart Association[7] reached essentially similar conclusions. They stated "Exercise testing is of little or no value, inappropriate or contraindicated" for "asymptomatic, apparently healthy men or women with no risk factors for coronary artery disease."

The Canadian viewpoint was that a two- or even a three-tiered system of screening should be adopted.[8] The initial triage should be based on a simple questionnaire, completed by the person who was contemplating exercise. Trial of various questions in Saskatoon (Bailey and Shephard, unpublished data, 1974) and at the Pacific National Exhibition in Vancouver[9] led to introduction of a simple, 7-item Physical Activity Readiness Questionnaire. Research subjects who gave a positive response to any one of the seven items in the questionnaire were advised to consult their physician before embarking on an exercise program. Twenty years' experience of this approach in Canada has shown it to be very safe. It is also fairly successful in making a preliminary triage of candidates for exercise, but greater specificity remains desirable. Some 20% of those completing the questionnaire are still directed to their physicians. One of the most common reasons is a positive response to the question about high blood pressure.[10] In most instances, the individual thus identified is normotensive—either the physician has been misunderstood or the report is caused by "white-coat hypertension," a temporary increase of blood pressure induced by anxiety in the doctor's office. We have recently revised the Physical Activity Readiness Questionnaire (PAR-Q) in an attempt to make it more specific. Guidance has been added for paramedical professionals so that they can assist users in responding correctly to the test

TABLE 1.—Guidelines for the Supervision of Exercise Tests (Ontario Medical Association, 1980)

SUBJECT	ECG MONITOR	SUPERVISION
Well, < 35 yr	For HR only	Paramedical
Well, > 35 yr	For HR only	Paramedical (doctor available)
Well, high-risk	Exercise ECG	Physician present
Known CVD	Exercise ECG	Test in specialized facility

Abbreviations: HR, heart rate; *CVD*, coronary vascular disease.
(Courtesy of Dr. Shephard.)

TABLE 2.—Major Coronary Risk Factors Influencing Level of Exercise Test Supervision

Sedentary lifestyle
Blood pressure > 160/90 mm Hg, 2 occasions
Fasting serum cholesterol > 6.2 mmol/L
Current cigarette smoking
Insulin-dependent diabetes mellitus
Sudden death of coronary vascular disease in parent or sibling < 55 yr

(Courtesy of Dr. Shephard.)

instrument.[11] Because there is no unequivocal "gold standard" against which the validity of responses to the revised questionnaire can be judged, we will now have to accumulate another decade of experience to decide how far the revised instrument combines the safety of the original PAR-Q instrument with a greater specificity in detecting contraindications to exercise.

It must be recognized that the legal situation in Canada is very different from that in the United States. In Canada, lawyers cannot bring claims of malpractice or negligence against health professionals on a contingency basis. In consequence, health care providers in Canada face fewer lawsuits, and it has been easier to introduce innovative approaches to both exercise clearance and exercise testing. Nevertheless, stimulated in part by Canadian developments, the U.S. policy has also changed substantially during the past two decades.[12] One reason for the high number of false positive tests with the original approach of the American College of Sports Medicine (ACSM) was the low incidence of ischemic pathologies in a population of healthy young adult exercise volunteers. Again, applying the principles of Bayes' theorem, we find that as the prevalence of abnormalities in a population rises, the proportion of false positive diagnoses diminishes. Accordingly, an important first step in the revised ACSM protocol (19951) is to undertake a stratification of risk, based on the presence of major cardiac risk factors (Table 2) or of major symptoms and signs suggestive of cardiopulmonary or metabolic disease (Table 3) in the test candidate. A second issue, again overlooked in the original protocol, is the intensity and

TABLE 3.—Major Symptoms or Signs Influencing Level of Exercise Test Supervision

Ischemic chest pain
Excessive dyspnea in relation to exercise load
History of dizziness or syncope
History of orthopnea or nocturnal dyspnea
Presence of ankle edema
History of cardiac palpitations or tachycardia
Intermittent claudication
Clinically significant heart murmur

(Courtesy of Dr. Shephard.)

duration of the exercise that the subject is proposing to undertake. Often, a person's intent is to do no more than begin a modest program of fast walking. The hazard associated with this is plainly much less than if a person is planning to complete a marathon at a fast pace, or indeed, to persist with a sedentary lifestyle. The ACSM now distinguishes an intensity of exercise that is less than 60% of the individual's maximal oxygen intake, a level that is well within a person's current capacity and at a level that can be tolerated for an hour or longer. Based on risk factors and the proposed intensity of activity, a much more realistic triage of candidates for detailed screening has been developed (Table 4).

Assuming that exercise screening is required, it still remains debatable whether this should be undertaken by a physician or a certified exercise test technologist with extensive experience in exercise testing. The reality of the situation is that the decision will be based on local legislation, but we should nevertheless approach the issue critically and ask whether existing legislation needs to be changed. The key issues are: (1) what type of competency will enable the person conducting the test to derive the most useful information from it?; (2) if the test candidate has an increased risk of an adverse test outcome, what type of competency will minimize the risks of testing?; and (3) what types of competency will provide the greatest chances of a successful resuscitation should a cardiac emergency develop?

Some physicians—particularly those who are members of the ACSM—have had extensive experience in exercise testing, and their combination of general clinical skills with detailed knowledge of normal exercise responses enables them to derive subtle information from patient symptoms and signs that would escape the attention of a person who lacked prolonged clinical training. However, the average family physician has had

TABLE 4.—Current Guidelines of the American College of Sports Medicine (1995) Indicating Need for Medical Pre-exercise Screening and Recommended Level of Exercise Test Supervision

PATIENT & Proposed Ex. Intensity	MED. SCREENING, Diagnostic Exercise Test	MEDICAL TEST SUPERVISION	
		Submaximal	Maximal Test
Well male < 40 yr			
Well female < 50 yr			
(moderate ex.)	NO	NO	NO
(vigorous ex.)	NO	NO	NO
Well male > 40 yr			
Well female > 50 yr			
(moderate ex.)	NO	NO	YES
(vigorous ex.)	YES	NO	YES
2 or more risk factors			
(moderate ex.)	NO	NO	YES
(vigorous ex.)	YES	NO	YES
Symptoms, signs of disease			
(moderate ex.)	YES	YES	YES
(vigorous ex.)	YES	YES	YES

little or no exposure to the evaluation of exercise responses, either normal or pathologic during medical training, and it is hard to support claims that such a person is better qualified to conduct an exercise test than a person who has worked for many years as a certified exercise specialist or exercise test technologist. Recent law cases suggest that a physician who chooses to engage in the practice of exercise testing will be held to the level of knowledge and the competencies expected of those certified by professional groups such as the ACSM.

The presence of an ill-informed and anxious doctor can in itself add to the dangers of a test, increasing the blood pressure and catecholamine output of the test candidate. A lack of knowledge on the part of a supervising physician will often show itself as a premature halting of a test or a misinterpretation of what is essentially a normal ECG, rather than in the pushing of an unhealthy individual to an excessive level of physical activity. Legal sequelae to such malpractice are unlikely, and often errors will pass unrecognized. However, if the false positive diagnosis of a cardiac abnormality has led to an unnecessary restriction of a person's habitual activity, the physician who has made this judgment is just as guilty of shortening the test candidate's life as if he or she had precipitated an immediate cardiac emergency. Lack of adequate exercise can shorten the life span of a young adult by as much as two years, not to mention the impact on mood state and quality-adjusted life expectancy.

An exercise test technologist now has clearly defined levels of competency that are required for certification. In terms of specific knowledge of exercise protocols and their likely influence on the body, one may argue that such specialists are often better prepared than general physicians. Their weaknesses are likely to be a little less intuition regarding unspoken messages from the demeanor of the exerciser and a little less experience in exploring symptomatic responses. Many ACSM-certified exercise specialists are also fitter than the average physician, and they are accustomed to pushing themselves to all-out effort. For this reason, they may expect an equally rigorous effort from an untrained sedentary individual, who is likely to be much less tolerant of such maximal stimulation. The incidence of exercise-induced events depends on the type of population tested and the period of observation: during the test or for 1 or 6 hours afterward. However, it is no more than 1 in 10,000 tests, sufficiently rare that it is difficult to compare risks between tests with differing patterns of supervision.

If an emergency does arise, quick, instinctive action is needed. The majority of exercise specialists have annually renewed certification in cardiac resuscitation and may thus be more aware of the latest procedures than a physician who has not had recent training in this skill and has only had occasion to attempt cardiac resuscitation a few times many years previously while serving as an intern. However, if the situation is not immediately critical, the instincts of a physician may be better than those of an exercise specialist.

This can be illustrated by an incident that occurred in our university a few months ago when a patient experienced angina while exercising. Previous exercise tests had all been normal, without evidence of ST segment depression. Exercise was halted, and after a few minutes the person claimed to feel fine. The exercise specialist who was supervising the test thus allowed this person to take a shower and then return home in a taxi, after advising him to consult his doctor the next day. In fact, the subject had a massive but nonfatal heart attack while in the taxi. It is easy to criticize handling of the event in retrospect, but most physicians, particularly those with experience in cardiology and exercise testing, would have recognized that cardiac pain in a previously normal heart is a serious warning of an impending crisis.[4, 5, 8] Further, their instinct would have been to suggest that the patient lie on the floor with his legs raised, inhaling oxygen, until he could be transported to the hospital for a thorough clinical evaluation. Whether this would have prevented or reduced the size of the resulting infarct is more debatable.

One final comment on this issue. If all of the adult population were to be tested, it plainly would be uneconomical to require extensive medical training as a condition for the supervision of such tests. However, the more the tests are restricted to the sick individuals who need such examination, the greater becomes the requirement for close supervision by an experienced physician. Thus, the key element in the process of ensuring an appropriate use of medical expertise is a sensitive and specific initial triage of risk.

References

1. Lalonde M: *A New Perspective on the Health of Canadians.* Ottawa, Health & Welfare Canada, 1974. This governmental paper, written by the (then) federal Minister of Health, set out the notion that in order to have an effective system of universal medical care, governments should invest increasingly in preventive medicine.
2. Cooper KH: Guidelines in the management of the exercising patient. *JAMA* 211:1663–1667, 1970. This paper presents the traditional U.S. view on clearance for exercise, including the recommendation of an ECG on all candidates over the age of 30 years, and a stress ECG on those over the age of 35 years.
3. American College of Sports Medicine: *Guidelines for Graded Exercise Testing and Exercise Prescription and Behavioral Objectives for Physicians, Program Directors, Exercise Leaders and Exercise Technicians,* ed 1. Philadelphia, Lea & Febiger, 1975. The original views on exercise testing, with a strong requirement for medically supervised exercise testing of almost all potential exercisers.
4. Shephard RJ: Sudden death: A significant hazard of exercise. *Br J Sports Med* 8:101–110, 1974. This was one of the first papers to attempt to quantify the risks associated with exercise testing and exercise participation. Based on a retrospective questioning of those surviving a first heart attack, it estimated that there was a fivefold increase of risk while the person was actually engaged in exercise.
5. Shephard RJ: *Ischemic Heart Disease and Exercise.* London, Croom Helm, 1981. This mongraph provides a detailed review of the risks and benefits of both exercise testing and exercise participation, both for the average adult and for those who have already sustained a first heart attack.
6. Public Health Committee, Ontario Medical Association: *Exercise Prescription. A physician's guide to assessment of patients who plan to exercise.* Toronto, Ontario

Ministry of Health, 1980. A compact and practical guidebook helping doctors to devise an appropriate exercise prescription for their patients. Points out categorically that preliminary medically supervised exercise testing is unnecessary for most patients who wish to begin exercising.

7. American College of Cardiology/American Heart Association: Guidelines for exercise testing. *Circulation* 74:653A–667A, 1986. Key paper marking a liberalization of policies in the United States.
8. Shephard RJ: Can we identify those for whom exercise is hazardous? *Sports Med* 1:75–86, 1984. This review examines screening options, and makes suggestions as to how the Physical Activity Readiness Questionnaire might be modified to increase its specificity in detecting those individuals at high risk from exercising.
9. Chisholm DM, Collis ML, Kulak LL, et al: Physical activity readiness. *British Columbia Med J* 17:375–378, 1975. This paper describes the development of a simple, seven item questionnaire, to be completed by patients contemplating beginning a programme of moderate exercise. If positive answers are made to any of the questions on the sheet, the person concerned is advised to consult his or her doctor before beginning to exercise.
10. Shephard RJ, Cox M, Simper K: An analysis of Par-Q responses in an office population. *Can J Public Health* 72:37–40, 1981. This paper compares the responses to the original PAR-Q questionnaire against the results of a direct medical screening for exercise. It notes that the PAR-Q questionnaire excludes about 20% of candidates from exercise participation, mainly because of a mistaken belief that blood pressures are elevated.
11. Thomas S, Reading J, Shephard RJ: Revision of the Physical Activity Readiness Questionnaire. *Can J Sport Sci* 17:338–345, 1992. This paper compares the original PAR-Q questionnaire with a revised version, designed to maintain the safety of the original version, but to increase its specificity.
12. American College of Sports Medicine: *Guidelines for graded exercise testing and exercise prescription,* ed 5. Philadelphia, Lea & Febiger, 1995. This book provides the current consensus of the College's wisdom on procedures for exercise testing and prescription. There has been a marked reduction in the demand for preliminary medical screening. Specific information is given on the levels of competency required for the supervision of testing in various categories of individual, and indications for the halting of tests.

1 Biomechanics, Epidemiology, and Injury Prevention

Cross-section Areas of Calf Muscles in Athletes of Different Sports

Strojnik V, Apih T, Demsar F (Univ of Ljubljana, Slovenia; Jozef Stefan Inst, Ljubljana, Slovenia)

J Sports Med Phys Fitness 35:25–30, 1995 1–1

Objective.—Because most sports activities load the ankle joint in a sport-specific manner, the cross-section areas of calf structures were quantified by MRI in 21 well-trained male athletes at the national and international levels. Seven sprinters, 6 long-distance runners, and 8 free climbers were examined. Seven healthy men not active in sports served as a control group.

Methods.—All the athletes were training regularly at the time of the study, had practiced their sport for at least 3 years, and had no current injury. For all athletes, T1-weighted cross-section MR images were acquired.

Findings.—Individual muscle areas did not differ significantly in the various groups. The only significant difference was a much smaller area of subcutaneous fat in all groups of athletes than in controls.

Conclusion.—To demonstrate the effects of activity on cross-section calf muscles, it will be necessary to individually load the foot and ankle joint.

► These authors began with the assumptions that muscles functionally adapt themselves to the loading they are exposed to and that the muscle's cross-section area is 1 of the important factors for muscle force production. Another assumption was that the loading in a certain sports discipline is relatively homogeneous and diverse enough between sports to be recognized in adapted morphologic structures of the muscles. However, their data do not support these assumptions. They learned that maybe changes in cross-section areas, especially those of single calf muscles, are just 1 of many possible mechanisms in adaptation processes to increased loading, and perhaps they are not as "sport specific" as one might expect. I must admit that I would have expected significant differences in the cross-section areas of the calf muscles between sprinters and distance runners.

Col. J.L. Anderson, PE.D.

The Relationship Between Cadence and Lower Extremity EMG in Cyclists and Noncyclists

Marsh AP, Martin PE (Arizona State Univ, Tempe)

Med Sci Sports Exerc 27:217–225, 1995 1–2

Objective.—Differences in steady-state pedaling cadences between experienced cyclists and noncyclists have been attributed to the individual's cycling experience. Thus, competitive cyclists are thought to adapt to the high cadences at which they train and race, whereas noncyclists select significantly lower cadences. The hypothesis that preferred cadence selection is related to electromyographic (EMG) activity of lower limb muscles was tested.

Methods.—Eight male cyclists and 8 male noncyclists took part in the study. The noncyclist group included 7 distance runners and 1 middle-distance swimmer, but none rode a bicycle as part of their training regimen. A Velodyne trainer was used to stimulate the inertial and noninertial loading of riding on the road during the maximal test and the cadence manipulation trials. In the EMG session, both groups used the same bike frame and crank length (170 mm). Muscles selected for EMG data were those shown to be important contributors to the cycling movement: the vastus lateralis, rectus femoris, biceps femoris, lateral soleus, and medial gastrocnemius. Both groups pedaled under 6 randomly ordered cadences (50, 65, 80, 95, and 110 rpm and the individual preferred cadence) at 200 W.

Results.—The average preferred cadences did not differ significantly between experienced cyclists (85.2 rpm) and noncyclists (91.6 rpm). Substantial changes in average and peak EMG were recorded only for the medial gastrocnemius muscle, for which EMG activity increased systematically as cadence increased. Both the rectus femoris and vastus lateralis showed only small EMG differences between cadences. Although there was a trend for soleus and gastrocnemius EMG to be higher in noncyclists than in experienced cyclists, the 2 groups did not differ significantly in patterns of muscle activity.

Conclusions.—Little support was found for the hypothesis that the average and peak EMG amplitude of the 5 tested muscles display minima at the preferred cadence in cyclists and noncyclists. Thus, preferred cadence selection appears to be unrelated to minimization of muscle activation, and lower extremity EMG does not help to explain why the preferred cadences tend to be significantly higher than the most economical cadences, reported to be between 50 and 60 rpm.

► This study is a good example why we should not automatically accept the results of even well-designed and well-conducted studies without replication and further examination by other investigators. Although it makes sense and has been generally accepted, cycling experience alone does not appear to explain why the average preferred cycling cadences of experienced cyclists tend to be significantly higher than the most economical cadences, if we accept the results of this study. It was also accepted, by observation and data collection in the laboratory environment, that the experienced cyclists prefer higher cadences than noncyclists at a constant power output. However, these authors demonstrated that when noncyclists who have equal aerobic capacity to the cyclists are tested, their preferred cadences were similar to the preferred cadences of the experienced cyclists.

Col. J.L. Anderson, PE.D.

The Influence of Hand Guards on Forces and Muscle Activity During Giant Swings on the High Bar

Neal RJ, Kippers V, Plooy D, Forwood MR (Univ of Queensland, Australia)

Med Sci Sports Exerc 27:1550–1556, 1995 1–3

Objective.—Various aids have been developed to help gymnasts maintain contact with the high bar during the giant swing, which is the basic skill required by male gymnasts. One device that has become the standard guard for use on the high bar is doweled hand guards (DHG), which form a hook over the bar to artificially increase grip strength. The impact of DHG on hand biomechanics has yet to be defined, however. The effects of DHG and other hand guards on bar forces and forearm muscle swing during giant swings on the high bar were investigated.

Methods.—Ten experienced male gymnasts were studied while completing at least 3 backward giant swings on a high bar. The high bar used was instrumented with strain gauges in a way that permitted estimation of the horizontal and vertical shear forces at each hand and the torque around the bar. The gymnasts were studied while swinging with bare hands, with webbing hoops, with DHG, and with a wind-up swing using DHG. The hand guards' effect on the load experienced by the gymnasts during giant swings, the forces applied to the bar by each hand, and the muscle activity of the extrinsic finger flexor and wrist extensor muscle groups were determined.

Results.—Peak reaction forces on the hands exceeded 2 times body weight for each hand. These forces were significantly lower when the gymnasts swung bare-handed than when they used hand guards. The use of hand guards made no difference in wrist flexor and extensor muscle activity, according to integrated electromyograms.

Conclusions.—By wearing hand guards during giant swings on the high bar, gymnasts can achieve greater tensile forces across the wrist with no measurable increase in forearm muscle activity. The use of hand guards may place additional stress on the wrist ligaments or epiphyseal plates. In young gymnasts, the additional tension on the distal radial and ulnar epiphyses could have implications for bone growth or injury.

▶ These authors not only identify a potential problem, primarily for younger men who are gymnasts, from the use of the DHG when performing on the high bar, but they also propose a possible solution. When doing giant swings on the high bar, the DHG allows the gymnast to swing faster and thus greatly increases the forces that cross the wrist. This causes passive structures such as ligaments of the hand and wrist to contribute a greater proportion of the total force required to prevent wrist separation. Because the distal epiphyseal plate does not normally close until between 17 and 19 years of age, younger male gymnasts can be placed at risk from using the present DHG.

These authors suggest a possible redesign of the DHG by attaching a forearm sleeve extending from a point distal to the elbow to a point that is proximal to the epiphyseal plates. The sleeve should be held in place by 3 or more Velcro straps. The longitudinal palmar band should be increased in width to spread the tensile forces over a larger area, compared with current designs. The authors surmise that the forearm sleeve will reduce tension and compression over the epiphyseal plates and distribute compression forces over most of the forearm, instead of concentrating them in the wrist. It is not clear whether these authors have actually tested this new design for the DHG.

Col. J.L. Anderson, PE.D.

Discriminant Analysis of Biomechanical Differences Between Novice, Good and Elite Rowers

Smith RM, Spinks WL (Univ of Sydney, Australia; Univ of Technology, Lindfield, Australia)

J Sports Sci 13:377–385, 1995 1–4

Background.—It can be difficult to recognize the most important predictors of sport performance and to discriminate between athletes of different ability levels while minimizing the number of variables used. Rowing ergometer tests are commonly used to assess rowing performance and even to select athletes for competition. However, most of these units only provide information on work output and stroke rate, neglecting consistency, technique, and other skill factors. Oar force and oar angle data were analyzed to identify biomechanical performance variables that could distinguish between rowers of differing ability levels and provide useful feedback for rowers and their coaches.

Methods.—Data on oar force and oar angle were collected during a 6-minute maximal rowing ergometer test performed by 9 novice, 23 good, and 9 elite-level male rowers (Fig 1). Work capacity variables analyzed were the mean propulsive power output per kg of body mass and propulsive work consistency. The skill variables analyzed were stroke-to-stroke

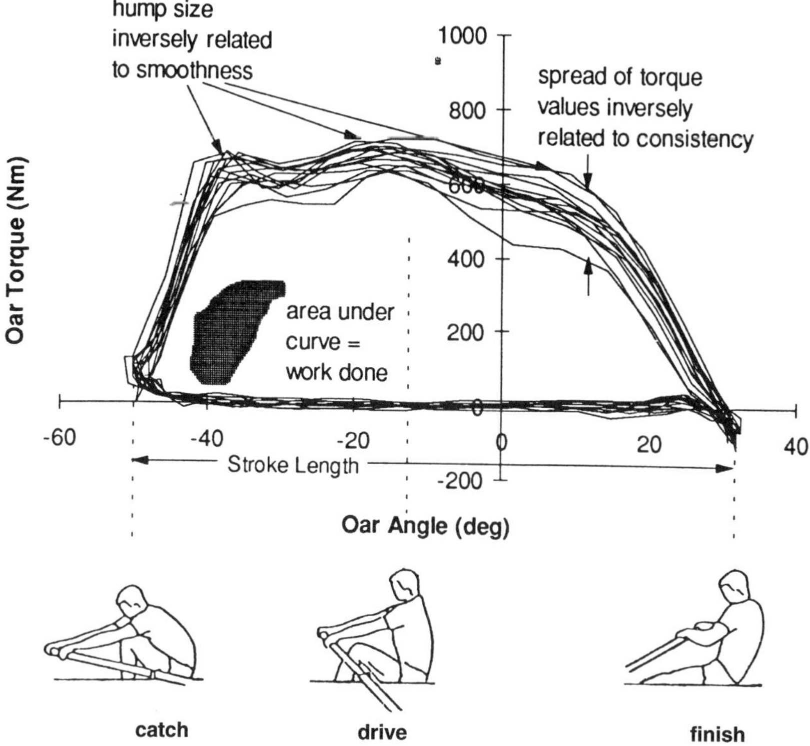

FIGURE 1.—Information provided by oar force and oar angle analysis in rowing. (Courtesy of Smith RM, Spinks WL: Discriminant analysis of biomechanical differences between novice, good, and elite rowers. *J Sports Sci* 13:377–385, 1995.)

consistency and stroke smoothness. Discriminant analysis was performed to identify performance variables that could differentiate among rowers at different levels of ability.

Results.—This analysis identified 2 functions, both of which illustrated that mean propulsive power output per kg of body mass was an important discriminating variable. Function 1 was a more powerful discriminator than function 2, which was more heavily weighted toward stroke-to-stroke consistency and stroke smoothness. The classification procedures used to predict the rowers' ability level involved defining the "distance" between each rower and the centroid of each ability level and then assigning the rower to the "nearest" ability level. This procedure resulted in the correct classification of 83% of all rowers, including 100% of the elite rowers, 74% of the good rowers, and 89% of the novice rowers. The most important variable on stepwise discriminant analysis was mean propulsive power output per kg of body mass, followed by stroke-to-stroke consistency, stroke smoothness, and propulsive work consistency.

Conclusions.—Biomechanical performance variables can be used to discriminate between rowers at various levels of ability. Mean propulsive power output per kg of body mass appears to be the most effective discriminator variable; propulsive work consistency is the least effective. The biomechanical performance data obtained from the rowing ergometer appear to be useful in predicting rowing capacity and skill and improving information feedback to rowers and coaches.

► The authors recognized that there are some statistical problems with the unequal sample sizes between the good and elite rowers and the novice rowers. However, they also know other authors have shown that in tests of significance, discriminant analysis is a robust technique that can tolerate some deviation from normality. Although the computed probabilities may not be exact, they are still quite useful if carefully interpreted.

In this situation, the percentages of correct classifications may be considered to be the best guide. Because the percentages were quite high, the authors recognized that any violation of normality assumptions was not very harmful.

Col. J.L. Anderson, PE.D.

Hitting a Baseball: A Biomechanical Description

Welch CM, Banks SA, Cook FF, Draovitch P (Human Performance Technologies, Inc, Jupiter, Fla; Good Samaritan Med Ctr, West Palm Beach, Fla)

J Orthop Sports Phys Ther 22:193–201, 1995 1–5

Purpose.—A great deal of research attention has focused on the development of conditioning, mechanics, and rehabilitation regimens for throwing athletes. In contrast, there has been little attention to the needs of hitting athletes. Progress in this area will require an understanding of the mechanics of hitting and the demands placed on the body during the swing. Quantitative biomechanical data were used to develop an understanding of the baseline mechanics of hitting a baseball.

Methods and Findings.—Three-dimensional kinematic and kinetic data from 7 professional baseball players—all right-handed hitters—were used to define the biomechanics of the baseball swing (Fig 2). At the start of the swing, the hitters shifted their weight toward the rear foot and generated a trunk coil. They strode forward a mean of 85 cm, or 380% of hip width, applying front foot force equal to 123% of body weight. This force promoted segment acceleration around the truncal axis. After hip segment rotation to a maximum speed of 714 degrees/sec, the shoulder segment accelerated to a velocity of 937 degrees/sec. This kinetic link led to a maximum linear bat velocity of 31 m/sec, which occurred in unison with a right-arm maximum extension velocity of 948 degrees/sec.

Conclusions.—An initial biomechanical description of the act of hitting a baseball was determined. Quantitative studies of the hitting motion should permit a more educated approach to rehabilitation, strength, and conditioning programs for hitting athletes. The data reflect the body's natural motion and coordination. Further studies will look at the link

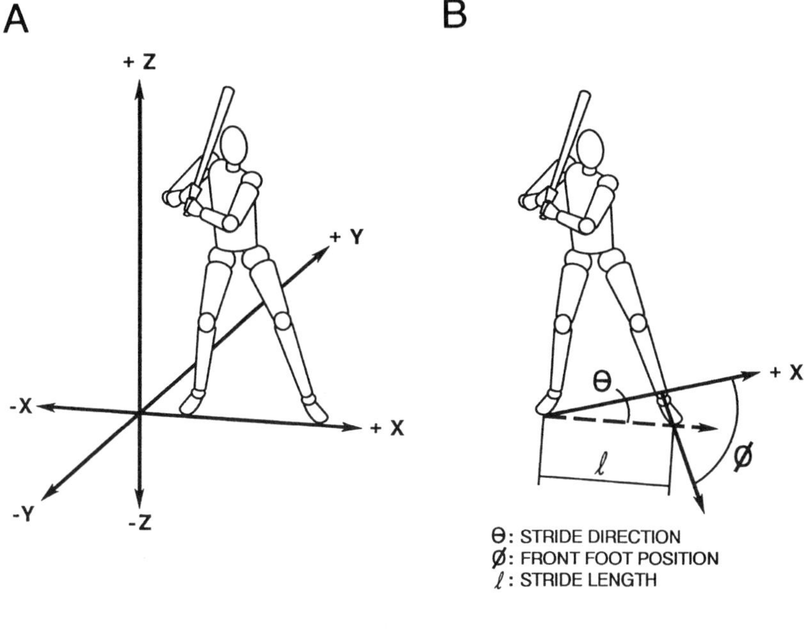

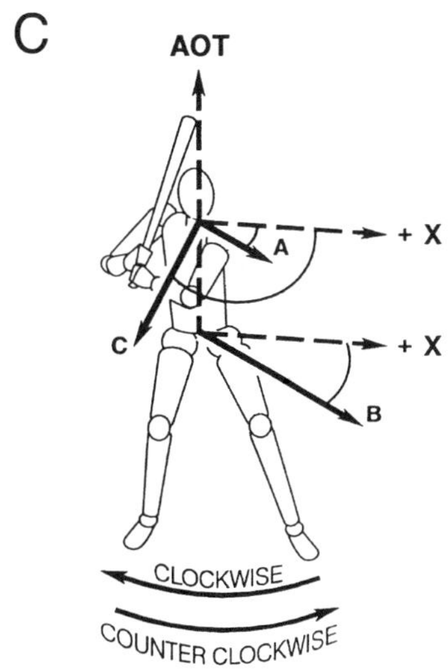

FIGURE 2.—Batter orientation and movement. **A,** global reference frame. **B,** stride parameters. **C,** segmental rotation around axis of the trunk (*AOT*). (Courtesy of Welch CM, Banks SA, Cook FF, et al: Hitting a baseball: A biomechanical description. *J Orthop Sports Phys Ther* 22:193–201, 1995.)

between the rotational and linear components of weight transfer, the specific interactions of segments involved in the kinetic link, and the acceleration and power with which the bat meets the ball.

▶ It has often been said that hitting a baseball that is coming at you at speeds of 80–95 mph may be 1 of the most difficult athletic skills to master. Likewise, doing a biomechanical analysis that will be useful to batting coaches will be equally difficult.

In this study the ball was hit off a batting tee. The issue of recognition of the pitch and adjustment to the location of the ball was not a problem here. However, in future studies the authors intend to bring those variables together, and an entirely new set of difficulties will be introduced. It may take a lifetime of work to fully analyze the baseball swing at a pitched baseball.

Col. J.L. Anderson, PE.D.

A Comparison of the High and Low Backspin Backhand Drives in Tennis Using Different Grips

Elliott B, Christmass M (Univ of Western Australia, Nedlands)

J Sports Sci 13:141–151, 1995 1–6

Objective.—Using 3-dimensional, high-speed cinematography, the backspin backhand techniques of state-ranked and international-ranked tennis players hitting low- and high-bouncing balls with different racket grips were compared.

Methods.—Study participants were 10 male and 3 female tennis players, 9 state-ranked and 4 playing at the international level. All were selected for their ability to play a high-performance-level backspin backhand drive. Players used their own rackets during the study condition and were filmed with identical camera positions. The preferred grip of all players was the eastern backhand or continental grip with the hand generally on top of the handle; also evaluated was the "behind the handle" grip, which was not preferred. The Direct Linear Transformation method was used for 3-dimensional reconstruction from the cameras' 2-dimensional images.

Results.—All players lifted their racket-hand to approximately shoulder height at the start of the backswing, producing the looped motion identified as a common feature of advanced play. The nonpreferred grip impacted the ball further in front of the body compared with the preferred grip, and this difference was significant. In addition, a significantly lower peak of racket-shoulder speed was recorded for a high-bouncing ball when using the nonpreferred grip. When hitting a high-bouncing ball (41.6 cm above hip height), players using both grips adopted a more upright trunk, a more rotated shoulder alignment, a larger front knee angle, and a more abducted upper arm. Racket velocity remained relatively constant whatever the grip condition or height of impact. The height of impact, however, had a significant influence on racket trajectory and racket-face angle. For all conditions, the racket-tip speed was approximately 50% of its pre-impact value during the early part of follow-through.

Conclusion.—High-level tennis players can still hit an effective backspin backhand to balls of various heights using the "behind the handle" grip. The only significant differences between this nonpreferred grip and the preferred grip were that the ball was impacted further forward of the front ankle and that the peak racket-shoulder speed was lower.

▶ Although these authors say there appears to be very little research concerning the mechanics of the backspin 1-handed backhand drive, I want to add that there has been very little scientific discovery involving the mechanics of anything having to do with tennis. Does anyone else feel that way? It appears that the mechanics of tennis strokes have been developed over years of trial-and-error practice. Those mechanics were then passed on from teacher to student, and only the most creative teacher tried to make significant changes in those mechanics. In recent years we have seen the hard-swinging and big topspin players dominate. Smaller players are again finding a role in tennis because of the change in stroke mechanics and the change in the tennis racket.

Col. J.L. Anderson, PE.D.

Optimizing the Determination of the Body Center of Mass

Kingma I, Toussaint HM, Commissaris DACM, Hoozemans MJM, Ober MJ (Vrije Universiteit, Amsterdam)

J Biomech 28:1137–1142, 1995 1–7

Background.—When studying translational motions, the entire mass of the body is viewed as being concentrated in the so-called center of mass (COM). The chief error in estimating body COM arises when apportioning mass over body segments and in estimating the positions of local centers of mass of the various segments. Because the trunk is a substantial part of total body mass, any error in locating its COM significantly affects the whole-body COM.

Objective and Methods.—An attempt was made to minimize error in estimating the body COM trajectory during movement through a simple static optimization of the position of the trunk COM. Five men picked up a barbell weighing one fifth of their body weight at a level of 14% of body height and lifted it vertically to the level of the acromion. They used both a back technique in which the knees are straight and the trunk is flexed and a leg technique with the knees flexed and the trunk kept as straight as possible. Three different postures, with the trunk at 0, 45, and 90 degrees of forward flexion, were each maintained for a few seconds. The position of the trunk COM was optimized by relating the center of pressure of the ground reaction force to the vertical projection of the body COM during the various postures. The validity of this estimation was determined by relating the external moment of the ground reaction force (with respect to the body COM) to the rate of change in angular momentum of the whole body.

Results.—After optimizing the trunk COM, the external moment of the ground reaction force corresponded more closely to the rate of change in angular momentum. This was the case for both lifting techniques. For the leg technique, optimization led to a mean regression slope closer to unity. Errors in absolute mean moment were less marked when the trunk COM was optimized, but this was significant only for the back technique of lifting.

Conclusion.—This procedure is a simple, rapid, and valid means of improving estimates of body COM when a precise estimate of the COM trajectory during movement is needed.

▶ This optimization procedure takes into account many sources of error that investigators must be aware of in doing biomechanical research. This is especially true when whole-body movements are being analyzed. We all realize that it is our ability to locate and control for measurement error that gives validity to our research findings. The authors have presented us with what appears to be a reasonable proposal.

Col. J.L. Anderson, PE.D.

The Extended Transentropy Function as a Useful Quantifier of Human Motion Variability

Hatze H (Univ of Vienna)

Med Sci Sports Exerc 27:751–759, 1995 1–8

A New Concept.—It is possible to quantify the variability of iterated human motions (as well as other recurring biological phenomena) by viewing variations in repeated stereotyped motions as manifestations of a regular stochastic process on which chaotic excursions are infrequently superimposed. The extended "transentropy" of such a process is a dimensionless quantitative expression of motion variability. Extended transentropy functions may be used to monitor changes in variability during the execution of various motions.

Application.—This approach was used to quantify the variability in repeated kip motions on the horizontal bar. In 2 of the 32 gymnasts studied, the learning process was monitored using this technique. The gymnasts were photographed while executing 3 sequences of 6 motion repetitions at baseline, after 3 weeks of practice, and again after 3 more weeks of training. Successive configurations of the motion were represented by computer graphics (Fig 2). The reference motion was defined as the best of all the successful motions executed.

Conclusion.—Transentropy is an appropriate means of quantifying motion variability, and in this way it may serve to depict the convergence properties of various motor-learning tasks.

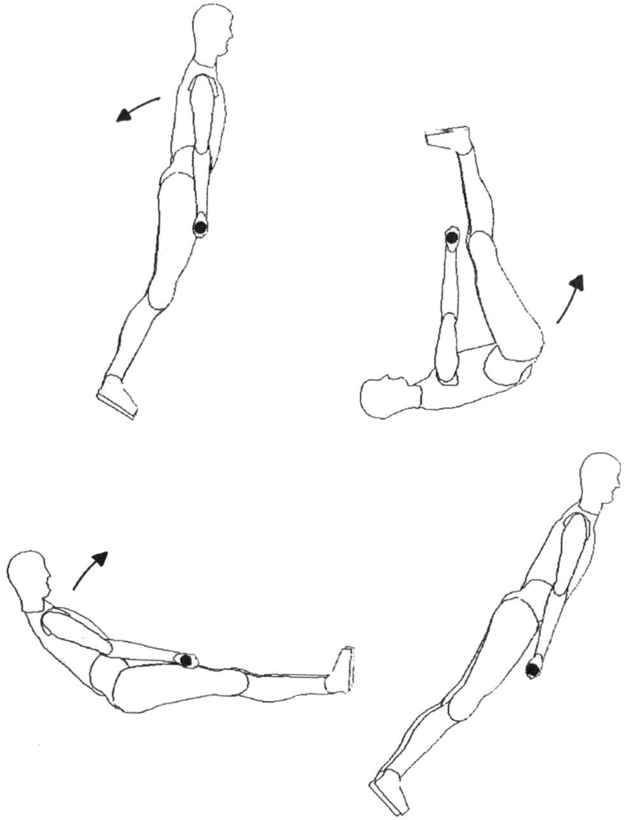

FIGURE 2.—Computer-graphical representation of 4 successive configurations of the type of kip on the horizontal bar investigated in the study. **Top left,** initial configuration. **Bottom right,** terminal configuration. (Courtesy of Hatze H: The extended transentropy function as a useful quantifier of human motion variability. *Med Sci Sports Exerc* 27:751–759, 1995.)

► The author explains that the transentropy concept is a dimensionless variability quantifier using the fixed and data-invariant chaotic excursion variances as normalizing quantities. He contends that the transentropy measure reflects solely the variability properties of the data set and does not depend on any other properties such as mean values. He also states that the transentropy concept may enable us to establish direct connections between the observed motion variations and their underlying causes. This method can be applied equally well to any biological phenomenon that is of a recurrent nature and that can be described by time functions of generalized coordinates. This method appears to have great promise as a useful tool in many areas of motion analysis.

Col. J.L. Anderson, PE.D.

Critical Characteristics of Technique in Throwing the Discus

Hay JG, Yu B (Univ of Iowa, Iowa City)
J Sports Sci 13:125–140, 1995 1–9

Objective.—A model of discus throwing was developed in an effort to learn which technical aspects of this activity determine the distance thrown. The chief components of the model are d_L, the distance lost, which is the horizontal extent over which the discus travels in flight for which

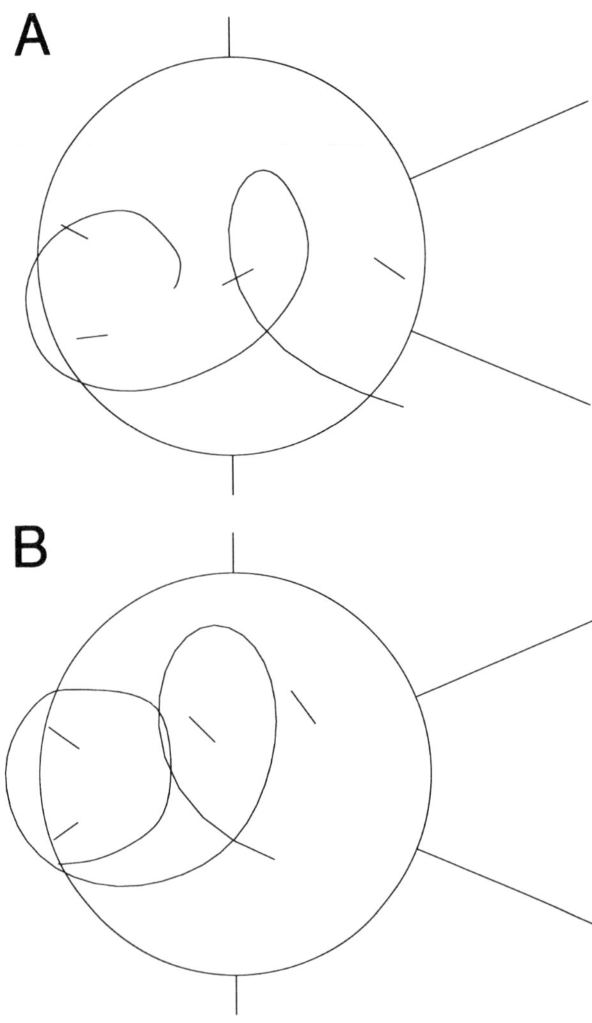

FIGURE 4.—The path followed by the center of gravity of the discus and the location of the point of release for the throws in which (**A**) the minimum and (**B**) the maximum values of distance lost were recorded. (Courtesy of Hay JG, Yu B: Critical characteristics of technique in throwing the discus. *J Sports Sci* 13:125–140, 1995.)

credit is not given in estimating the official length of the throw; and d_F, or flight distance—the horizontal extent from the center of the discus when released to the landing mark.

Methods.—Two video cameras recorded the performance of men and women competing in discus-throwing events at 2 major meetings. The direct linear transformation procedure provided 3-dimensional performance data.

Results.—Values of d_L were small compared with the overall distance thrown (less than 1%), but this parameter is not a negligible one (Fig 4). For male throwers, the change in discus speed in the second double support phase was a more important determinant of distance than the change in speed during any other phase. For women, changes in speed during both the flight phase and the second double support phase were important. The speed of release was by far the most outstanding determinant of the distance thrown. For both men and women, approximately two thirds of the speed at release was generated in the second double support phase.

Conclusions.—The emphasis placed on the final discus-throwing motion is well placed. Elite women throwers might usefully attempt to increase the discus speed in the flight phase of their throws.

▶ This is an excellent demonstration and discussion of the biomechanical techniques necessary to produce accurate analyses of the many variables involved in throwing events. The authors point out that we must be aware that we should not overgeneralize from our data. For instance, if the data are from a cross-section research design, taken from the best trial by each of a number of individuals, generalizations can only be made about the technique factors that influence the distances recorded by those individuals. Likewise, in a longitudinal analysis, involving analysis of many throws by 1 athlete, generalizations can only be drawn about the factors that influence the distances recorded by that 1 individual.

This study was a cross-section study. Because this study included both elite women and men throwers, it is of interest to see that the techniques of the men and women, although apparently the same, produce different results. For instance, for the men, the change in speed of the discus during the second double support phase was most influential in accounting for differences in the distances of the throws recorded. For the women, the change in speed of the discus during the flight phase—which is measured from the end of the first single support phase to the instant the athlete's right foot regains contact with the ground—and during the second double support phase were about equally influential in accounting for differences in the distance of the throw. Do coaches encourage women to do something differently, or does the difference come about by trial and error?

Col. J.L. Anderson, PE.D.

Modelling of Rational Variants of the Speed-skating Technique

Voronov AV, Lavrovsky EK, Zatsiorsky VM (All Union Research Inst of Sport, Moscow; Univ of Moscow; Pennsylvania State Univ, University Park)

J Sports Sci 13:153–170, 1995 1–10

Objective.—An attempt was made to model the various phases of speed skating, including the free-skate phase starting at push-off, the single support push-off phase ending when the swing foot touches the ice, and the double support push phase.

Methods.—An 11-segment planar model was computerized to estimate net joint moments, reaction moments, and mechanical energy expenditure. Initially, a 2-dimensional mechanical model of speed skating was constructed. Experimental data on aerodynamic forces and kinematics were applied. Finally, the known average velocities in the 3 phases and body positions at the phase boundaries were used to estimate instantaneous velocities and accelerative forces.

Findings.—When a skater is skating the straight parts of a circuit, the most efficient technique is the run without arm swing and use of the sideward push-off. No active swing is made by the recovery leg. It is most efficient for the skater to place the recovery leg on the ice and "load" it as rapidly as possible. An increased wind speed opposing the skater increases mechanical energy expenditure and reduces the efficiency of the technique. Sideward push-off with a small swing movement lessens the negative value of the horizontal reaction force in the final part of the single support push-off.

▶ Most of us who enjoy watching speed skating are probably amazed at the small time differences that determine the winners. These authors have studied the skating techniques on the straight parts of the skating oval to determine the most efficient technique by computing the mechanical energy expenditure. This is a very complicated, well-done, biomechanical study. The 3 phases of the study include developing the 2-dimensional mechanical model; conducting experiments to determine the aerodynamics forces and develop the kinematics data to include step length, length of phases, form of touchdown, and average velocity in phases; and finally, solving the inverse dynamics problems and making a comparison of the possible variants of the speed-skating techniques. I would imagine that a similar study of the skating techniques around the curves will be even more challenging.

Col. J.L. Anderson, PE.D.

The Assessment of Mechanical and Neuromuscular Response Strategies During Landing

Caster BL, Bates BT (Western Oregon State College, Monmouth; Univ of Oregon, Eugene)

Med Sci Sports Exerc 27:736–744, 1995 1–11

Objective.—To gauge the relative roles of mechanical and neuromuscular mechanisms in controlling landing, studies were performed in 4 male university students who participated recreationally in sports involving landing activities.

Methods.—Vertical ground reaction forces were recorded on a force platform as the study participants performed numerous landings from a height of 2 ft with and without ankle weights attached. Masses of 1,024 and 1,800 g were used on different test days. Electromyographic data were recorded from 5 lower-limb muscles.

Results.—Fourteen of 32 single subject comparisons were significant in a mechanically predicted direction, indicating that both mechanical and neuromuscular response strategies were used. Rearfoot impact responses were consistent with a model predicting altered mechanical force. More than protective neuromuscular responses may be involved, as suggested by the presence of mechanical responses for forefoot impact that were not totally explained by the model. Multiple regression analyses showed the integrated electromyographic data of the vastus medialis to be the most common independent variable.

Conclusions.—Different individuals use multiple strategies entailing mechanical and neuromuscular responses during landing activities. Future studies should take perceptual parameters and cognitive characteristics into account.

▶ This study was done using 4 men in a 25-trial design that was deemed adequate for both individual subject and group analyses. The authors pointed out that this study identified multiple response strategies among research subjects and that the nature of the response patterns was consistent with the types of strategies observed in response to the addition of mass in running. They then went on to generalize their results to the population of young adults.

I suggest that it would be far safer to conduct a similar study using women as research subjects before generalizing these data to the population of women. My own observation is that women demonstrate different landing patterns than men, especially from greater heights than those used in this study.

Col. J.L. Anderson, PE.D.

Predicting the Kinematics and Kinetics of Gait Based on the Optimum Trajectory of the Swing Limb

Chou LS, Song SM, Draganich LF (Univ of Chicago; Univ of Illinois, Chicago)
J Biomech 28:377–385, 1995 1–12

Background.—Human locomotion is a highly complex, organized, and efficient activity. Self-determined walking results in maximum gross efficiency, suggesting that body motion during locomotion is controlled as to minimize mechanical energy expended. Much of the energy demand that occurs during gait comes from the swing limb. To predict the minimum energy consumption trajectory of the swing limb, an algorithm was developed, and the predictions were compared with actual measurements.

Methods.—The study modeled the lower extremities during the swing phase as an open-chain manipulator system. The multistage optimization method known as dynamic programming was used to determine the optimum swing ankle trajectory that would minimize the mechanical energy required to generate the joint moments of the lower extremities during the single support phase of gait. Six healthy individuals provided gait measurement data for comparison with the predictions.

Results.—For most hip and knee flexion angles in the swing limb, the predicted values were not significantly different from the measured ones. The only significant differences were noted in hip flexion at times greater than 75% of the swing period. The predicted and measured ground reaction forces were similar. In addition, the joint moments measured were comparable to those calculated from the measured ground reaction forces and the kinematics of the limbs.

Conclusions.—Predictive equations based on the optimum trajectory of the swing limb support the hypothesis that human gait is energy efficient in terms of the mechanical energy generated by the joints. The muscles and joints of the hip, knee, and ankle are controlled such that the resulting joint loads minimize the energy required during gait.

▶ The purpose of this study was to develop an algorithm to predict the minimum energy consumption trajectory of the swing limb and then to compare its accuracy by using 6 healthy individuals. The authors began by hypothesizing that the human gait is energy efficient. They used the criterion of minimum energy consumption to predict the most energy-efficient trajectory of the swing limb between toe-off and heel strike. In comparing the predicted and measured results, no statistical differences were found in hip flexion angles except at times greater than 75% of the swing period; no statistical differences were found between the predicted and measured knee flexion angles; no statistical differences were found between the predicted and measured ground reaction forces; and no statistical differences were found between the predicted and measured moments of the stance ankle and knee, moments of the stance hip, or moments of the swing hip. It appears that the hypothesis that human gait is energy efficient must be accepted.

Col. J.L. Anderson, PE.D.

Determinants of the Gait Transition Speed During Human Locomotion: Kinematic Factors

Hreljac A (Human Movement Research Ctr, San Diego, Calif)
J Biomech 28:669–677, 1995 1–13

Background.—Gait transitions may be a means of saving energy, but recent studies suggest that both human beings and horses prefer to change their gait at speeds that are not ergonomically optimal. If metabolic energy consumption is not the chief determinant of the preferred transition speed (PTS), kinetic factors are an alternative possibility. The human locomotor system shows very consistent kinematic patterns.

Objective and Methods.—An attempt was made to learn whether kinematic factors are determinants of the PTS during human locomotion. For 20 active and physically fit individuals, 10 men and 10 women, the PTS was determined at 0%, 10%, and 15% treadmill inclination. Four criteria were specified that must be satisfied by a given variable to accept it as a determinant of PTS. Three of them were examined by literature search as well as being experimentally tested.

Findings.—Values of PTS differed significantly with the degree of inclination. All variables increased with walking speed under each condition, and they decreased abruptly when the study participant began running. The only variable that met all 4 criteria was maximum angular velocity at the ankle. Maximum angular acceleration at the ankle came close to meeting all the criteria.

Conclusion.—The chief reason why humans change gait at the PTS is to prevent overexertion and injury of the small dorsiflexor muscles, which may work close to peak capacity during walking at speeds at or near the PTS.

▶ The PTS can best be explained as that speed at which an individual goes from a fast walk to a slow running gait. This study is a continuation of a number of studies to discover the determinants of the gait transition speed or the PTS. This author believes it is probable that the localized discomfort experienced in the dorsiflexor muscles, including the tibialis anterior, the extensor digitorum longus, and the extensor hallucis longus, was responsible for the change in gait because the study participants reported a higher perceived exertion when walking at the PTS than when running at the same speed.

Col. J.L. Anderson, PE.D.

Footswitch System for Measurement of the Temporal Parameters of Gait

Hausdorff JM, Ladin Z, Wei JY (Boston Univ; Beth Israel Hosp, Boston; Harvard Med School, Boston)

J Biomech 28:347–351, 1995 1–14

Background.—Accurate measures of initial and end foot contact times are essential in gait analysis. These contact times serve as a reference for correlating all other data on gait and as a way to distinguish normal from abnormal gaits. To provide accurate estimates of the beginning and end of the stance phase for sequential steps, a simple, inexpensive footswitch system was developed.

Methods.—Five men and 5 women volunteered for a study to validate the new system. The system, which can be easily reproduced for laboratory use for less than $50, was based on a commercially available transducer. The start and end of the stance phase were estimated, which did not necessitate custom footwear, extensive calibration, or exact placement of the sensor in the shoe. Footswitch-based estimates of initial and end foot contact times were compared with those acquired as each volunteer took 30 steps across a force platform. Ten steps each were taken at slow, normal, and fast walking speeds.

Findings.—The estimates coincided within ± 10 msec for the start of the stance phase and ± 22 msec for the end. The differences ranged from − 24 to 28 msec for the duration of stance. Combined, these measures were able to estimate stance duration to within 3% of values determined by force platform for steps with stance durations of 446–1,594 msec. Swing and stride duration estimates were also within 5% of the values determined by force platform.

Conclusions.—This new footswitch system provides continuous, sequential estimates of the temporal parameters of gait and can therefore supplement platform-based measures limited to isolated steps. The analogue voltage signal included in the new system permits the use of other thresholds and provides a step-by-step qualitative description of the time history of the forces in the shoe. Estimates of initial foot contact are highly accurate. Initial foot contact time determined by this system can serve as a well-defined reference point for other data on gait. The main advantage of this system is its easy, cost-effective reproducibility.

► Any time someone develops an easier and cheaper way to collect data accurately, we should pay attention to it. Here is such a case.

Col. J.L. Anderson, PE.D.

Comparison of 2-Dimensional and 3-Dimensional Rearfoot Motion During Walking

Cornwall MW, McPoil TG (Northern Arizona Univ, Flagstaff)

Clin Biomech 10:36–40, 1995 1–15

Background.—The relationship between rearfoot motion and injury has made video-based motion assessment systems popular. Two-dimensional analysis is increasingly used in clinical settings, probably because it is not as costly as 3-dimensional systems. To determine the validity of the 2-dimensional system, 2-dimensional and 3-dimensional analyses of foot inversion and eversion during walking were compared.

Methods and Findings.—Seven women and 4 men (mean age, 26.7 years) volunteered for the study. All individuals underwent 2- and 3-dimensional analyses while walking (Fig 1). Rearfoot motion assessed with either system was essentially the same for the first 60% of the stance phase. The 2 methods did not differ significantly in variables that are usually assessed in studies on rearfoot motion. Although stance duration and heel strike angle differed significantly between the 2 analyses, no significant differences were found in time to heel off, maximum pronation, or time to maximum pronation. Stance-phase durations in the 2 analyses were very strongly correlated.

Conclusions.—Assessing rearfoot motion during walking often provides useful information in a clinical setting. However, the high cost of equipment needed for 3-dimensional analysis and the time required make this type of analysis impractical. Rearfoot motion determined by either 2- or 3-dimensional analysis in this study was essentially the same for the initial 60% of the stance phase. Also, the 2 methods were comparable in vari-

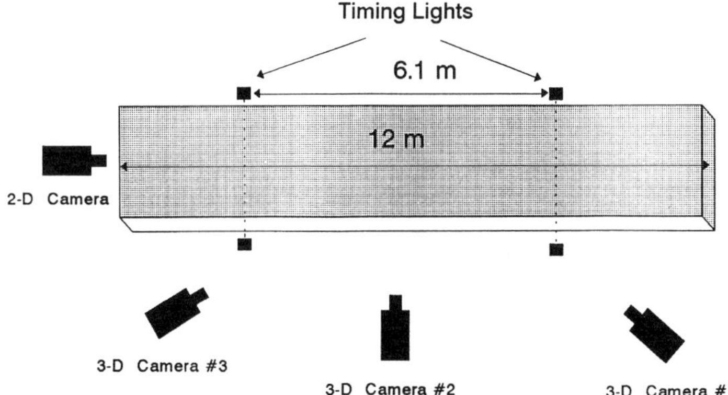

FIGURE 1.—Diagram of the walkway, timing lights, and camera placement used during filming of each walking trial. (Reprinted from Cornwall MW, McPoil TG: Comparison of 2-dimensional and 3-dimensional rearfoot motion during walking. *Clin Biomech* 10:36–40, Copyright 1995, with kind permission from Elsevier Science Ltd, The Boulevard, Langford Lane, Kidlington OX5 1GB, UK.)

ables typically included in studies of rearfoot motion. Thus, 2-dimensional analysis is an accurate, feasible way to measure rearfoot motion in the clinic.

► In a clinical setting, there appears to be no justifiable reason to use 3-dimensional analysis for recording rearfoot motion during walking when the less expensive and less time-consuming 2-dimensional method gives results that are about as accurate within the first 8% to 60% of the stance phase.

Col. J.L. Anderson, PE.D.

Incline, Speed, and Distance Assessment During Unconstrained Walking

Aminian K, Robert P, Jéquier E, Schutz Y (Swiss Fed Inst of Technology, Lausanne, Switzerland; Univ of Lausanne, Switzerland)

Med Sci Sports Exerc 27:226–234, 1995 1–16

Introduction.—The use of accelerometers allows various aspects of the complex mechanism of walking to be assessed. To record body accelerations during walking, a portable measuring device was used. A new method for parameterizing the body acceleration signals and determining patterns of different forms of walking at a variety of inclines and speeds also was outlined.

Methods.—Six healthy volunteers, 3 men and 3 women with a mean age of 21 years, took part in the study. A period of treadmill acclimatization was provided because only 2 participants were accustomed to treadmill walking. The volunteers then walked at their own preferred speeds on the level and at positive and negative inclines. Experiments were repeated with participants walking below and above their own preferred speed at 0%, +10%, and −10% inclines. These treadmill exercises were followed by self-paced walking on an outdoor test circuit involving roads of various inclines.

A total of 20 parameters obtained during walking were averaged over the number of gait cycles to obtain mean values. Parameters computed from the accelerations recorded on the treadmill formed a set of 360 training patterns. Neural networks designed to recognize patterns of walking and estimate speed and incline were first "trained" by known patterns of treadmill walking. Estimates were then produced for the inclines, speeds, and distances covered during the outdoor circuit.

Results.—Ten of the 20 parameters demonstrated an appreciable correlation with speed and incline. For all participants, the median value of the forward acceleration, the covariance between vertical and heel acceleration, and the covariance between lateral and heel acceleration showed a strong correlation with incline; variance of the vertical acceleration and gait cycle time were strongly correlated with speed. For the other 5 parameters, the correlation with speed or incline was related to each participant's gait characteristics. Actual and predicted variables showed good agreement.

Conclusion.—This new method of parameterization of body accelerations during walking used 2 neural networks to estimate the incline, speed, and covered distance of walking. After treadmill data were obtained, individual estimations of these variables were made for level and slope overground walking. This method provides a new tool for the assessment of walking and other daily physical activities.

► With the increased popularity of walking for exercise, it is time that investigators begin a more complete assessment of walking as a daily exercise. However, because many if not most of the individuals who are using walking as a daily exercise are in the chronologically superior category, we should know whether this new tool is equally applicable to them.

Col. J.L. Anderson, PE.D.

Influence of Shoes and Heel Strike on the Loading of the Hip Joint

Bergmann G, Kniggendorf H, Graichen F, Rohlmann A (Free Univ, Berlin)

J Biomech 28:817–827, 1995 1–17

Background.—The forces and moments acting at the hip joint affect the long-term stability of endoprosthetic fixation and the course of coxarthrosis. These loads may rely on the type of footwear being used as well as walking or running styles. To determine whether the peak values of the forces and moments acting at the hip joint during walking and slow jogging are affected by shoe type or heel strike intensity, 1 patient with arthritis was studied.

Methods.—A patient with severe arthritis with instrumented hip implants was studied. This man was in excellent physical condition and was 82 years of age. He was assessed while wearing different sports shoes, normal leather shoes, hiking boots, and clogs with soft, normal, and hard heel strikes. He was also assessed while walking barefoot (Fig 1).

Findings.—Loads were lowest when the patient was walking and jogging barefoot. All shoes increased the joint force and the bending moment slightly at the implant. The torsional moment increased by as much as half. No association was found between shoe type and load increase. Only shoes with very hard soles were clearly a disadvantage. No advantages were associated with soft heels, soles, or insoles.

Conclusions.—Gait stability apparently plays the most important role in increasing joint loading. Therefore, this should be the criterion for choice of footwear. The only way to decrease joint loading during slow jogging is by smooth gait patterns with soft heel strikes.

► This study was selected because it is an excellent demonstration of a biomechanical procedure to determine whether the peak values of the

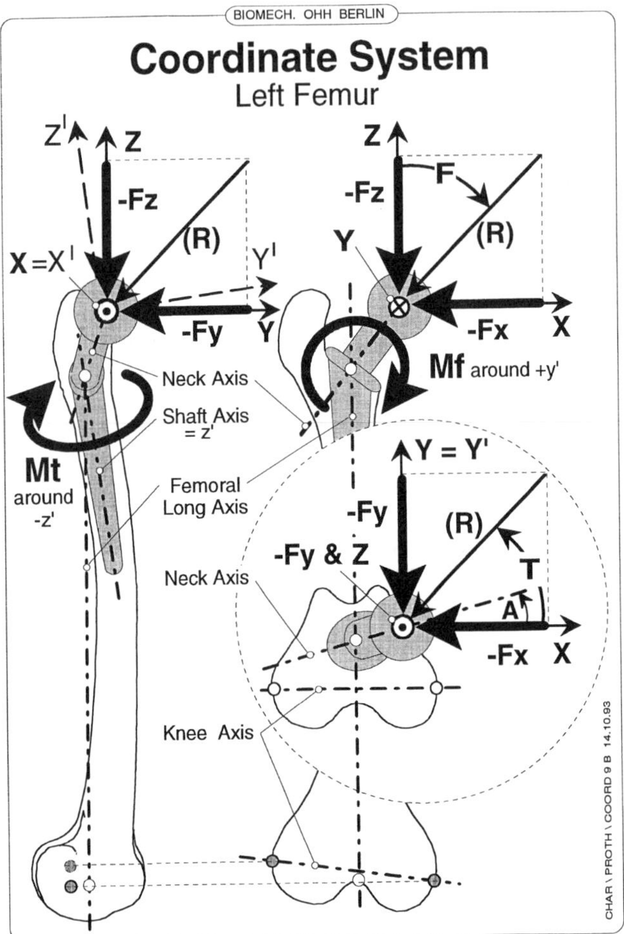

FIGURE 1.—Coordinate systems and measured loads and angles. The coordinate system *x-y-z* is femur-based. The *z* axis is parallel to the long femoral axis, *x* lies in the plane *z*/knee axis. The resultant force *R* consists of the components $-F_x$, $-F_y$, $-F_z$, which points toward the center of the head. The direction of *R* is described by the angles *F* in the frontal plane *x-z* and *T* in the transverse plane *x-y*. The bending moment M_f and the torsional moment M_t are given in the implant-based coordinate system *x-y-z'*. M_f acts around the intersection of the stem and the neck axis, M_t acts around the stem axis. The direction *z'* is parallel to the stem axis. *A* is the anteversion angle of the implant. (Reprinted from Bergmann G, Kniggendorf H, Graichen F, et al: Influence of shoes and heel strike on the loading of the hip joint. *J Biomech* 28:817–827, 1995. Courtesy of Bergmann G, Graishen F, Rohlmann A: Is staircase walking a risk for the fixation of hip implants? *J Biomechanics*, in press, with kind permission from Elsevier Science Ltd, The Boulevard, Langford Lane, Kidlington OX5 1GB, UK.)

forces and moments acting at the hip joint during walking and slow jogging are influenced by the kind of shoes or by the intensity of the heel strike. Other authors have shown that the mechanical interaction between foot, shoe, and floor is extremely complex and is influenced by a variety of parameters. I imagine that 1 of those parameters is foot placement. It has been my experience and observation that individuals whose foot placement exaggerates the toe-out position experience more injuries to the knees and ankles. It could therefore follow that the same could apply to the hip joint.

Col. J.L. Anderson, PE.D.

Influence of Heel Height on Ankle Joint Moments in Running

Reinschmidt C, Nigg BM (Univ of Calgary, Alta, Canada)

Med Sci Sports Exerc 27:410–416, 1995 1–18

Introduction.—Heel height is 1 of the parameters of shoe design that can affect the kinetics or kinematics of the lower extremities during running. Heel lifting is thought to decrease the Achilles tendon forces, thereby serving to prevent and treat Achilles tendinitis. To determine the effect of heel height on resultant ankle flexion moments during running, 5 physically active men were studied.

Methods.—The 5 men had a mean age of 31.6 years and a mean weight of 72.7 kg. Standard running shoes were used, all identical except in their heel height. Each participant took part in 5 running trials, during which it was assumed that plantarflexion moments at the ankle joint would indicate Achilles tendon loading. Running was performed so that the research subjects would contact a force plate with their right foot; running speed was controlled by photo cells. The study was limited to analysis of axial or average Achilles tendon loading within the sagittal foot plane.

Results.—In 4 of the 5 study participants, a small dorsiflexion moment occurred during the first 20% of the stance phase; the average magnitude of this initial dorsiflexion moment was 12.6 nm. Plantarflexion moments were present in all research subjects and trials after 20% of the stance phase. For all research subjects and trials, the maximum plantarflexion

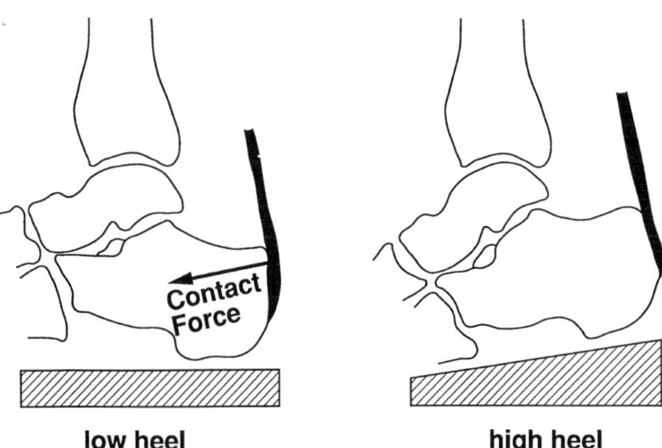

FIGURE 5.—Representation of the idea of friction between Achilles' tendon and calcaneus (superior calcaneal tuberosity) in low- and high-heel running shoes. (Adapted from Hintermann B, Holzach P: Die Bursitis subachillea: Eine Biomechanische Studie [Bursitis subachillea: A biomechanical study]. *Der Orthopäde* 130:114–119, 1992. Courtesy of Reinschmidt C, Nigg BM: Influence of heel height on ankle joint moments in running. *Med Sci Sports Exerc* 27:410–416, 1995.)

moment averaged 240 nm. Changes in heel height had a significant effect on the variables associated with the maximum flexion/extension moment. A lifting of the heel changed the relative position of the calcaneus with respect to the tibia (Fig 5). Maximum plantarflexion moment and its time of occurrence were not significantly affected, however, indicating that heel lifts do not generally decrease the Achilles tendon loading during running.

Conclusion.—Changes in heel height of running shoes primarily affected the beginning of the stance phase. Because maximum plantarflexion moments were not significantly altered, changes in heel height do not appear to be able to reduce Achilles tendon forces in most individuals.

▶ These authors did not find that increasing the heel height in running shoes will lessen the strain on the Achilles tendon, thus reducing the chance for Achilles tendinitis. I have found that most cases of Achilles tendinitis can be prevented or controlled with the use of rear foot controls, which correct for excessive pronation of the feet.

Col. J.L. Anderson, PE.D.

Direct Dynamics Simulation of the Impact Phase in Heel–Toe Running

Gerritsen KGM, van den Bogert AJ, Nigg BM (Univ of Calgary, Canada)

J Biomech 28:661–668, 1995 1–19

Background.—The relationship between the causes of running injuries and the mechanics of running is not clear. The effects of muscle activation, position, and velocities of body segments at touchdown and surface properties on impact forces during heel–toe running were studied.

Methods and Findings.—A direct dynamics simulation technique was used. A 2-dimensional, 4-segment, musculoskeletal model represented the runner (Fig 1). Activation dynamics and the force-length and force-velocity characteristics of 7 major muscle groups of the lower extremities were incorporated into the muscle model. The muscle groups were the glutei, hamstrings, rectus femoris, vasti, gastrocnemius, soleus, and tibialis anterior muscles. Vertical force-deformation characteristics of the heel, shoe, and ground were simulated with a nonlinear viscoelastic element. A typical simulated impact force was a maximum of 1.6 times body weight.

The effects of muscle activation were assessed by generating muscle stimulation combinations producing the same resultant joint moments at heelstrike. With these different combinations of muscle stimulation levels, simulated impact peak forces varied less than 10%. Muscle activation had a potentially much greater effect on impact force without this restriction on initial joint moments. Plantarflexion and vertical velocity of the heel at touchdown heavily influenced impact peak force. Also, initial knee flexion played a role in impact absorption. Increased surface stiffness produced greater impact peak forces.

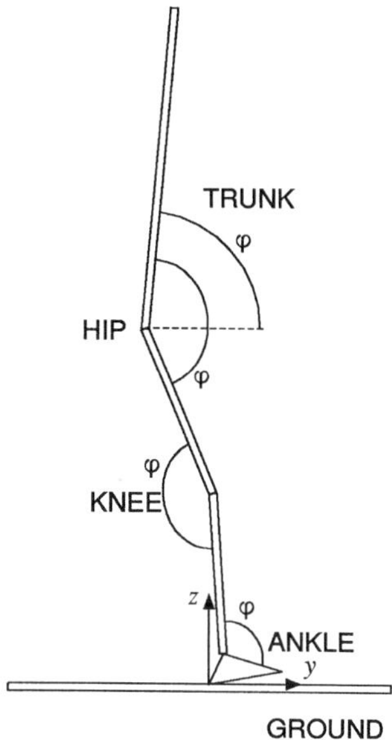

FIGURE 1.—The 4-segment model of the runner and the ground. (Courtesy of Gerritsen KGM, van den Bogert AJ, Nigg BM: Direct dynamics simulation of the impact phase in heel–toe running. *J Biomech* 28:661–668. Copyright 1995, with kind permission from Elsevier Science Ltd, The Boulevard, Langford Lane, Kidlington OX5 1GB, UK.)

Conclusions.—Changes in initial kinematic conditions are primarily responsible for variations in impact forces. Muscular co-contraction does not play a major role.

▶ Although the relationship between the causes of running injuries and the mechanics of running may not be clear, we will agree, I think, that the amount of running is a major cause of many of the injuries. Even our best runners become injured as they add more and more miles to their training. It also seems that women runners experience as many if not more injuries than male runners as their mileage increases.

Impact peak forces alone apparently also are not the answer because those forces vary so greatly depending on the runner. Do we know the relationship between impact peak forces and body mass? It would appear to be a direct correlation, but do well-conditioned heavy individuals exerience more running injuries per mile run than do well-conditioned individuals who weigh less? Is it not possible that the amount of running is the best predictor of running injuries for the average runner?

Col. J.L. Anderson, PE.D.

Muscle Damage Following Repeated Bouts of High Force Eccentric Exercise

Nosaka K, Clarkson PM (Yokohama City Univ, Japan; Univ of Massachusetts, Amherst)

Med Sci Sports Exerc 27:1263–1269, 1995 1–20

Background.—Strenuous eccentric exercise is known to damage muscle tissue, but repeated bouts of the same exercise have not resulted in more than modest changes in indicators of damage. Most studies, however, have focused on the period of adaptation and have not examined the effect of a second bout of exercise preceding full recovery of muscle function.

Study Plan.—Whether several days of rest are needed for strenuous repeat exercise not to exacerbate initial muscle damage was determined in 12 young adult men who had not participated in weight training. High-force eccentric exercise was repeated 3 and 6 days after the initial bout, which consisted of 3 sets of 10 eccentric elbow flexor actions using a dumbbell set at 80% of baseline maximal isometric force.

Observations.—Significant muscle soreness was demonstrated by palpation and by extending the forearm after initial exercise; it gradually diminished after 4 days. Force generation was decreased by 50% after the first bout of exercise and by nearly as much after the subsequent 2 episodes. Loss of force did not exceed 50% of baseline at any time. The relaxed elbow angle was significantly reduced after initial exercise, and the flexed angle increased. Subsequent exercise did not lead to significantly greater changes in range of motion. Changes in creatine kinase and glutamic oxaloacetic transaminase activities were not exaggerated after the second or third bouts of exercise. Ultrasonography showed increased echo intensity after initial exercise but no signs of increased damage subsequently.

Interpretation.—Strenuous exercise of "damaged" muscles did not lead to more marked damage in this study and did not delay repair. Changes after the initial bout may have made the muscles less vulnerable to damage from subsequent exercise. Motor units may be more efficiently recruited when muscle fibers are injured.

▶ The authors' choice of the term "muscle damage" appears to be inappropriate. What they have determined is that there is loss of muscle strength and range of motion, increase in muscle proteins in the blood, and development of muscle soreness after the first exercise session. This study indicates that the muscle subsequently adapts, and these findings are not reproduced with subsequent bouts of intense exercise. What the authors really described—rather than damage—is muscle adaptation after repeated bouts of high-force eccentric exercise.

J.S. Torg, M.D.

Do Selected Kinanthropometric and Performance Variables Predict Injuries in Female Netball Players?

Hopper DM, Hopper JL, Elliott BC (Curtin Univ of Technology, Shenton Park, Wash; Univ of Melbourne, Australia; Univ of Western Australia, Nedlands)

J Sports Sci 13:213–222, 1995 1–21

Background.—Netball is a popular sport among women and girls. More than 28 countries are affiliated with the International Federation of Netball Association. However, this sport is known to be injurious to the knee and ankle joints. Ligamentous structures are the tissues most damaged. To determine which selected kinanthropometric and performance variables best predicted injuries, female netball players were studied.

Methods.—Seventy-two grade A female netball players volunteered for the prospective study. Ages ranged from 15 to 36 years. Before the start of the 14-week netball season, hypermobility, somatotype, static balance, jumping abilities, and anaerobic fitness were measured.

Findings.—Twenty-two injuries occurred in 22 players. The injuries affected the ankle joint lateral ligament complex in 59% of players, the knee ligaments in 19%, the back in 18%, and the Achilles tendon in 5%. Fifty-four percent of the injuries occurred among grade A1 players, compared with only 19% among the other grades. The proportion of injuries in grade A1 players declined with age. Injuries were more likely to occur among players with better jumping ability and better anaerobic fitness and in those who were low on the endomorphy somatotype scale. After adjustment for jumping ability and endomorphy, the difference between A1 and non-A1 players in the risk of injury was no longer significant.

Conclusions.—Young, high-performance netball players, who have better jumping ability and anaerobic capacity and a lower endomorphy component, are more susceptible to lower-limb and back injuries than older players whose performance is not as great. Prevention strategies should be focused on younger elite players to minimize the risk of injury during netball. The strongest independent predictor of injury was jumping ability.

▶ Although netball is not widely known in the United States, it is a very popular sport in many other countries around the world. It shares many of the characteristics of basketball and also, apparently, many of the same injuries. The high incidence of anterior cruciate ligament injuries among women basketball players has caused some to question whether anatomical differences between men and women at the juncture of the pelvis and femur lessen the stability of the female knee. Others point to less emphasis on teaching jumping, stopping, and turning skills or poorer conditioning for female players.

At first glance, it seems odd that netball players with better jumping skills had the highest rates of injury, but injury occurs during the landing, not the jump. Australian netball players were able to reduce the risk of ankle injuries by taping the ankle and practicing jumping and other quick movements.

Whether similar drills designed specifically for basketball could reduce anterior cruciate ligament injuries remains to be seen.

B.L. Drinkwater, Ph.D.

Kinetics of Baseball Pitching With Implications About Injury Mechanisms

Fleisig GS, Andrews JR, Dillman CJ, Escamilla RF (American Sports Medicine Inst, Birmingham, Ala)

Am J Sports Med 23:233–239, 1995 1–22

Introduction.—The large forces and torques exerted at the shoulder and elbow joints during pitching are believed to be responsible for overuse injuries, resulting from accumulated microtrauma developed during repetitive use. Building on Atwater's work and subsequent insights, shoulder and elbow joint kinetics were analyzed to determine critical instants during the pitching motion.

Methods.—Twenty-six healthy, elite pitchers (mean age, 22 years) underwent kinetic evaluation of shoulder and elbow joint during 10 fastball pitches. Reflective markers were attached to the: distal end of the mid-toe, lateral malleolus, lateral femoral epicondyle, greater trochanter, tip of the acromion, lateral humeral epicondyle, and wrist bilaterally. Motion of the whole body was digitalized. Pitches were thrown from a portable pitching mound toward a strike zone ribbon located at 60.5 feet over home plate. Ball speed was recorded with a radar gun. The 3 fastest pitches were analyzed.

Results.—Two critical instances were observed. The first critical instant occurred at maximum internal rotation torque during arm cocking, when 64% of the time from foot contact until ball release had been completed. The second critical instant occurred at maximum compressive force during arm deceleration, when 108% of the foot contact to ball release time interval had been completed.

Conclusion.—Kinetic data supported the theory that most overuse injuries to the shoulder occur at, or during the short time between, elbow flexion torque and shoulder compressive force. A need for balance between joint laxity and flexibility was observed. Further investigation of the biomechanical differences between groups of pitchers of varying skill levels and of pitchers with ineffective mechanics would help improve understanding of injury etiology.

▶ The relevance of this article lies in its explanation of injury mechanisms incurred by the throwing athlete. Explained are the forces involved in the cocking phase, which could lead to an anterior glenoid labral tear. After a ball release, posterior and compressive forces combined with horizontal abduction torque are suggested to result in cuff tensile failure. Horizontal adduction, internal rotation, and superior translation of the abducted humerus may cause subacromial impingement. Finally, the authors point out that biceps contraction for elbow flexion torque may tear the anterosuperior labrum.

J.S. Torg, M.D.

The Abductor and Adductor Strength Characteristics of Professional Baseball Pitchers

Wilk KE, Andrews JR, Arrigo CA (HEALTHSOUTH Sports Medicine & Rehabilitation Ctr, Birmingham, Ala; Alabama Sports Medicine & Orthopaedic Ctr, Birmingham)

Am J Sports Med 23:307–311, 1995 1–23

Background.—The abductor and adductor muscles of the shoulder are critical to overhead throwing. Professional baseball pitchers generate large stresses at rapid angular velocities. The shoulder muscles must be able to stabilize the glenohumeral joint dynamically, and they also must aid arm propulsion in the accelerative phase of throwing.

Objective.—An attempt was made to quantify the isokinetic performance of the shoulder adductor and abductor muscles in 83 healthy pitchers whose average age was 23 years.

Methods.—The shoulders were assessed using the Biodex Multi-Joint isokinetic dynamometer with the pitcher seated. The throwing and nonthrowing arms were tested concentrically at 180 and 300 degrees per second. Ten maximal repetitions were performed at each speed.

Results.—At both speeds, a significant difference was found in adductor muscle peak torque between the dominant and nondominant extremities. No such difference was noted for the shoulder abductors. Peak torque output for both muscle groups decreased as contraction speed increased. Abductor-to-adductor muscle ratios were significantly different in the 2 extremities at both test speeds, and they also decreased as contraction speed changed. Trends for mean peak torque-to-body ratios followed those for mean peak torque.

► The clinical relevance of this article lies in the resulting specific, isokinetic criteria that should be accomplished before the initiation of throwing or the return to competitive pitching. "The authors believe that it is imperative to evaluate dynamic shoulder strength before throwing is initiated."

J.S. Torg, M.D.

The Mathematical Relationship Between the Number of Events in Which People Are Injured and the Number of People Injured

Uitenbroek DG (Univ of Edinburgh, Scotland)

Br J Sports Med 29:126–128, 1995 1–24

The Problem.—Two different ways of counting may be used when determining the number of injuries and establishing rates of injury. Very different results are obtained when counting those occasions when individuals are injured, such as accidents, in a particular time frame, and when counting those injured in a similar time frame. If the number of individuals injured is counted, including those injured more than once, the total will be lower than for "events." When the number of individuals injured is counted in a retrospective survey, the number must be multiplied with the average number of events per injured individual to estimate the total number of events for the population.

A Solution.—A mathematical modeling approach to describing injuries may be taken to learn whether sustaining injury is a random process or whether other factors must be taken into account. The Poisson distribution may be used to clarify the relationship between the number of individuals injured and the number of injury-causing events in a population. This approach was tried for analyzing running-related injuries. It appeared that these injuries are not, in fact, randomly distributed but that there is a "proneness" to injury implying that some factor—personal or situational—must be associated with an increased risk of injury.

Transmission of Disease Through Transplantation of Musculoskeletal Allografts

Tomford WW (Massachusetts Gen Hosp, Boston)

J Bone Joint Surg (Am) 77–A:1742–1754, 1995 1–25

Introduction.—There is always the risk of disease transmission from the donor to the recipient during human allograft transplantation. Diseases transmitted during transplantation were reviewed and strategies to reduce the risk of disease transmission were explored.

Bone and Soft-tissue Allografts.—Human immunodeficiency virus has been transmitted twice in the United States through transplantation of musculoskeletal allografts. In the first instance, a young woman received a diagnosis of AIDS 4 years after receiving a femoral-head allograft from a 52-year-old man who had a routine primary total hip arthroplasty. Both donor and recipient died of AIDS. The donor had not been tested for HIV status before donation. In a second report, another recipient of a femoral-head allograft tested positive for HIV 7 years after transplantation. Four other recipients of an organ from this donor were also HIV-positive after receiving kidney, liver, and heart donations. Recipients of freeze-dried bone chips and freeze-dried segments of fascia lata, tendon, and ligament from this same donor did not test positive for the HIV antibody. The 3 procedures used in the bone grafts that did not transmit the virus were removal of blood and bone marrow from the bone allografts, treatment with ethanol, and freeze-drying of the bone grafts.

Transmission of homologous-serum hepatitis was first reported in 1954 by transplantation of a bone allograft. Three cases of transmission of hepatitis C through transplantation of musculoskeletal allografts have been reported. These reports confirm the necessity of screening tissue donors for hepatitis C. These were the same type of allografts that transmitted HIV—frozen unprocessed femoral heads and patellar ligament complexes.

The most significant advance for testing donors for viral disease is the polymerase chain reaction (PCR) assay. The strength of PCR assays is their ability to amplify rare target sequences in a background of genomic DNA. They have been useful in detecting hepatitis C.

Other Tissue and Organ Transplantations.—Viral disease has not been reported subsequent to cartilage transplantation. Cartilage tissue is avascular and is not likely to be infected with viral agents found in plasma. Heart valves and corneas have been transplanted from donors infected with hepatitis B, with no evidence of transmission. Transplantation of organs has resulted in transmission of HIV, hepatitis B virus, hepatitis C virus, cytomegalovirus, and Epstein-Barr virus.

Risk of Transmission.—The risk of disease transmission is higher when fresh tissues are transplanted and when recipients of banked tissue grafts are immunosuppressed. It is also higher when screening techniques are not followed and when unprocessed femoral heads are used. The risk of viral transmission through transplantation of allografts can be reduced by obtaining tissue from banks that follow the standards of the American Association of Tissue Banks.

Processed allografts should be used whenever possible. These tissues have been thoroughly cleaned of blood, bone marrow, soft tissues, and periosteum. The most common is freeze-dried bone chips. Tissues that cannot be freeze-dried can be sterilized by other methods, such as gamma irradiation and ethylene oxide.

Donor screening is another important facet of decreasing disease transmission. Physicians must inform patients about the risk of viral transmission associated with musculoskeletal allografts and obtain informed consent.

Conclusions.—Although the risk is low, musculoskeletal allografts can transmit viral diseases. Orthopedic surgeons must be familiar with suppliers of grafts they use to ensure adherence to current tissue-banking standards. Some types of grafts are associated with a higher risk than others. Low-dose irradiation can give a margin of safety with insignificant adverse effect on the graft. Informed consent is crucial.

▶ This is a comprehensive, current concepts review of the subject matter. The original paper is strongly recommended for orthopedic surgeons who use musculoskeletal allografts. It should be pointed out that, to my knowledge, there have been 3 cases of HIV transmission through transplantation of musculoskeletal allografts. The authors point out that since 1985, at least 500,000 allografts have been transplanted in the United States, with no reports of infection resulting from the transmission of HIV. However, in view of the natural history of HIV, that is, a protracted interval between infection and clinical manifestations, determining risks in this manner is flawed. Specifically, what is needed to determine the true risk of HIV transmission from allografts would be to test for HIV a population of individuals who have previously received an implant.

J.S. Torg, M.D.

Acute Injuries in Off-road Bicycle Racing

Kronisch RL, Chow TK, Simon LM, Wong PF (San Jose State Univ, Calif; Loma Linda Univ, Calif; Pleasanton, Calif)

Am J Sports Med 24:88–93, 1996 1–26

Background.—Off-road, or mountain bike, racing is growing in popularity. In a descriptive study, injuries sustained at a major race were reported.

Methods.—The race took place at Mammoth Mountain, California, July 6–10, 1994. There were 4,027 individual starts in 5 race events, including cross-country, downhill, dual slalom, and hill climb. The total number of competitors was 3,624. Some cyclists participated in several events. Injuries were defined as significant if they occurred during competition and prevented the rider from finishing the event.

Findings.—Sixteen cyclists had serious injuries, for an overall injury rate of 0.4%. Forty-four injuries occurred in the 16 cyclists. The most common injury was abrasions, followed by contusions, lacerations, fractures, and concussions. The mean Injury Severity Score was 3 on a 1-to-5 scale. Eighty-one percent of the injuries occurred when the cyclists were going downhill. More severe injuries occurred when the cyclists were thrown from their bikes. A different mechanism of injury was noted in each event, suggesting that the risk factors associated with these events may be different as well.

Conclusions.—Most of the injuries in these off-road bicycle race participants occurred when the cyclists were going downhill. Cyclists thrown from their bicycles tended to be injured more seriously than those falling from their bikes to the side. The risk factors associated with the various events in this race may differ.

► This is a well-documented study, the results of which are opposite what one would expect. Specifically, the injury rate was surprisingly low, and the specific injuries sustained by those 16 cyclists cited were all relatively benign. This is in contrast to previously reported studies. Chow et al. reported a 51% acute injury occurrence in the recreational off-road cyclist.[1] Kronisch and Ruben, in a retrospective survey, reported an 85.7% injury occurrence in competitive off-road cyclists.[2] However, the injury rates reported in these 2 studies were based on self-reports using loosely defined inclusion criteria and were subject to the biases inherent in retrospective surveys.

J.S. Torg, M.D.

References

1. Chow TK, Bracker MD, Patrick K: Acute injuries from mountain biking. *West J Med* 159:145–148, 1993.
2. Kronisch RL, Ruben AL: Traumatic injuries in off-road bicycling. *Clin J Sport Med* 4:240–244, 1994.

Ski Injury Statistics, 1982 to 1993, Jackson Hole Ski Resort

Warme WJ, Feagin JA Jr, King P, Lambert KL, Cunningham RR (Teton Village Clinic, Jackson Hole, Wyo)

Am J Sports Med 23:597–600, 1995 1–27

Introduction.—The epidemiology of alpine skiing injuries has been studied extensively in previous decades. To identify the current trends in skiing injuries, the skiing injuries occurring between the 1981–1982 and 1992–1993 seasons in Jackson Hole, Wyoming, were retrospectively analyzed.

Methods.—Injured skiers were examined clinically and with appropriate radiographs to establish diagnoses. Ticket sales determined the population at risk, used to analyze injury rates, which were analyzed over time. The trends in injury rates were studied over 12 seasons.

Results.—A total of 9,749 skiing injuries occurred during the 2.55 million skier-days studied, for an overall injury rate of 3.7 injuries per 1,000 skier-days. This injury rate remained steady over the 12 seasons. The ratio of lower extremity to upper extremity injuries decreased significantly, from 4:1 in the 1981–1982 season to 2:1 in the 1992–1993 season. Soft-tissue knee injuries accounted for 34% of all skiing injuries, and 30% of all injuries were ligamentous knee injuries. The most commonly diagnosed injury was medial collateral ligament sprains. Injury to the anterior cruciate ligament (ACL) accounted for 49% of all soft-tissue knee injuries. The frequency of ACL injuries per 1,000 skier-days increased significantly during the study period. The most common upper extremity injury was the ulnar collateral ligament injury of the thumb (33% of all upper extremity injuries and 7% of all skiing injuries).

Discussion.—The rate of lower extremity injuries decreased during the study, following the trends of the late 1970s and early 1980s. However, knee sprains are still common, with ACL injuries increasing.

▶ The interesting statistics provided by this study are that the incidence of ACL tears has increased as a function of time, accounting for 16% of all injuries during the study period. On the other hand, ankle injuries are now relatively uncommon, accounting for only 5% of the total skiing injuries. It appears from a historical standpoint that ACL disruptions have replaced the "boot top fracture" as the primary skiing nemesis. This is a classic example of how a change in equipment or environment can result in a change in injury type and pattern.

J.S. Torg, M.D.

Severe Skiing Injuries: A Retrospective Analysis of 361 Patients Including Mechanism of Trauma, Severity of Injury, and Mortality

Furrer M, Erhart S, Frutiger A, Bereiter H, Leutenegger A, Rüedi T (Kantonsspital Chur, Switzerland)

J Trauma: Injury Infect Crit Care 39:737–741, 1995 1–28

Study Population.—An apparent increase in serious head injuries and multiple injuries in skiers prompted a review of 2,053 patients seen from 1984 to 1992 whose injuries necessitated admission to a hospital. The 361 patients considered to have serious injuries included 179 who had either multiple injuries with an Injury Severity Score of at least 18 or multiple fractures; 58 having a single thoracic or abdominal injury; and 124 with isolated head injury. Patients in the latter groups had an Abbreviated Injury Scale score of 2 or greater.

Injuries.—Two thirds of patients were injured in a fall, whereas nearly one third collided with an obstacle—often another skier. Nearly two thirds of patients were transported by helicopter. Patients with multiple injuries tended to have somewhat more severe injuries in the latter years of the period under review.

Outcome.—Eighty percent of patients were severely disabled or vegetative when admitted to hospital, and 4% died within a month of injury. Mortality increased from 2% to 7% over the study period. Patients having isolated injuries of the abdomen or thorax had the best outlook; none of them have died. Severe head injury carried the poorest prognosis. The 4 patients with multiple injuries who died had an average Injury Severity Score of 44. Associated brain injury was the greatest problem in these cases.

Prevention.—Better transport capability will limit overpopulation of the downhill runs. Runs should not be groomed to the extent of encouraging high-speed skiing. Obstacles and crossings must be well marked. Particular efforts are needed to improve safety for children on ski lifts and chairlifts.

▶ As the authors point out, the epidemiology of ski injuries has been studied extensively; however, only a few reports have dealt with the more seriously injured skier. This article succeeds in this effort. Two important observations are that major head injuries increased from 11.6% during the period of 1984 to 1988 to 19.3% during 1989 to 1992 and that "... death after a skiing accident is practically always due to a severe head and brain lesion." In view of this, one unanswered question is why it was not stated that skiing is a helmet sport.

J.S. Torg, M.D.

Left-handedness as an Injury Risk Factor in Adolescents
Graham CJ, Cleveland E (Univ of Arkansas, Little Rock)
J Adolesc Health 16:50–52, 1995 1–29

Introduction.—One of the leading causes of adolescent morbidity and mortality is injury. Left-handedness has been implicated as a risk factor for unintentional injury, particularly in older adolescents and adults. A survey of junior and senior high school athletes explored the significance of left-handedness as a risk factor for injury.

Methods.—Data on handedness and past injuries were gathered on 634 junior and senior high school students, using a questionnaire administered during preparticipation physical examinations. Handedness was determined with 4 questions that asked the respondents to identify the hand used to write, hold a toothbrush, erase, and throw a ball.

Results.—Of the respondents, 65.6% were male, and they had a mean age of 13.6 years. Fifty-five percent were white and 45% were black. Left-handers comprised 9.9% of the respondents. No differences were found in the frequency of left-handedness associated with age, sex, or race. Injuries during the past year were reported by 62% of the left-handers and 43% of the right-handers. Past hospitalization for injuries was reported by 14% of the left-handers and 4.4% of the right-handers. Injuries requiring surgery were reported by 7.9% of the left-handers and 2.6% of the right-handers.

Discussion.—A higher incidence of unintentional injury was found among left-handed than among right-handed adolescents. A significantly higher risk of more serious injuries also was found among the left-handed adolescents. The reasons for this increased risk are unclear and require additional study focusing on the mechanism of injury in various types of trauma sustained by left-handers.

► In 1991, investigators shocked the scientific world by publishing data from California death certificates suggesting that "lefties" die 9 years earlier than "righties."[1] Earlier research had suggested that lefties were more susceptible to accident-related injuries.[2] The conclusion that lefties die early was soon debunked as a classic fallacy, based on comparing the mean ages at death, that is, comparing only the numerators of rates, not the rates themselves.[3] Using this same approach, one would conclude that nursery school is more dangerous than paratrooper school, because the mean age at death of children in nursery school is lower than that of paratrooper trainees. So lefties do not die early.[4]

But the notion that lefties are at risk in a right-handed world—that lefties have more accidents—remains alive. In a survey of nearly 1,900 college students, lefties were almost twice as likely as righties to report an injury needing medical attention.[2] In a case-control study, left-handedness was a risk factor for unintentional trauma in a pediatric emergency department population.[5] Now this report extends to athletes the perils of being a southpaw. In short, left-handedness appears to be a risk factor for injury among adolescent school athletes. A sinister implication!

E.R. Eichner, M.D.

References

1. Halpern DF, Coren S: Handedness and lifespan. *N Engl J Med* 324:998, 1991.
2. Coren S: Left-handedness and accident-related injury risk. *Am J Publ Health* 79:1040–1041, 1989.
3. Salive ME, Guralnik JM, Glynn RJ: Left-handedness and mortality. *Am J Publ Health* 83:265–267, 1993.
4. Cerhan JR, Folsom AR, Potter JD, et al: Handedness and mortality risk in older women. *Am J Epidemiol* 140:368, 1994.
5. Graham CJ, Dick R, Rickert V, et al: Left-handedness as a risk factor for unintentional injury in children. *Pediatrics* 92:823–826, 1993.

Trampoline-related Injuries

Larson BJ, Davis JW (Logan Regional Hosp, Utah)
J Bone Joint Surg (Am) 77–A:1174–1178, 1995 1–30

Objective.—A total of 217 injuries resulting from recreational trampoline use were assessed at a single emergency department in a 2-year period. The patients ranged in age from 18 months to 45 years, but the average was 10 years of age. Injuries were most prevalent in children aged 5–9 years.

The Injuries.—The elbow or forearm was injured in 26% of cases and the head/neck region in 21%. The ankle or foot and the knee or leg were the next most frequently involved sites. Younger children tended to have upper-limb injuries, whereas older adolescents most often had leg injuries. Fractures were present in 39% of patients, and a sprain or strain was found in 25%.

Mechanisms of Injury.—Fifty-seven percent of injuries occurred while the individual was on the trampoline and 29% when falling from the device. In nearly two thirds of 72 evaluable cases, there had been more than 1 individual on the trampoline at the time of injury. The most common mechanisms were a collision with the trampoline frame and a fall from the trampoline. Roughly half of the 72 patients from whom information was obtained at follow-up were beginners, and only 11% had advanced skills. When asked, the patients suggested allowing no more than 1 individual at a time on the trampoline, and they also proposed enforcing family rules about using the trampoline.

Suggestions.—Using the trampoline entails a high risk of injury. It seems advisable to have the bars and springs padded; to prohibit more than 1 individual at a time from using the device; and to place the trampoline in a hole so that the jumping surface will be at ground level. In addition, somersaults and other high-risk maneuvers should be avoided. Parental supervision is very important.

► Unfortunately, because of the universally unorganized use of both the trampoline and the mini-trampoline, it has been impossible to present data from these devices in terms of injury rates. However, it would appear that 217 injuries requiring attention in 1 hospital emergency department in a 2-year period is indicative of a problem activity. Several years ago, in a review of the world's literature, we identified 114 catastrophic cervical spine injuries with associated quadriplegia resulting from use of the trampoline and mini-trampoline.[1] It was our conclusion that both the trampoline and mini-trampoline are dangerous devices when used in the best of circumstances and that their use has no place in recreational, educational, or competitive gymnastics. I stand by this opinion.

J.S. Torg, M.D.

Reference

1. Torg JS, Das M: Trampoline-related quadriplegia: Review of the literature and reflections on the American Academy of Pediatrics' position statement. *Pediatrics* 74:804–812, 1984.

Injury Profile of Amateur Australian Rules Footballers

Shawdon A, Brukner P (Olympic Park Sports Med Ctr, Melbourne, Australia)

Aust J Sci Med Sport 26:59–61, 1994 1–31

Background.—Australian Rules Football (ARF), a popular sport throughout the winter months in Australia, involves a considerable amount of physical contact. Studies of the injury profile in professional and semi-professional ARF players report the most common injury to be hamstring strain/tear. To document injuries at the amateur level, a club competing in the Victorian Amateur Football League was followed during the 1993 season.

Methods.—The club's squad consisted of 80 players from which 2 teams were selected weekly during the 18-game season. Recorded injuries were those that caused the player to miss at least 1 game, as well as all fractures, lacerations, and concussions. Data collected included the nature and site of the injury, games missed, and the mechanism of the injury.

Results.—Fifty injuries occurred among the 80 players, resulting in a rate of 96 injuries per 1,000 player-hours. Most injuries were traumatic in origin (65%) and resulted in at least 1 game being missed (69%). Surgery was required in 11 cases. The most common head and neck injuries were concussions (50%) and facial lacerations (31%). Almost one third of the injuries were fractures, and 50% of these involved bones in the hand. The most common site of injury was the lower limb (40%).

Discussion.—Compared with professional and semi-professional clubs, these members of an amateur ARF club had a considerably lower injury rate (96% vs. 63%). Overuse injuries were less frequent in amateur than in semi-professional and professional clubs, whereas concussions were more common among amateur players. Reasons for these differences include lower levels of preseason training and of technical skill in the amateur clubs. Athletic trainers are encouraged to assess injured players for the degree of concussion and, because of the frequency of lacerations, to recommend immunization against hepatitis B for ARF players at all levels.

▶ The authors conclude that with regard to injuries in Australia, "... more work is required to establish what injuries are most common, and importantly, what measures can be taken to decrease their incidence." It must be pointed out that although it is not mentioned in this article, the major injury problem of Australian Rules Football in terms of severity is cervical spine injuries with resulting quadriplegia. The most comprehensive study of spinal cord injuries resulting from Australian Rules and Rugby Union Football was reported by Taylor and Coolican.[1] They reviewed 107 spinal cord injuries that occurred between 1960 and 1985 and emphasized the need for preventive measures.

J.S. Torg, M.D.

Reference

1. Taylor TK, Coolican MR: Spinal-cord injuries in Australian footballers, 1960–1985. *Med J Aust* 147:112–118, 1987.

Epidemiology of Rugby Football Injuries

Garraway M, Macleod D (Edinburgh Med School, Scotland; St John's Hosp, Livingston, Scotland)

Lancet 345:1485–1487, 1995 1–32

Purpose.—Most previous studies of rugby injuries have focused on spinal cord injuries. A prospective cohort study sought to define the frequency, nature, circumstances, and outcome of rugby injuries.

Methods.—The study included all players who were members of the senior rugby clubs in 1 district of the Scottish Rugby Union during the 1993–1994 season. The study design included weekly visits to the clubs by physiotherapists, who confirmed the details of each reported injury. Complete data, including any new or recurrent injuries occurring in matches or rugby-related training, were available for 1,169 of 1,216 eligible players.

Results.—There were 584 injuries occurring in 512 episodes in 361 players. Eighty-four percent of the injuries occurred in matches. Match injuries occurred at a period prevalence rate of 13.95/1,000 playing hours, or 1 injury episode every 1.8 matches. Twenty-two percent of the episodes were classified as transient in nature, 38% as mild, 24% as moderate, and 16% as severe. No spinal injuries occurred. The most common injuries were dislocations, strains, and sprains of the knee, although fractures were most likely to occur in the upper extremity. Each episode of injury caused the player to miss an average of 39 days from rugby. Twenty-eight percent of the episodes caused the player to miss an average of 18 days' time from work or school. Tackling was a major factor in the injuries; tackling accounted for 18% of lost time from work and being tackled, for 43%.

Conclusions.—Rugby injuries are common and an important source of morbidity. Continued follow-up would be needed to determine the amount of degenerative disease that might occur in rugby players over time. The frequency and circumstances of tackling must be studied further so that players can be coached in safer tackling techniques.

▶ Perhaps the most interesting statistics discerned from these data are that a rugby player can expect to be injured every 2.7 seasons while playing an average of 20 matches per season and, once injured, will be out for approximately 6 weeks. As the authors have concluded, "Rugby injuries are an important source of morbidity in young men. They need to be better understood if their frequency and consequences are to be reduced."

J.S. Torg, M.D.

Injuries in Junior A Ice Hockey: A Three-year Prospective Study

Stuart MJ, Smith A (Mayo Clinic Sports Medicine Ctr, Rochester, Minn; Mayo Clinic and Found, Rochester, Minn)

Am J Sports Med 23:458–461, 1995 1–33

Introduction.—Because of the speed, equipment, and frequent collisions associated with playing ice hockey, there is a great potential for injury in athletes participating in this sport. The incidence and types of injury sustained in practice and in games were studied in a United States Junior A hockey team over 3 consecutive seasons.

Methods.—All injuries sustained by team players over the 3 seasons spanning 1990 to 1993 were reported, using a standardized form that described the activity, player position, time of occurrence, mechanism, type, anatomical location, and severity. Pre-existing injuries were identified and a musculoskeletal baseline was obtained during a preseason screening examination.

Results.—During the study period, the team had 540 hours of on-ice practice, resulting in 13,500 player-practice hours, and played 144 games, resulting in 864 player-game hours. A total of 142 injuries were documented, with 58% occurring during games, 37% occurring during practice, 3% occurring during weight training, and 2% occurring during off-ice training. The injury rate was 9.4 per 1,000 player-hours overall, 96.1 per 1,000 player-game hours, and 3.9 per 1,000 player-practice hours.

The practice injury rate was highest during the earliest third of the season, whereas the game injury rate was relatively constant throughout the season. The game injury rate was highest in the third period of the games.

Collision with other players and with the boards, but not with the ice, were the most common mechanisms of injury in both practice and games, followed by stick- and skate-related injuries. Strains (25%), lacerations (24%), contusions (18%), and sprains (16%) were the most common types of injuries. The face was the most common site of injury (26%), followed by the shoulder (20%) and hip (11%). The severity of the injuries was rated as mild in 58%, moderate in 36%, and severe in 6%.

Discussion.—Hockey players are at substantial risk of injury caused by both biomechanical and equipment factors. The higher rates of game injuries during the third period may be attributed to fatigue and aggression, whereas the higher rates of practice injury during the first third of the season may be attributed to inflexibility and increased workout intensity. The lack of full facial protection for players in the Junior A league may contribute to the high rate of facial trauma. Stretching programs for the hip flexor, adductor, and lumbar paraspinal musculature are recommended to reduce the incidence of muscle strains in these areas. Improved shoulder-pad design may reduce the incidence of acromioclavicular joint injuries.

▶ It is concluded that "Further research is necessary to determine if injuries in Junior A amateur ice hockey can be reduced by mandatory full facial protection ...." It should be pointed out that requiring all Canadian junior hockey players to wear a helmet with partial face protection correlated with an increase in cervical spine injuries associated with permanent paralysis.[1] Thus, it would appear that any equipment changes affecting head and face protection should be approached with caution.

J.S. Torg, M.D.

Reference

1. Tator CH: Neck injuries in ice hockey: A recent unsolved problem with many contributing factors. *Clin Sport Med* 6:101–114, 1987.

Tobogganing Injuries in Children

Kim PCW, Haddock G, Bohn D, Wesson D (Hosp for Sick Children, Toronto)
J Pediatr Surg 30:1135–1137, 1995 1–34

Background.—Despite the popularity of tobogganing in Canada, there is little information on injuries sustained in tobogganing accidents. One experience with tobogganing-related injuries was reviewed.

Patients and Findings.—Twenty-two children with tobogganing-related injuries treated between December 1991 and December 1993 were included in the review. The patients were 13 boys and 9 girls, aged 3–17 years. Nine patients had struck a tree, 8 had struck other objects, and 5 had fallen from the toboggan. Only 1 child was wearing protective headgear at the time of the accident. In 13 children, the initial site of impact was the head; in 5, the trunk; and in 4, the extremities. Major injuries occurred in all systems of the body. Fifty-nine percent of the children needed surgery. Two children died, 1 of cerebral edema and 1 of acute renal failure and subsequent multiple-organ failure.

Conclusions.—Injuries sustained while tobogganing comprise a small percentage of all injuries in hospitalized children. However, these injuries can be serious. Significant morbidity and mortality can result. Public awareness of the risks associated with tobogganing needs to be increased. Several precautions should be stressed: tobogganing where there are trees, posts, and other stationary objects is dangerous and should be avoided. Tobogganing in the prone, head-first position also should be avoided. Wearing protective headgear seems a reasonable precaution. Towing toboggans behind a motor vehicle, a dangerous practice, should be banned. Children who are tobogganing need close supervision, especially when the hill is crowded.

▶ As would be expected, the head is most at risk when one is tobogganing in the prone, head-first position. Although in a published report by Hedges and Greenberg[1] the severity of head injury in sledding accidents was the same among patients wearing and not wearing helmets, it would seem that protective headgear is indicated in these activities.

J.S. Torg, M.D.

Reference

1. Hedges J, Greenberg MI: Sledding injuries. *Ann Emerg Med* 9:131–133, 1980.

Goal Post Injuries in Soccer: A Laboratory and Field Testing Analysis of a Preventive Intervention

Janda DH, Bir C, Wild B, Olson S, Hensinger RN (Inst for Preventative Sports Medicine, Ann Arbor, Mich; Catherine McAuley Health Systems, Ann Arbor, Mich; Univ of Michigan, Ann Arbor)

Am J Sports Med 23:340–344, 1995 1–35

Introduction.—Soccer is the most popular team sport worldwide and is the fastest-growing team sport in the United States. The most common cause of fatal injury in soccer occurs after impact with goalposts. In 2 case studies, young players were injured when a movable goalpost system fell on them. A laboratory and field-testing summary of preventive intervention was described.

Case 1.—Boy, 10 years, sustained a C4-5 fracture when he was struck by a goalpost that was blown over by the wind. He experienced C5 radiculopathy but was otherwise neurologically intact. He underwent a posterior cervical fusion of C3–C5. After immobilization in a halo for 8 weeks, his C5 radiculopathy resolved and he was asymptomatic at follow-up.

Case 2.—Boy, 11 years, lost consciousness after being struck on the head by a goalpost unseated by another child. Both lower extremities were pinned under the crossbar. The patient was treated for a closed head injury and a Salter III condylar fracture of the left distal femur and a right distal femoral shaft fracture. After his leg fractures healed, he required physical therapy. At follow-up, his legs were pain free and functioning well. However, he was experiencing difficulties with short-term memory, short attention span, behavioral difficulties, and falling grades. None of these were present before injury.

Preventive Intervention.—Results of laboratory testing of horizontal and vertical impact testing showed that impact force was significantly reduced when stationary goalposts were covered with protective padding. In a pilot field-testing phase, 4 soccer fields were equipped with padded goalposts. Over a 3-year period, 471 soccer games played by youth, teen, and adult leagues were monitored for collisions with goalposts. Seven player collisions with the padded goalposts occurred in the 3 years of monitoring. No injuries were recorded.

Conclusion.—Preventive measures in recreational softball and baseball have yielded significant reductions in injuries and related health care costs. The use of padded stationary goalposts should reduce injuries without altering the flow or enjoyment of the game.

► The conclusion that "the use of padded goal posts within the game of soccer has been documented to reduce the possibility of injury, both in the laboratory phase and in the pilot field testing phase" is not supported by the research design or data obtained. With regard to injury reduction, there is no control group and, statistically, it is doubtful that the numbers involved would have had the power to demonstrate a difference. Although the laboratory study demonstrated that impact force was diminished when the posts were covered with protective padding, this was not correlated with injury occurrence.

J.S. Torg, M.D.

In-line Skating Injuries

Malanga GA, Stuart MJ (Mayo Clinic Rochester, Minn)

Mayo Clin Proc 70:752–754, 1995 1–36

Introduction.—The popularity of in-line skating is increasing rapidly. The technology and materials used to manufacture in-line skates can now allow high speeds, which, combined with inexperience in the skater and the difficulty of the braking technique, can result in an increased risk of injury. The medical records of patients treated for in-line skating injuries in an emergency department during an 18-month period were reviewed to illuminate the frequency and type of injuries associated with this sport.

Methods.—Patients treated in the emergency department between July 1992 and December 1993 for injuries associated with in-line skating were identified through a computer search. Their medical records were reviewed to obtain data on the patient's sex, age, type of injury, and injured body part.

Results.—Thirty-two injuries occurred in 32 patients. Nineteen (59%) of the patients were women and 13 (41%) were men. Their ages ranged from 6 to 46 years, with a mean of 17 years. Injury occurred most frequently in the upper extremity (78%), followed by the lower extremity (16%) and the head (6%). The most common site of injury was the wrist (56%), followed by the elbow (19%). The knee was the most frequently injured site in the lower extremity. The most common type of injury was fracture, occurring in 62% of the patients. Of these, 2 of the fractures were severe, both in the lower extremities, and 1 required surgical treatment.

Discussion.—The severe lower extremity injuries may have been caused by the tight fit of the skates and the linear wheels, producing a long lever arm and forces seen in skiing injuries. Recommendations for reducing in-line skating injuries include the use of protective equipment and training in braking and protective falling techniques. Future studies should investigate the roles of protective equipment, the skater's experience, and the action at the time of injury.

▶ Considering that 9.3 million individuals were estimated to have participated in in-line skating in 1992, with 30,863 treated injuries documented by the National Electronic Injury Surveillance System,[1] this current report is a modest representation of the problems that this activity presents. Also, it should be pointed out that the National Electronic Injury Surveillance System data indicate that 5% of all the injured in-line skaters had a head injury. Thus, protective equipment must certainly include a bicycle helmet. With regard to other principles of prevention, my own experiences with these devices has resulted in adherence to this simple principle: Do not lean back!

J.S. Torg, M.D.

Reference

1. Schieber RA, Branche-Dorsey CM, Ryan GW: Comparison of in-line skating injuries with rollerskating and skateboarding injuries. *JAMA* 271:1856–1858, 1994.

A Method to Help Reduce the Risk of Serious Knee Sprains Incurred in Alpine Skiing

Ettlinger CF, Johnson RJ, Shealy JE (Univ of Vermont, Burlington; Rochester Inst of Technology, NY)

Am J Sports Med 23:531–537, 1995 1–37

Background.—Since the 1970s, the overall injury rate among skiers has declined, but the proportion of injuries involving serious knee sprain has increased. Through prospective monitoring of injuries at a Vermont ski area during a 22-year period, injuries involving the anterior cruciate ligament (ACL) were found to result from 2 main mechanisms of injury: the phantom-foot mechanism, in which the tail of the ski functions as a lever that points in a direction opposite that of the foot (Fig 1), and the boot-induced mechanism, caused by hard landings while off balance (Fig 2).

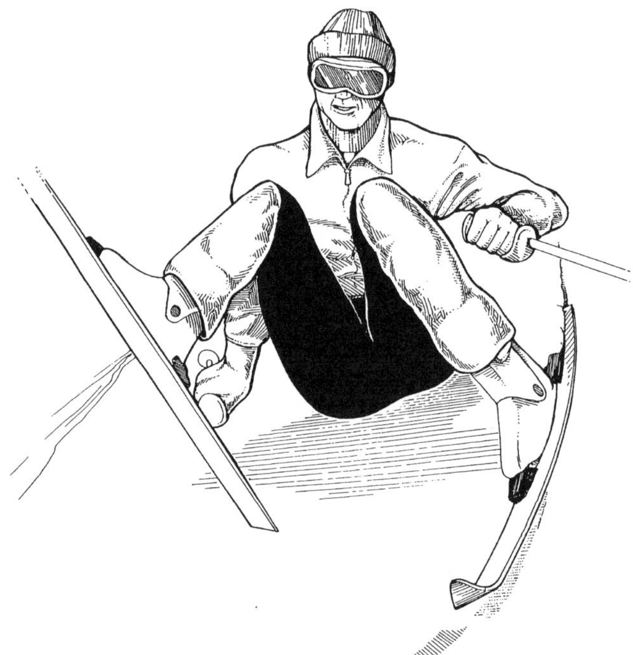

FIGURE 1.—"Because this injury involves the tail of the ski, a lever that points in a direction opposite that of the human foot, we have termed this mechanism of injury the phantom-foot ACL injury mechanism and believe it to be the most common and insidious ACL injury scenario in alpine skiing today. In all the cases we have observed in our video analysis, the skier is off balance to the rear, with all his or her weight on the inside edge of the tail of the downhill ski and the uphill ski unweighted. The hips are below the knees with the upper body generally facing the downhill ski. The uphill arm is back and the injury is sustained in each case by the downhill leg." *Abbreviation: ACL,* anterior cruciate ligament. (From Ettlinger CF, Johnson RJ, Shealy JE: A method to help reduce the risk of serious knee sprains incurred in alpine skiing. *Am J Sports Med* 23:531–537, 1995. Courtesy of *ACL Awareness Training—Phase II.* Copyright Vermont Safety Research 1994. Illustration is copyrighted by William Hamilton, 1988. Reprinted with permission.)

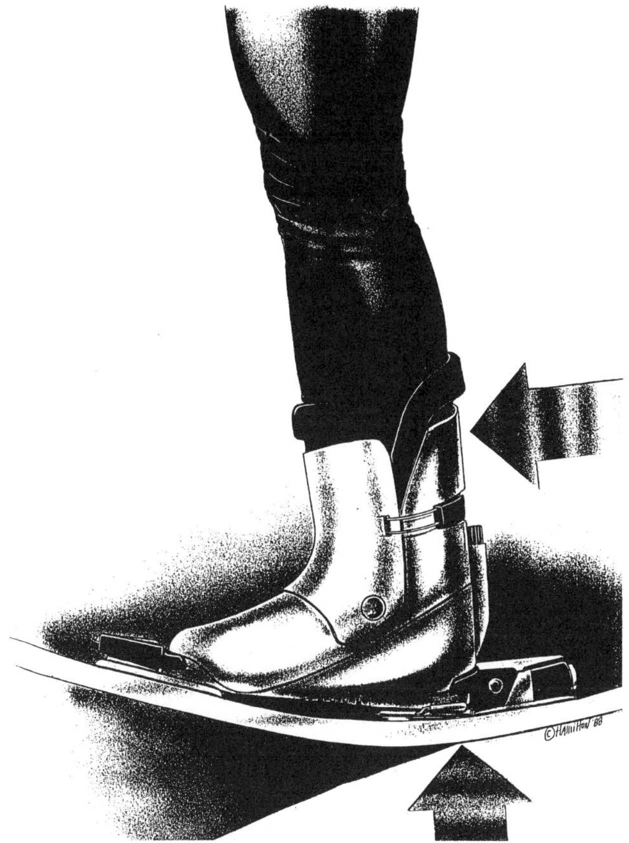

FIGURE 2.—"The boot-induced ACL injury mechanism occurs during hard landings by off balance skiers. In the typical case, the skier, after beginning a jump off balance to the rear, rotates one arm upward and rearward and fully extends the opposite (contralateral) knee. When the skier lands, the tail of the ski hits first. By the time the ski directly under the boot heel contacts the snow surface, everything that can be stretched and everything that can be compressed has been compressed. With no capacity remaining to absorb the jarring impact of the boot heel, the stiff back of the modern alpine boot is able to drive the tibia out from under the femur, thereby tearing or completely severing the ACL." *Abbreviation: ACL,* anterior cruciate ligament. (From Ettlinger CF, Johnson RJ, Shealy JE: A method to help reduce the risk of serious knee sprains incurred in alpine skiing. *Am J Sports Med* 23:531–537 1995. Courtesy of *ACL Awareness Training—Phase II.* Copyright Vermont Safety Research 1994. Illustration is copyrighted by William Hamilton, 1988. Reprinted with permission.)

An experimental training program was developed for experienced skiers, and its impact on ACL injury rates was studied.

Methods.—Videotapes showing accidents resulting in knee injuries were shown to ski instructors and ski patrols. Open-ended discussion was then used to identify a profile of the skiing behaviors and situations that increase the risk of ACL injury and to develop strategies for responding to the threat of injury. Analysis of these discussions led to a cognitive training program including instruction in guidelines to avoid high-risk behavior, recognition of potentially dangerous situations, and specific strategies to address the elements of the phantom-foot injury mechanism. After this 2-year phase, the cognitive training program was used in preparation for the next skiing season at 25 ski areas. Anterior cruciate ligament injury rates were compared between these ski areas and 22 control ski areas not using the awareness training program.

Results.—The average incidence of ACL sprains among the instructors and patrollers was 31 during the 2 seasons preceding the intervention and 16 during the season of the intervention, a 62% reduction. At the control ski areas, the incidence of ACL sprains among the instructors and patrollers averaged 23 for the first 2 years and 29 for the third year. Analysis of the injuries in the experimental group during the third year revealed that there were other injury mechanisms not addressed by the program.

Conclusions.—Educational awareness training can reduce the risk of ACL injury among skiing professionals in a cost-effective manner.

▶ With education, the number of ACL injuries in skiing can be reduced. This study could have a major impact on reducing injuries not only in skiing but also in other sports.

The authors isolated the "phantom-foot" mechanism as being the cause of most ACL injuries, followed by the "boot-induced" mechanism. Other sports should be closely scrutinized to determine whether causative injury factors can be isolated. If so, an educational program may be developed to instruct athletes in other aspects of injury prevention. We have tried strengthening and agility programs, bracing, shoe and equipment modifications, and rules changes to help prevent injuries.

Videotaping of games and practice sessions has become a part of many different sports. With this technology and our better understanding of biomechanics, this additional method of injury prevention should be introduced. In skiing, it has been proven to be effective and cost-efficient. Educating athletes to prevent injuries is a wonderful concept.

F.J. George, A.T.C., P.T.

Basketball Shoe Height and the Maximal Muscular Resistance to Applied Ankle Inversion and Eversion Moments

Ottaviani RA, Ashton-Miller JA, Kothari SU, Wojtys EM (Univ of Michigan, Ann Arbor)

Am J Sports Med 23:418–423, 1995 1–38

Background.—Ankle inversion injuries are common among athletes. Peroneal muscle resistance to inversion rotations is only significant when the muscles are already activated; otherwise, the peroneal muscle responses are delayed by neuromuscular latencies. Therefore, resistance can only be provided passively by bone, soft tissue, or shoes. High-top athletic shoes are often used to improve ankle support, although reports of their efficacy vary. The resistance offered by a ¾-top basketball shoe was studied with the ankle joint close to the neutral position in the frontal plane.

Methods.—Twenty healthy, young adult men with no ankle injuries in the 6 months preceding the study were tested wearing both low-top and ¾-top shoes. The active range of motion and strength in dorsiflexion, plantarflexion, inversion, and eversion of each ankle were measured with a goniometer and an isokinetic dynamometer. In addition, strength under unipedal weight-bearing conditions at 0 degrees, 16 degrees, and 32 degrees of plantarflexion was tested.

Results.—The measurements of range of motion demonstrated that no tests were conducted near any participant's maximal range of motion. Compared with the low-top shoe, the ¾-top shoe increased active resistance to an inversion moment by 29.4% (significant) with the foot at 0 degrees of plantarflexion, by 20.4% (significant) with the foot at 16 degrees of plantarflexion, and by 11% (nonsignificant) with the foot at 32 degrees of plantarflexion. Active resistance to an eversion moment with the ¾-top shoe was increased only at 0 degrees of plantarflexion, by 6.8%. No significant correlations were found among calf circumference, isokinetic peak torque, isokinetic time to peak torque, and performance in the weight-bearing unipedal strength test.

Conclusions.—Wearing ¾-top shoes allows increased active resistance to external moments at low degrees of ankle plantarflexion and to inversion moments, particularly at higher degrees of ankle plantarflexion, compared with wearing low-top shoes.

► A good deal of controversy continues regarding the relationship of athletic-shoe height and the frequency of ankle sprains. Will a high-top shoe help to prevent an ankle sprain? Will it affect performance? Will it be accepted by the athletic population as an "in" shoe? Many factors must be considered before a blanket statement that high-top shoes help prevent ankle sprains can be made.

Please read the abstract by Barrett et al.[1] and the comments of Dr. Joseph S. Torg in the 1994 YEAR BOOK OF SPORTS MEDICINE.[2] Dr. Torg made some interesting comments, comparing this study to studies done in the past. Dr. J.G. Garrick, commenting on this study, stated, "Tightly laced shoes may be the key words here. Our experiences would suggest that tight lacing might not be the norm and may indeed explain the absence of apparent protection documented in the study by Barrett et al."[3]

F.J. George, A.T.C., P.T.

References

1. Barrett JR, et al: High-versus low-top shoes for the prevention of ankle sprains in basketball players: A prospective randomized study. *Am J Sports Med* 21:582–585, 1993.
2. 1994 *YEAR BOOK OF SPORTS MEDICINE*, pp. 18–19.
3. *Athletic Training: Sports Health Care Perspectives* 2:95–96, 1995.

2 Head and Neck, Spine

The Classification of Anatomic- and Symptom-based Low Back Disorders Using Motion Measure Models

Marras WS, Parnianpour M, Ferguson SA, Kim J-Y, Crowell RR, Bose S, Simon SR (Ohio State Univ, Columbus; Ohio Spine Ctr, Columbus)

Spine 20:2531–2546, 1995 2–1

Introduction.—Despite the high prevalence and cost of low back disorders (LBDs), there are few quantitative techniques for objectively quantifying the extent of the problem in an individual patient. Having such techniques would aid in determining a patient's progress, in prescribing adequate treatment, and in avoiding treatments that would worsen the problem. Previous research has suggested that measurement of trunk angular velocity is a promising approach to quantifying the extent of LBD. The value of trunk motion measures as a quantifiable tool for classifying LBDs was assessed.

Methods.—Two groups of men and women, ranging in age from 20 to 70 years, were studied. Three hundred thirty-nine healthy individuals had no history of significant back pain, and 171 patients had various chronic LBDs. The angular position, velocity, and acceleration of the trunk was measured with a tri-axial electrogoniometer in each individual as the research subjects flexed and extended their trunks in all 5 planes of motion. The trunk angular motion measurements of the LBD group were normalized by sex and age to those of the healthy individuals. Various models of trunk motion interactions were then constructed to classify the individuals in both groups into 1 of 10 anatomical and symptom-based LBD classification categories (Fig 2).

Results.—For the most part, the trunk motion measurements were highly repeatable. The measures served as a quantifiable indicator of the functional limitations associated with LBD as a percentage of expected normal ability. A stage 1 model with 8 variables proved capable of correctly classifying more than 94% of the individuals as either healthy or having an LBD, according to conservative cross-validation measures. In addition, 1 of the stage 2 models with 8 variables was reasonably good at classifying the patients with LBD into 1 of 10 LBD classification categories.

Conclusions.—Higher-order trunk motion characteristics could be very useful in quantifying the musculoskeletal status of the trunk in patients

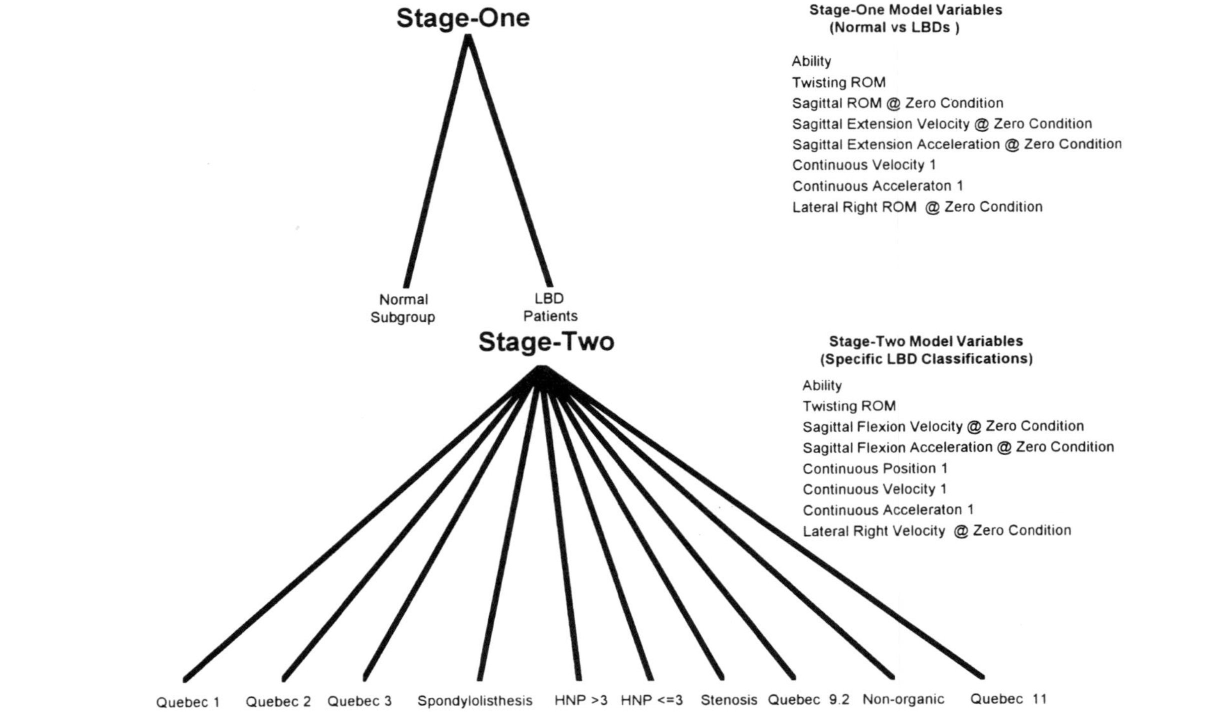

FIGURE 2.—The stage 2 model used to categorize patients with low back disorders (*LBDs*). The stage 1 model separates healthy individuals from patients with LBD (as a group), whereas the stage 2 model categorizes the patients with LBD into 1 of 10 LBD classifications. (Courtesy of Marras WS, Parnianpour M, Ferguson SA, et al: The classification of anatomic- and symptom-based low back disorders using motion measure models. *Spine* 20:2531–2546, 1995.)

with LBD. These measurements may give valuable information on the extent of LBD and the progress of rehabilitation efforts. Diagnostic applications could be possible once the interactions among the trunk motion characteristics are determined. The findings need to be validated in independent samples.

▶ These authors have developed a 2-stage model for assessing and categorizing LBD. They recognized that the current socioeconomic climate demands increased quality of health care delivery while maintaining costs. They see their model as a beginning in an effort to quantify trunk performance and eventually to quantify the rehabilitation process. They envision that the task of LBD management will consist of several stages—objectively measuring the present state of trunk performance, making a diagnosis, quantifying the functional deficits, planning a definite goal, selecting the optimal effective treatment, prescribing a quantifiable dose of therapeutic exercise, and providing feedback for positive reinforcement of progress and functional restoration with an operant conditioning behavioral approach. They believe that this study contributed to the first 3 stages of the rehabilitation process, but more studies are needed to validate their work.

Col. J.L. Anderson, PE.D.

A Cineradiographic Study on the Lumbar Disc Deformation During Flexion and Extension of the Trunk

Kanayama M, Tadano S, Kaneda K, Ukai T, Abumi K, Ito M (Hokkaido Univ, Sapporo, Japan)

Clin Biomech 10:193–199, 1995 2–2

Introduction.—One reason the human lumbar spine is vulnerable to degenerative disk disease may be that it is relatively mobile and sustains relatively large loads from the upper extremities and the trunk. Most past studies have used simple radiography, which demonstrates only discontinuous motion.

Objective.—To document the deformation of normal lumbar disks, cineradiography was done during flexion/extension movements of the trunk in 8 healthy young men.

Methods.—The neutral spinal position was defined as upright standing with the occiput and the thoracic and sacral regions aligned vertical to the floor. Participants flexed the trunk actively from the neutral to the fully flexed position in 6 seconds and extended it. A system of local coordinates was used to express deformation on each disk (Fig 1). Deformation was assessed by displacement of the superior corners of the disk, which were measured against the upper surface of the next lower vertebra. The strain distribution of each lumbar disk was determined by the finite element method.

Results.—Lumbar disk deformation increased rapidly during spinal flexion after a delay, and it peaked before trunk motion was completed.

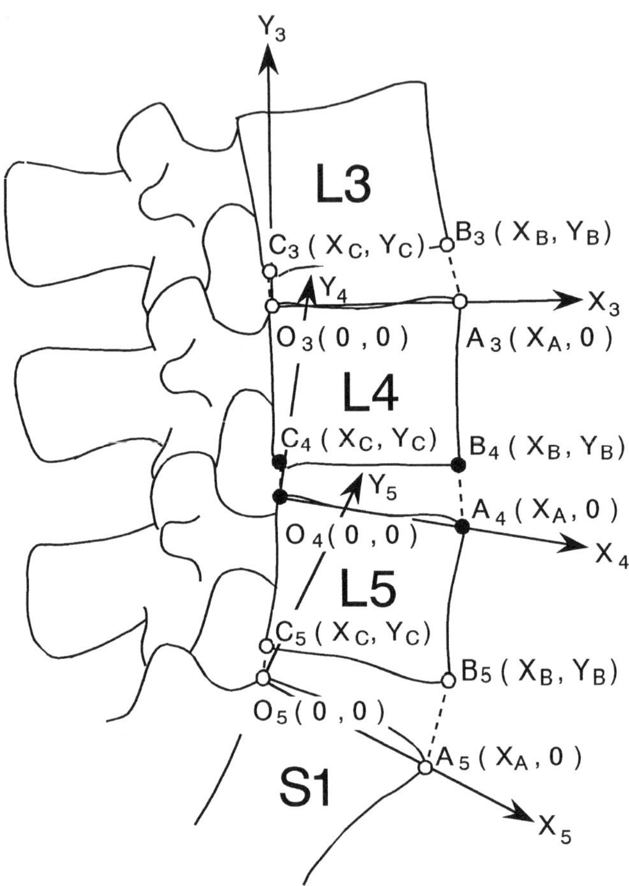

FIGURE 1.—Local coordinate systems of the intervertebral disks. (Reprinted from *Clinical Biomechanics,* Vol. 10, Kanayama M, Tadano S, Kaneda K, et al: A cineradiographic study on the lumbar disc deformation during flexion and extension of the trunk, pp 193–199, Copyright 1995, with kind permission from Elsevier Science Ltd, The Boulevard, Langford Lane, Kidlington OX5 1GB UK.)

The disks did not deform simultaneously, but rather in a stepwise manner from the upper to the lower level. At the time the lower disk began deforming, strain at the adjacent upper disks had reached more than half of the value at full flexion. No significant deformation of the L3–L4 and L4–L5 disks was found during extension.

Conclusion.—After an initial delay, the lumbar intervertebral disks deformed rapidly during spinal flexion.

► Although the finding of deformation of the lumbar disks with back flexion is not surprising, this study does demonstrate that the deforming is sequential from the lower- to the higher-numbered vertebrae. This does follow common sense, but it is the first time investigators have been able to confirm it. I wonder whether there is any relationship between the strength of the erector spinae and the amount of the deformation of the disks. Also, look at Abstract 2–9 by Nelson et al., because they have found that when lifting and lowering weights of 9.5 kg in extension, the deformation is more likely to be sequential, and in flexion, deformation is more likely to be simultaneous. Is it possible that flexing and extending with weights causes the difference, or is it measurement error?

Col. J.L. Anderson, PE.D.

Trunk Muscle Strength in and Effect of Trunk Muscle Exercises for Patients With Chronic Low Back Pain: The Differences in Patients With and Without Organic Lumbar Lesions

Takemasa R, Yamamoto H, Tani T (Kochi Med School, Japan)

Spine 20:2522–2530, 1995 2–3

Objective.—Patients with chronic low back pain (CLBP) appear to have reduced trunk muscle strength, and trunk muscle exercises appear to be an effective treatment for such patients. However, there are no data on the differences in trunk muscle strength or the effectiveness of trunk muscle exercise in patients with and without organic lumbar lesions. The impact of organic lumbar lesions on trunk muscle strength and on the effectiveness of trunk muscle exercises in patients with CLBP was assessed.

Methods.—Trunk muscle strength was evaluated in 123 patients with CLBP and 126 healthy controls. Of the patients with CLBP, 68 had organic lumbar lesions identified as the cause of their pain, and 55 had no evidence of such lesions. Seventy-two patients—41 with and 31 without organic lumbar lesions—were instructed in trunk muscle–strengthening exercises (Fig 2). Correlations were sought between the patients' improvement in low back pain and their increase in trunk muscle strength.

Results.—Both groups of patients had significantly lower trunk flexor and extensor strengths than controls. The patients with organic lumbar lesions had a significantly greater flexor/extensor ratio of maximum torque than the controls; this value was similar in the patients without organic lumbar lesions and controls. Both groups of patients had reductions in low back pain with trunk muscle exercise, but the exercises were more effective in patients without organic lumbar lesions. The patients without organic lesions also showed a greater degree of correlation between the increase in trunk muscle strength and the degree of improvement in low back pain.

Conclusions.—Among patients with CLBP, those with organic lumbar lesions show a significantly greater flexor/extensor ratio, perhaps arising from reduced extensor strength caused by neurogenic muscle weakness. In these patients, increasing trunk muscle strength through exercise improves low back pain but does not eliminate it completely. By comparison, increasing trunk muscle strength in patients with CLBP without organic lumbar lesions is very effective in decreasing low back pain. Patients with CLBP should undergo a comprehensive study of the cause of their pain before trunk muscle exercises are recommended.

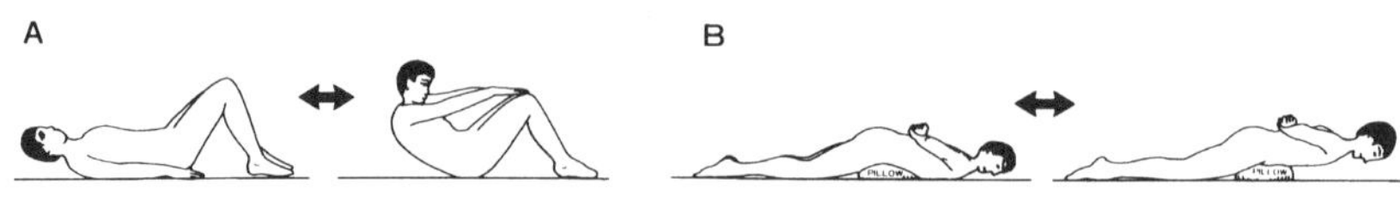

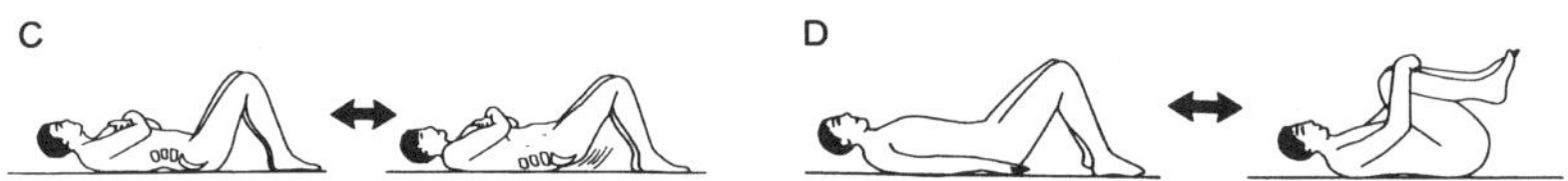

FIGURE 2.—Trunk muscle exercises. **A**, supine trunk raising (sit-up exercise). **B**, prone trunk extension exercise. **C**, pelvic tilting exercise. **D**, double-knee-to-chest (low back stretching) exercise. Patients were instructed to continue the exercises daily at home. (Courtesy of Takemasa R, Yamamoto H, Tani T: Trunk muscle strength in and effect of trunk muscle exercises for patients with chronic low back pain: The differences in patients with and without organic lumbar lesions. *Spine* 20:2522–2530, 1995.)

▶ It is good to see investigations done that try to correlate CLBP with trunk muscle strength. At West Point it has been our experience that trunk extension exercises are effective in treating CLBP. The 2 most effective methods have been the Backmate protocol and the Life Circuit trunk extension and abdominal machine. A number of patients who have tried the exercises in Figure 2 have complained that the exercises do not help them. I do not know whether that is because the patients were not diligent in doing the exercises; however, I am convinced that back extension and flexion exercises using machines with adjustable weights do strengthen the trunk flexor and extensor muscles and do eliminate low back pain for many patients.

Col. J.L. Anderson, PE.D.

Measurement of Muscle Strength of the Trunk and the Lower Extremities in Subjects With History of Low Back Pain

Lee J-H, Ooi Y, Nakamura K (Jichi Med School, Tochigi-ken, Japan; Univ of Tokyo)

Spine 20:1994–1996, 1995 2–4

Background.—Patients with low back pain are assumed to have weaker trunk muscles than healthy individuals. However, no studies have been done of lower extremity muscle strength in patients with low back pain. Muscle strength of the trunk and lower extremities was therefore assessed and correlated with low back pain.

Methods.—Ninety-eight men, aged 17–49 years, volunteered for the study. Sixty-one volunteers with some history of low back pain formed 1 group, and 37 with no such history comprised the control group. Total trunk strength was defined as the sum of peak torques of trunk extension, flexion, and rotation. Total knee strength was defined as the sum of peak torques of bilateral knee extension and flexion.

Findings.—Total trunk strength was a mean 281 nm and knee strength was a mean 301 nm in the group with low back pain. These values were significantly lower than the corresponding 543 and 441 nm in the control group. In both groups, total trunk strength was correlated linearly with total knee strength.

Conclusions.—The trunk and lower extremity muscles were affected similarly in these volunteers with low back pain. This finding can be explained by generalized muscular weakness resulting from disuse atrophy or poorly developed musculature by nature or by psychological factors, such as fear of injury.

▶ There is no doubt that individuals who experience low back pain will immediately cease exercising and will eventually become sedentary because no one gives them a program to rid them of the low back pain. A very simple treatment, which we have found to be effective once skeletal structural problems have been ruled out, is a relatively simple exercise program to include back extension exercises to strengthen the erector spinae muscles. Two methods that have been effective are the Backmate protocol and the use of the Life Circuit back extension machine. There are probably other pieces of equipment that can be used to strengthen the erector spinae muscles that will produce the same positive results.

Col. J.L. Anderson, PE.D.

Influence of Weight and Frequency on Thigh and Lower-trunk Motion During Repetitive Lifting Employing Stoop and Squat Techniques

Hagen KB, Sørhagen O, Harms-Ringdahl K (Norwegian Forest Research Inst, Ås, Norway; Karolinska Inst, Stockholm)

Clin Biomech 10:122–127, 1995 2–5

Objective.—Lifting activities are unrestrained dynamic movements, and movements during lifting may change because of fatigue during repetitive activity. Kinematic changes were examined in relation to lift frequency and weight in 10 experienced forest workers, men whose average age was 31 years.

Methods.—The men repeatedly lowered and lifted a box with side handles in a sagittal and symmetric manner, starting while standing straight with the arms hanging. Five submaximal bouts were performed at different combinations of weight and frequency at 6-day intervals, in ascending order of work intensity. The men initially were trained to lift using the squat and stoop techniques. Kinematic data were collected using electrolytic liquid level sensors within cylinders (Fig 1).

Results.—Nearly 6,400 lifts were analyzed. Lifting weight and frequency did not influence range of motion in stoop lifting. In contrast, lift frequency significantly affected the range of thigh motion during squat

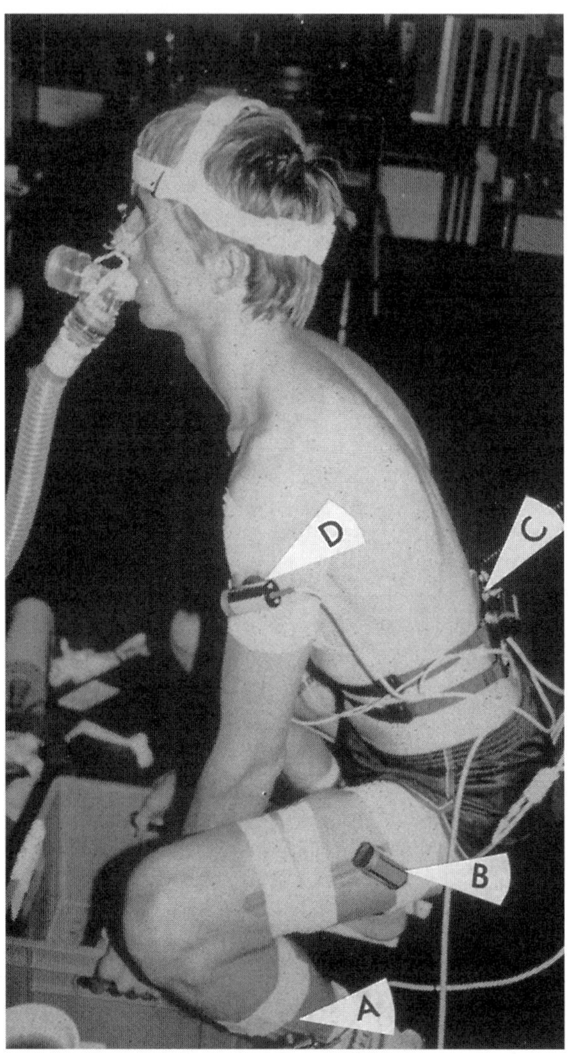

FIGURE 1.—Cylinders attached to the patient's lower leg (*A*), thigh (*B*), trunk (*C*), and upper arm (*D*) during the lifting experiments. (Reprinted from *Clinical Biomechanics,* Vol. 10, Hagen KB, Sørhagen O, Harms-Ringdahl K: Influence of weight and frequency on thigh and lower-trunk motion during repetitive lifting employing stoop and squat techniques, pp 122–127, Copyright 1995, with kind permission from Elsevier Science Ltd, The Boulevard, Langford Lane, Kidlington OX5 1GB UK.)

lifts, with motion decreasing as the frequency increased. The decreased thigh motion usually was accompanied by increased motion of the lower trunk. Motions of both the thigh and lower trunk varied significantly more during squats than in stoop lifting.

Conclusion.—Lifting a weight using the stoop technique entails an attempt to reduce demand on the quadriceps muscles.

▶ It has been well established that occupational lifting often results in low back disorders. It is also well established that most low back pain is not the result of skeletal structural problems but more likely the result of the imbalance in muscular strength and inappropriate lifting techniques for the job at hand. This study demonstrated that even experienced workers will shift from the appropriate to the inappropriate lifting technique as fatigue begins to set in. It appears that these workers would benefit from an exercise program to strengthen the quadriceps. Most workers that I have spoken with believe that they get enough exercise from their jobs. However, those who train athletes know that athletes do not get enough or proper conditioning just by playing the game.

Col. J.L. Anderson, PE.D.

Lumbar Spine Maximum Efforts and Muscle Recruitment Patterns Predicted by a Model With Multijoint Muscles and Joints With Stiffness
Stokes IAF, Gardner-Morse M (Univ of Vermont, Burlington)
J Biomech 28:173–186, 1995 2–6

Background.—Analyzing load transmission through the lumbar spine is complicated. The spine anatomy includes many joints and many muscles that cross several of these joints. A 3-dimensional lumbar spine model with realistic anatomy was studied. In this model, equilibrium had to be satisfied simultaneously at all joints crossed by multijoint muscles. The model included both forces and moments associated with their deformations.

It was hypothesized that the need to maintain equilibrium simultaneously at all vertical levels would preclude simultaneous maximum activation of synergistic muscles. It also was suggested that the maximal loads that could be carried by the spine and the degree of muscle activation would increase as motion segment stiffness increased.

Methods.—The maximum moments applied to T12 were determined for moments in 3 principal directions. They were subjected to equilibrium at all 6 joints and constraints on the maximum muscle strength and intervertebral displacements (Fig 3).

Findings.—Compared with a "ball-and-socket" joint model, the new model predicted maximum efforts increased by 1.4 to 3.3 times. The predictions of the model with the realistic motion segment stiffness were also more consistent with published results from maximum effort experiments. Compared with moments transmitted through the joints, the differences in maximal effort were greater. Although muscle activation levels were increased, submaximal activation was still observed in many synergistic muscles. Multijoint equilibrium was maintained through antagonistic muscles.

Conclusions.—In the commonly used 2-dimensional slice analyses of spinal forces, it is assumed that muscle forces need to satisfy equilibrium only at the 1 anatomical level being considered. However, this is generally not compatible with equilibrium at other levels, because so many lumbar

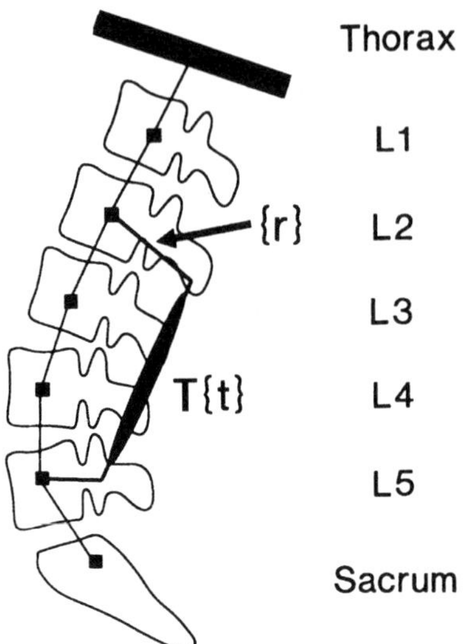

FIGURE 3.—Lateral view of lumbar spine model. The positions of vertebral body centers are shown by *squares*. A general muscle has a unit direction vector {*t*} and is activated with tension *T*. Its vertebral attachment is identified relative to the vertebral body center by the vector {*r*}. (Reprinted from *Journal of Biomechanics,* Vol. 28, Stokes IAF, Gardner-Morse M: Lumbar spine maximum efforts and muscle recruitment patterns predicted by a model with multijoint muscles and joints with stiffness, pp 173–186, Copyright 1995, with kind permission from Elsevier Science Ltd, The Boulevard, Langford Lane, Kidlington OX5 1GB UK.)

spine muscles cross multiple levels. Moment transmission in the joints of the stiffness model increased the predicted maximal efforts, bringing them closer to published values. The representation of the lumbar spine in this model may therefore be more realistic. Alterations in motion segment stiffness resulting from aging, injury, or degeneration may change the pattern of muscle activation and the trunk strength of an individual.

▶ These authors point out that previous biomechanical analyses of the spine have been done with a free body diagram created by a single transverse cutting plane through 1 vertebral level, which ignored the requirement that equilibrium must be satisfied at all of the spinal articulations and did not consider the implications of the numerous multijoint muscles. They have developed a 3-dimensional model of the lumbar spine with multijoint muscles to analyze lumbar spinal muscle recruitment and loading at all the lumbar joints simultaneously. In the analyses, 132 muscle forces and either the 6 displacements at each vertebra or the 3 forces between each pair of vertebrae were considered as variables. Linear programming was used to calculate the variables subject to the constraints on spinal equilibrium, muscle stress, and intervertebral displacements. This is a very nice piece of work.

Col. J.L. Anderson, PE.D.

The Psoas Major Muscle: A Three-dimensional Geometric Study
Santaguida PL, McGill SM (Univ of Waterloo, Ont, Canada)
J Biomech 28:339–345, 1995 2–7

Background.—Although the psoas major muscle is the largest muscle in the lower lumbar spine, there is little information about its mechanical capacity. Data from 1 MRI study suggest that the major line of action of the psoas major is better represented by a curve than by a straight line. The line of action and mechanical function of the psoas major muscle was studied using 3-dimensional data from cadavers and living individuals.

Methods.—The study included 7 cadaver dissections with measurement of the fiber/tendon architecture. In addition, 15 men underwent MRI scanning to determine centroid paths and area scales of the psoas major muscle over its entire length. The muscle's line of action and mechanical function were assessed in 3 dimensions around each level of the lumbar spine.

Results.—The MRI technique used in the study accommodated the curving path of the muscle's line of action and—combined with force and moment predictions—recognized the significant increase in stress related to the presence of a tendon at the lower lumbar levels. This tendon extended up to L3 in some men. As suggested by previous studies, the mechanics of the psoas could not be adequately represented by a series of

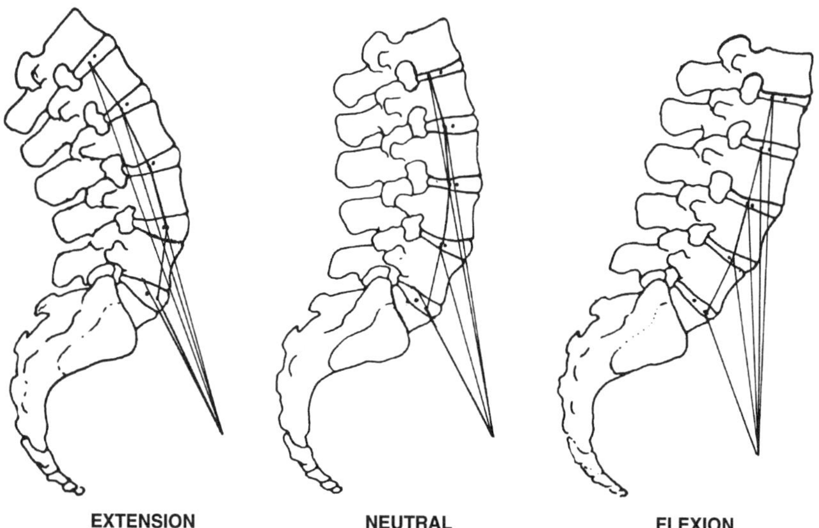

FIGURE 2.—A sagittal view of the centroid line of action based on MRI data is compared with a straight line of action in 3 lumbar postures. The *thick line* represents the centroid line of action, whereas each *thin line* represents a straight line of action from a vertebra. The centroid path used in this study suggests greater compression forces and increasing shear forces from upper to lower levels compared with the straight line approach. (Reprinted from *Journal of Biomechanics*, Vol. 28, Santaguida PL, McGill SM: The psoas major muscle: A three-dimensional geometric study, pp 339–345, Copyright 1995, with kind permission from Elsevier Science Ltd, The Boulevard, Langford Lane, Kidlington OX5 1GB UK.)

straight-line vectors running from the vertebral origins to the insertion (Fig 2). Its path of action changed with changes in spine posture, demonstrating that the mechanical action of the psoas major does not change as a function of lumbar spine lordosis. The psoas was not found to act as a functional "derotator" of the spine, was not responsible for major shear forces at any posture except L5–S1, and had no major effect in controlling lordosis. Its functional potential included stabilization of the lumbar spine with compressive loading and bilateral activation, lateral flexion of the lumbar spine, and creation of large anterior shear forces at L5–S1.

Conclusions.—The potential forces generated by the psoas major muscle appear to be greater than predicted on the basis of the muscle's cross-section area alone. Its mechanics are only adequately depicted by a curving line of action, not by a series of straight-line vectors from vertebral origins to insertion. The mechanical potential of the psoas major does not change with lumbar spine lordosis. The findings need to be validated in force measurement studies of the function of the psoas major muscle.

▶ These authors continue the ages-long discussions to determine the role of the psoas muscle. Just over 20 years ago,there was significant evidence that we should change from doing straight-knee sit-ups to bent-knee sit-ups because, by bending the legs, we are taking the psoas muscle out of play and thus reducing the potential of placing undue stress on the low back caused by the lumbar lordosis.

The results of this study seem to indicate that the location of the psoas muscle centroid is not significantly affected by changing the lumbar spine and hip position. Recent studies seem to suggest that the psoas is neurally activated during both straight- and bent-knee sit-ups. The current study, however, by representing the psoas major muscle with a curving line of action as opposed to a straight-line approach, has demonstrated that the compression and shear loads do not significantly differ as a result of changing lordosis and hip posture. These findings suggest that changes in forces during the performance of a bent-knee sit-up are not a result of changes in the moment arm but rather the change in muscle length.

Col. J.L. Anderson, PE.D.

The Effects of Lateral Trunk Bending on Muscle Recruitments When Resisting Nonsagittally Symmetric Bending Moments

Lavender SA, Chen I-H, Trafimow J, Andersson GBJ (Rush-Presbyterian-St Luke's Med Ctr, Chicago; Tsu-Chi Gen Hosp, Hua Lian, Taiwan)
Spine 20:184–191, 1995 2–8

Introduction.—Lateral bending of the torso may result from asymmetric material-handling tasks. Both lateral bending and asymmetric material handling have been associated with low back disorders. However, there are few data on the response of the trunk muscles when the trunk is bent to 1 side. The myoelectric responses of 8 trunk muscles to asymmetric loading of the laterally bent torso were evaluated.

Methods.—Fifteen individuals were studied as they stood in a reference frame, adjusting their trunk posture to achieve a 20-degree lateral bend to the right. The individuals then resisted symmetric and asymmetric moments applied to their torsos through weights connected to a chest harness. The moment magnitudes were 20 and 40 nm, with transverse plane directional components in 30-degree increments around the participants' torsos. Surface electromyographic activity was recorded from the erector spinae, latissimus dorsi, rectus abdominis, and external oblique muscles.

Results.—Electromyographic activity was greatest when the muscles were in opposition to applied sagittal and frontal plane moments. The response was greatest for the left external oblique muscle, which also was sensitive to the widest range of moment direction conditions. All but the left latissimus dorsi muscle sometimes contributed antagonistic moments in the sagittal or frontal plane or both. Compared with previous data recorded with individuals in the upright neutral posture, the responses of the external oblique and the left erector spinae muscles to the moment direction conditions were significantly different.

Conclusions.—Trunk muscle recruitment appears to rely heavily on the combination of the trunk posture and the direction of an applied moment. Larger moment magnitudes elicit recruitments of greater magnitude, but only for the more active parts of each muscle's response envelope. With the torso laterally bent, the response envelopes for many muscles shift such that the range of moment directions to which the muscle is sensitive lead to increased co-contraction.

▶ Several previous studies were concerned with the effects on the spine of various loading methods. I am certain we all know that the muscles are there to help protect the spine from dangerous distortion. These authors focus on the role of the muscles to accomplish their purpose. Would not a useful study be one that considered both the roles of the muscles and the effect on the spine at the same time? Possibly such a study could look at the strength of the erector spinae muscles and whether there is a correlation between their strength and protection of the spine.

Col. J.L. Anderson, PE.D.

Relative Lumbar and Pelvic Motion During Loaded Spinal Flexion/Extension

Nelson JM, Walmsley RP, Stevenson JM (Queen's Univ, Kingston, Ont, Canada)

Spine 20:199–204, 1995 2–9

Objective.—There is controversy as to whether rotatory movements of the pelvis and lumbar spine occur in sequence or simultaneously during bending and lifting tasks. Anecdotal evidence suggests that the direction of movement may affect the coordination of lumbar and pelvic motion. Lumbar-pelvic rhythm was evaluated during sagittal plane trunk motion, including an assessment of the effect of direction of lift.

Methods.—Thirty healthy women, ranging in age from 19 to 20 years, were studied with the 3Space Tracker System to measure differential lumbar and pelvic motion during trunk flexion and extension. Lumbar and pelvic rotation were compared as the women lifted and lowered a 9.5-kg box with the knees extended.

Results.—Simultaneous lumbar and pelvic motion was observed during flexion and extension. However, these motions showed greater separation during the upward lifts than the "down lifts." In most women, lumbar flexion increased during the initial stages of upward lift but did not peak at the same time as pelvic flexion.

Conclusions.—The characteristics of lumbar-pelvic rhythm appear to vary according to whether the trunk is in flexion or extension. As the trunk is flexing—that is, during down lift—lumbar and pelvic rotation are more likely to take place at the same time. In contrast, during trunk extension—that is, upward lifting—lumbar and pelvic rotation are more likely to be sequential. Although the lumbar-pelvic rhythm is consistent within individuals from day to day, it varies considerably among research subjects.

▶ In the study by Kanayama et al. (Abstract 2–2), they used the amount of deformation of the disks to determine what the authors of this study call "rhythm." They also found that the disk deformation is sequential from the lower- to the higher-numbered vertebrae as the trunk is flexed. Did the use of weights cause the difference, or is it measurement error?

Col. J.L. Anderson, PE.D.

Neuromuscular Coordination of Squat Lifting: I. Effect of Load Magnitude

Scholz JP, Millford JP, McMillan AG (Univ of Delaware, Newark)
Phys Ther 75:119–132, 1995 2–10

Purpose.—Despite all the attention paid to understanding lifting performance, lifting-related back injuries continue to be extremely common. Most studies have focused on the initial lifting posture alone, without considering the changes in neuromuscular coordination that might occur during the lift. Information on how the nervous system resolves the many task demands of lifting could be useful in setting realistic guidelines for worker performance and in developing effective programs for training workers in how to lift. Changes in kinematic and electromyographic (EMG) measurements of coordination during a squat-lifting task with increasing loads were evaluated.

Methods.—A convenience sample of 15 male industrial workers was studied while lifting a weighted crate containing 15% to 75% of the workers' peak lifting capacity. All workers used a symmetric squat-lift technique. Videography was performed to evaluate movement kinematics, and the relative phase between joint motions was derived from this assessment. In addition, EMG recordings were made from the vastus lateralis and erector spinae muscles for estimation of the relative timing of their onsets and peaks.

Results.—A quasilinear change was noted in the relative phase of movement between joints—such as the knee and lumbar spine—with increasing load during lifting only, not during lowering. The change in relative time of onset of erector spinae muscle EMG activity and its peak activity was consistent with the interjoint relative phase patterns. Increasing load had no significant effect on the timing of vastus lateralis EMG activity.

Conclusions.—For workers performing lifts from an initial squatting posture, relatively continuous changes occur in coordination between limbs as the load increases. The changes in relative timing of EMG changes in relevant muscles partially corroborate these changes. More research is needed to determine whether the coordination changes that occur during the lift are helpful or harmful to the musculoskeletal system. Clinically, performance of squat lifting should be evaluated under a range of task conditions.

▶ Unlike the previous 2 studies, this one uses the squat technique for lifting. The authors found that even though individuals may begin by using the squat technique, there is no assurance that they will lift the load in exactly the same manner regardless of the weight lifted or in the face of changing other task variables such as movement speed. Again, I repeat, does it not make sense to offer strength development training for workers who do heavy lifting, just as we do for our athletes?

Col. J.L. Anderson, PE.D.

Neuromuscular Coordination of Squat Lifting: II. Individual Differences

Scholz JP, McMillan AG (Univ of Delaware, Newark)

Phys Ther 75:133–144, 1995 2–11

Background.—Few studies have addressed the relative timing of joint movements and muscle activity of the task of squat lifting. Knowledge of the coordination of lifting may contribute to an understanding of the mechanisms of back injury. To determine whether individual differences observed qualitatively in lifting could also be identified quantitatively, 12 men were studied. The study also examined whether differences in patterns of knee–lumbar spine coordination during load acceleration were related to differences in other measures related to task performance.

Methods.—Fifteen men from 26 to 52 years of age were recruited for the study; data from 12 were available for analysis. The experimental procedure consisted of lifting a weighted crate to the height of the waist from a starting posture with the knees bent, the back relatively straight, and the feet positioned symmetrically. The crate contained 15% to 75% of the participants' lifting capacity. Various locations on the men and the crates had reflective markers attached, and videography was used to obtain movement kinematic data. Electromyographic (EMG) activity of the vastus lateralis and erector spinae muscles was recorded with surface EMG. Two dominant patterns of coordination during load acceleration were apparent in the 12 research subjects. Group differences were compared using the kinematic data and measurements of coordination derived kinematically and via EMG.

Results.—An equal number of the research subjects fell into each of the 2 coordination patterns observed. Six men limited lumbar spine motion more when lifting the heaviest loads, whereas the other 6 men limited lumbar spine motion during load acceleration for all loads lifted. These differences were apparent both qualitatively and quantitatively. After initial load acceleration, the effect of load on the coordination of the involved joints was the same for both groups. The 2 groups did not differ significantly in mean height or weight.

Conclusions.—Men of similar height and weight showed individual differences in the performance of squat lifting, even under the same lifting conditions and with identical and consistent instructions. Although men in both groups began the lift in a squatting posture, differences in knee–lumbar spine relative timing were greatest at early points in the lift. Subtle differences in coordination may need to be addressed when workers are trained to lift heavy loads from the floor.

► This is a continuation of the study preceding it (Abstract 2–10), by 2 of the same authors. Again, the authors had their research subjects use the squat technique for lifting loads that varied between 15% and 75% of their maximum lift capacity. In this study, they found that individual differences occur in how workers lift a load from an initial squatting position, despite identical and consistent instructions. They found that just demonstrating to workers how to perform the squat-lift technique does not ensure that they will perform it properly or that they will not experience low back pain. Instructors must pay more attention to the subtle differences in coordination when training workers to lift.

Col. J.L. Anderson, PE.D.

A Biomechanical Assessment and Model of Axial Twisting in the Thoracolumbar Spine

Marras WS, Granata KP (Ohio State Univ, Columbus)

Spine 20:1440–1451, 1995 2–12

Objective.—Considerable evidence from epidemiologic studies indicates that axial twisting of the torso is a risk factor for work-related low back disorders. An attempt was made to biomechanically model the loads imposed on the spine during dynamic torsional exertion.

Methods.—Twelve asymptomatic men, 21–31 years of age, with no history of low back problems were placed in a twisting reference frame and asked to apply axial torque to a yoke placed about the back, shoulders, and chest (Fig 1). Torsional exertions were performed at 100% and 50% of maximal voluntary contraction (MVC) effort in both the clockwise and counterclockwise directions. Normalized electromyograms (EMGs) were recorded from 10 trunk muscles using surface electrodes.

Results.—Despite an effort to produce purely torsional forces, significant forces developed about the other body axes. Full MVC exertions produced at least 25% greater EMGs than did 50% MVC exertions. Many vertically oriented trunk muscles altered their activity when the applied torsional direction changed. Torsional exertions led to significant flexion-extension and lateral moments. Muscular co-activity was signifi-

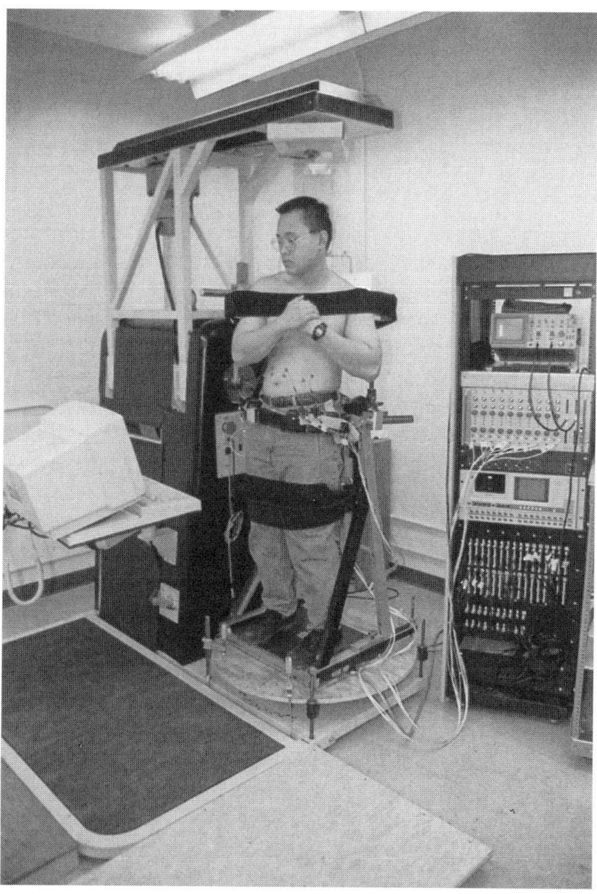

FIGURE 1.—A twisting reference frame was used to control and monitor static posture and dynamic motions of the individuals during torsional exertions. (Courtesy of Marras WS, Granata KP: A biomechanical assessment and model of axial twisting in the thoracolumbar spine. *Spine* 20:1440–1451, 1995.)

cantly less than that associated with lifting. Trunk moments were accurately predicted when EMG data were used to represent muscle co-activity.

Conclusion.—The finding that the load on the spine increases with torsional exertional load, velocity, and twist angle agrees with clinical observations that these factors influence the risk of low back pain.

▶ These investigators believe that the physiologically reasonable results generated by their model compared with other models can be attributed to 3 important differences in model design and assumption. First, their model includes the activity and contribution of the latissimus dorsi muscles. Second, they used the maximum cross-section area of the muscle to predict the maximum force contribution of each trunk muscle. Third, their model treats the trunk musculature as a series of vectors capable of changing their orientation and mechanical advantage during a twisting motion. Their analyses also have demonstrated that dynamic torsional trunk movements may be predicted from kinematics and EMG data within the constraints of physiologic validity. Compression and shear forces at the lumbosacral junction may be predicted from muscle equivalent forces scaled relative to the twisting movements. Therefore, qualitative if not quantitative loading may be compared as a function of exertion load, trunk rotation, and motion characteristics.

They also report that the predicted spine loadings indicated that when any twisting velocity was present, significant increases in compression resulted. Also, greater shear loading accompanied the higher compressive forces. This led them to the observation that twisting may create a situation where the combination of forces acting upon the spine places individuals at a higher risk of exceeding their tolerance of these forces. In the interest of preventive medicine, can we develop exercise programs to strengthen the trunk muscles and help protect the back?

Col. J.L. Anderson, PE.D.

The National Basketball Association Eye Injury Study

Zagelbaum BM, Starkey C, Hersh PS, Donnenfeld ED, Perry HD, Jeffers JB (Cornell Univ, Manhasset, NY; Albert Einstein College of Medicine, Bronx, NY; Northeastern Univ, Boston; et al)

Arch Ophthalmol 113:749–752, 1995 2–13

Objective.—A 1992 survey found that basketball accounted for the greatest prevalence of sports-related eye injuries in the United States. To determine the incidence and characteristics of eye injuries sustained by professional basketball players in the National Basketball Association (NBA), players were studied prospectively.

Methods.—Data forms were sent to all 27 NBA team athletic trainers, physicians, and ophthalmologists. Information was requested on any player who was examined for an eye injury of any severity between February 1, 1992, and June 20, 1993. Included in the study were practices and preseason games, regular season games, play-offs, and championships. All but 1 of the 27 teams responded to the study request.

Results.—During the 17-month period, 59 (5.4%) of the 1,092 injuries sustained by NBA players involved the eye and adnexa. The most common diagnoses were abrasions or lacerations to the eyelid (50.9%), contusions to the eyelid or periorbital region (28.8%), and corneal abrasions (11.9%). More than half of the injuries occurred while the player was rebounding (30.5%) or on offense (27.1%), and most were caused by the fingers (35.6%) or elbows (28.8%). The chief complaints after injury were bleeding, eye redness, and ocular pain. Only 2 of the 59 injured players were wearing safety goggles at the time of the eye injury. Nine players missed subsequent games because of the injury.

Conclusions.—The incidence of ocular injury for NBA players during the 17-month season was 1.44 per 1,000 game exposures. Few professional basketball players wear protective eyewear, despite the risk of disabling eye injury from frequent physical contact. It is recommended that players wear properly fitting sports goggles made of 3-mm-thick polycarbonate lenses and unbreakable frames.

Golf-related Ocular Injuries

Mieler WF, Nanda SK, Wolf MD, Harman J (Med College of Wisconsin, Milwaukee)

Arch Ophthalmol 113:1410–1413, 1995 2–14

Background.—Although sports-related activity accounts for a small proportion of all ocular injuries, patients injured while playing sports represent a high percentage of hospital admissions for ocular injuries. To determine the nature of golf-related eye injuries in the United States, all sports-related traumas treated at 1 institution were reviewed.

Methods.—The records of the institute were reviewed for an 8-year period (1986–1994). Data collected included clinical characteristics, mechanisms of injury, presence of eyewear, medical and surgical management, and visual outcome. Patients were followed for a minimum of 6 months after the injury; the average follow-up was 27 months.

Results.—Eight blunt ocular injuries caused by golf-related activities were identified during the study. Six patients were male; the average age of the group was 44 years. Two patients were struck by a golf club and 6 by a golf ball projectile. Ruptured globes were present in 4 patients, and 2 had an accompanying blowout orbital fracture. One patient was wearing sunglasses, but none had protective eyewear. Patients with ruptured globes underwent repair of the corneoscleral laceration on the day of injury. Three subsequently had enucleation surgery, and 1 experienced progressive hypotony after a pars plana vitrectomy, performed 12 days after the injury. All 4 trauma cases without rupture required surgical procedures to achieve anatomical stability. Final visual acuities at the latest follow-up ranged from 20/25 to 20/40.

Conclusions.—Golf-related eye injuries, although uncommon, often have serious consequences. A previous study reported that golf was the sport with the third highest incidence of enucleations per injury (71%), behind only hockey (80%) and use of BB guns (75%). Patients who had ruptured globes have not fared well visually, and those without rupture required intraocular surgery. Because of the high velocity of the golf ball, there appears to be no effective means of eye protection.

Catastrophic Injuries to the Eyes and Testicles in Footballers

Lawson JS, Rotem T, Wilson SF (Univ of New South Wales, Sydney, Australia; Royal North Shore Hosp, Sydney, Australia)

Med J Aust 163:242–244, 1995 2–15

Background.—Footballers in New South Wales, Australia, commonly experience injuries such as bone fractures and tears, bruises, and muscle and ligament strains. Although relatively rare, other catastrophic injuries causing permanent disability and death also have been reported, particularly among rugby league and rugby union footballers. The occurrence of catastrophic eye and testicular injuries to New South Wales rugby league and rugby union footballers was retrospectively investigated.

Methods.—The New South Wales Sporting Injuries Insurance Scheme, established to provide financial compensation to athletes who have been seriously injured during sports activities, prepares detailed medical assessments for all claimants. Assessments prepared between 1980 and 1993 were retrospectively reviewed to determine the incidence and nature of serious injuries. Injuries causing 50% or more permanent loss of function of 1 eye, and those causing 50% or more loss of 1 testicle, were defined as catastrophic. Although the findings of this review do provide an indication of the incidence and nature of very serious injuries, the number of catastrophically injured athletes is likely underestimated because not all footballers are members of the Insurance Scheme.

Results.—Each year, an average of 81,000 league and 23,500 union players were registered with the New South Wales Sporting Injuries Insurance Scheme. Twenty-one league and 5 union footballers had catastrophic eye injuries, including eye rupture, retinal impairment, and optic nerve damage. Overall, these injuries resulted in 90% to 100% vision loss in 1 eye (15 players), 75% vision loss in 1 eye (5 players), 75% vision loss in both eyes (2 players), and 50% vision loss in 1 eye (4 players). Common causes of eye injuries included gouging with fingers, kicking, and blows from fists, elbows, knees, or the ball. Injuries appeared to be intentionally caused in 5 instances.

One union and 13 league players also had testicular injuries, resulting in complete loss of 1 testicle in 11 players and partial loss of 1 testicle in 3 players. Testicular injuries were caused by kicking and kneeing during a tackle. In 3 instances, injuries appeared to have been deliberately inflicted.

Conclusions.—Football-related injuries to the eyes and testicles can have devastating consequences. Educating officials, players, parents, and the public may help garner support for the strengthening and strict enforcement of rules pertaining to tackles, kicks, and other assaults directed at the head and groin. Increased awareness and policing of these rules may, in turn, help prevent the occurrence of catastrophic injuries.

Sports-related Eye Injuries

Ghosh F, Bauer B (Univ Eye Hosp of Lund, Sweden)
Acta Ophthalmol 73:353–354, 1995 2–16

Objective.—The files of a Swedish university hospital were searched for records of all patients treated for blunt trauma between January 1991 and September 1993. Patients whose injuries were sports related were reviewed for type and mechanism of injury, patient age, and sex distribution.

Results.—During the 33-month study, 109 (40%) of 272 patients treated for eye injuries resulting from blunt trauma had been injured during sports activities. Eleven of 39 injuries requiring hospitalization were sports related. Floor ball, played with a hollow plastic ball the size of an orange and a hard plastic bat with a curved blade, was responsible for almost half (48%) of the sports-related injuries. Football accounted for 15% of the sported-related injuries, and tennis accounted for 13%. Most of those with eye injuries were boys or men (83 of 109 patients) between the ages of 10 and 29 years (64 of 109 patients). The most common injury (51% of the total) was blood in the anterior chamber. Retinal edema accounted for 28% of sports-related eye injuries and corneal erosion for 22%. The rate of permanent visual impairment was low. Six patients had visual acuity less than 0.5 3–6 months after injury.

Conclusion.—Sports-related injuries make up a large proportion of injuries to the eye caused by blunt trauma. In nearly all reported cases, a ball had struck the eye. Protective eyewear is needed during play. No injuries were reported for ice hockey, a sport that usually mandates the use of face and eye protection.

► These 4 articles (Abstracts 2–13 to 2–16) dealing with injuries to the eye, orbit, and adnexa cover areas rarely reported in the medical literature. Noteworthy is the variety of both pathology and severity of injuries seen. Although the prospective NBA eye injury study documented a relatively high injury rate, most of these injuries were of lesser severity. On the other hand, golf-related ocular injuries, while uncommon, had devastating sequelae.

In considering prophylactic protective devices, 3 questions must be addressed. First, in any given activity, are ocular injuries a problem from the standpoints of both occurrence and severity? Second, what type of protective device would be most effective? As pointed out by Zagelbaum, "open eye guards are of no value in racquetball and may increase injury by funneling a compressible ball into the orbit."[1] This funneling phenomenon also was a problem with the first-generation hockey goalkeeper mask. Third, will a particular protective device contribute to other injuries? Some evidence suggests that implementation of the requirement for hockey players to wear a helmet and eye shield has been responsible for an increase in cervical spine injuries.

J.S. Torg, M.D.

Reference

1. Zagelbaum BM: Sports-related eye trauma: Managing common injuries. *Physician Sportsmed* 21:25–42, 1993.

Head Injuries Incurred by Children and Young Adults During Informal Recreation

Baker SP, Fowler C, Li G, Warner M, Dannenberg AL (Johns Hopkins Injury Prevention Ctr, Baltimore, Md)

Am J Public Health 84:649–652, 1994 2–17

Objective.—Sports and recreation account for more than 40% of all head injuries in children and adolescents. Head injuries during informal recreational activities in children and young adults were investigated.

Methods.—Injuries related to playground equipment, children's vehicles, skateboards, and roller skates were examined using data from the 1991 emergency records of patients younger than 25 years included in the Consumer Product Safety Commission's surveillance of 91 hospitals in the United States. Head injuries included scalp lacerations, skull fractures, concussions, and other brain injuries, and excluded injuries to the face, mouth, eye, or ear.

Findings.—Head injury was the primary diagnosis among an estimated 58,480 (13%) of 464,000 individuals younger than 25 years who received emergency treatment for injuries related to playground equipment, children's vehicles, and roller skates. The percentage of injuries that involved the head significantly decreased with age for each major category of activity (Fig 1). For all ages combined, 74% of head injuries occurred in connection with playground equipment, particularly swings, slides, and monkey bars. Almost 6% of individuals with head injuries were admitted to the hospital, and head injuries associated with skateboards had an especially high proportion of hospital admission (12.7%). The number of head injuries from recreational activities exceeded those from bicycling, was more than twofold higher than head injuries for bicyclists younger than 5 years, and was 80% more frequent than head injuries for bicyclists aged 5–14 years (Fig 2).

Recommendations.—Although estimates based on emergency department data are conservative, a large number and a high rate of head injuries were found in children involved in informal recreational activities. Multipurpose helmets are an appealing approach to this problem, and currently, the Snell Memorial Foundation is developing a standard for mul-

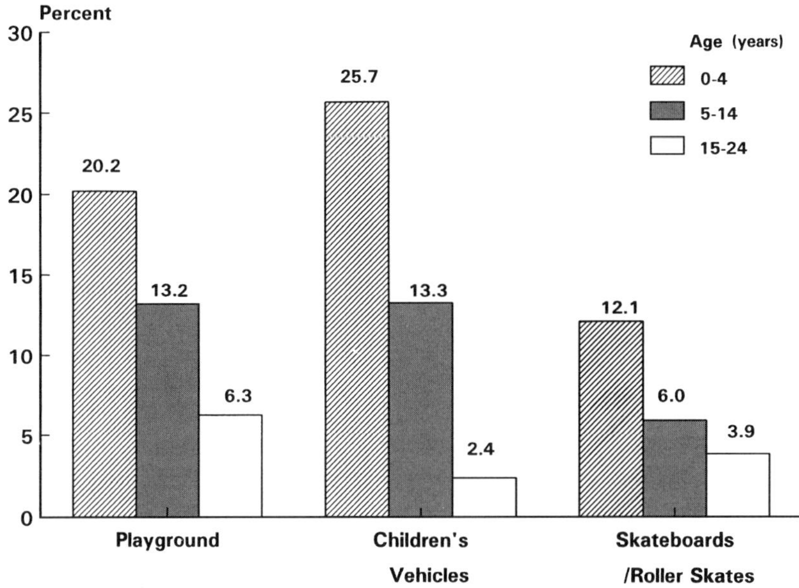

FIGURE 1.—Head injuries as a percentage of all injuries incurred during informal recreation, by age and activity, 1991. Data provided by the Consumer Product Safety Commission. (Courtesy of Baker SP, Fowler C, Li G, et al: Head injuries incurred by children and young adults during informal recreation. *Am J Public Health* 84:649–652, 1994, American Public Health Association.)

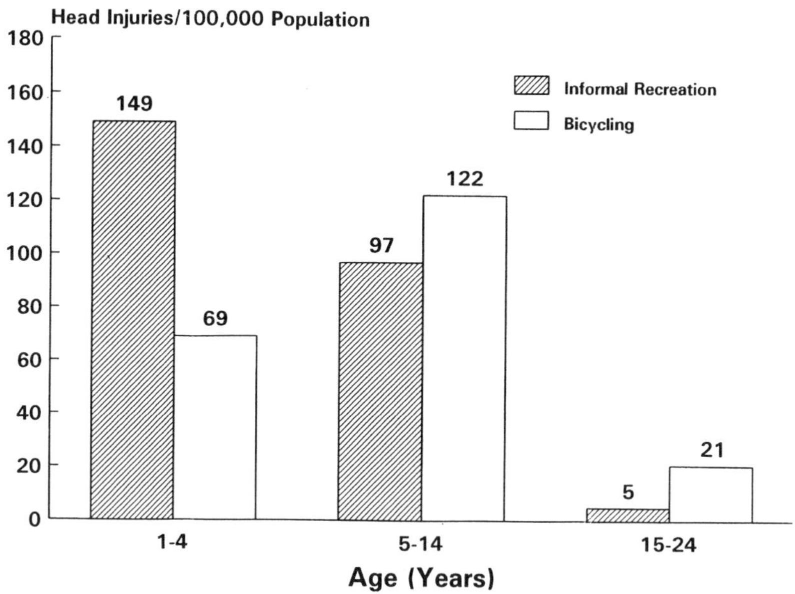

FIGURE 2.—Incidence rates of head injury from bicycling and informal recreation, by age, 1991. Data provided by the Consumer Product Safety Commission. (Courtesy of Baker SP, Fowler C, Li G, et al: Head injuries incurred by children and young adults during informal recreation. *Am J Public Health* 84:649–652, 1994, American Public Health Association.)

tipurpose helmets. Early emphasis on helmets may be more effective in preventing head injury in recreational activities than trying to make a later change in existing behavior.

► Of the more than 1,000 bicycling deaths each year, three fourths are caused by head injuries, and half of those killed are schoolkids.[1] Bicycling is the leading cause of recreational injury among children, and many studies have shown that use of helmets can reduce the risk of head injury among bicyclists and the severity of head injury when a crash occurs.[2] Alas, most children still do not wear a helmet while cycling.

This report reminds us that head injuries similar to those from cycling occur in connection with playground equipment (swings, slides, monkey bars), skateboarding, roller skating, and other recreational activities. In fact, such head injuries are twice as common as those from cycling in children younger than 5 years of age. Wide use of multipurpose helmets beginning early in life would save precious lives.

E.R. Eichner, M.D.

References

1. 1994 YEAR BOOK OF SPORTS MEDICINE, pp 8–10.
2. Li G, Baker SP, Fowler C, et al: Factors related to the presence of head injury in bicycle-related pediatric trauma patients. *J Trauma* 38:871–875, 1995.

Pathophysiology of Spinal Cord Injury: Recovery After Immediate and Delayed Decompression

Delamarter RB, Sherman J, Carr JB (Univ of California, Los Angeles)
J Bone Joint Surg (Am) 77–A:1042–1049, 1995 2–18

Introduction.—Motor vehicle accidents, sports injuries, falls, tumors, and infections are the most frequent causes of severely disabling spinal cord injuries. Although surgical stabilization is an accepted procedure, the role of decompression, as well as the timing of decompression, are questioned because the cord is believed to be irreversibly damaged at the initial trauma. A variety of animal models for spinal cord trauma result in variable durations of compression. Differing durations of compression and the timing of decompressive surgery were studied in dogs.

Methods.—Thirty beagles had a laminectomy at the L4–L5 level. The spinal cord was compressed to 50% of its original initial diameter by an electrical cable 2.8 mm wide. The animals were divided into 5 groups: decompression immediately after 3- to 5-second compression (group 1), compression for 1 hour after initial closure of the wound (group 2), and compression for 6 hours (group 3). All dogs in these groups stayed under some level of anesthesia during the compression. Groups 4 and 5 recovered from the anesthesia, and group 4 had the compression removed at 24 hours; group 5 had it removed 1 week later. Somatosensory evoked potentials were monitored before and after compression was applied. Neurologic evaluation was performed daily and graded according to the method of Tarlov. Six weeks after compression, the dogs were killed. Sections of the cord were fixed for histologic examination.

Results.—All dogs were paraplegic after spinal cord compression. Decompression that was performed immediately after compression or 1 hour later allowed the dogs to recover the ability to walk (Tarlov grade 4 or 5). In addition, the animals regained bladder and bowel control. Evoked potentials improved an average of 72%. No neurologic recovery was achieved if the compression lasted 6 hours or more. Progressive necrosis of the cord was seen. Evoked potential fell from 29% in group 3 to 26% in group 4 to 10% in group 5.

Conclusion.—The degree of damage and subsequent recovery of neural tissue is related to nonischemic compression, vascular ischemia, and an immune response. Injury may be a result of the initial compression or subsequent events. Spinal cord damage may, in large part, result not from the initial impact but from the duration of the compression. A "window of opportunity" seems to be open for neurologic recovery after spinal cord compression.

The Pathomechanics and Pathophysiology of Cervical Spinal Cord Injury

Torg JS, Thibault L, Sennett B, Pavlov H (Univ of Pennsylvania, Philadelphia; Cornell Med College, New York)

Clin Orthop 321:259–269, 1995 2–19

Background.—Cervical spine injuries occurring during American football games have led to neurologic deficits that are reversible, incompletely

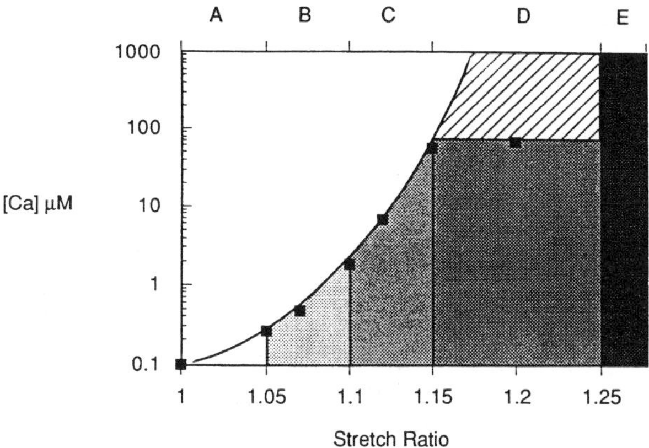

FIGURE 9.—The functional relationship between the magnitude of mechanical strain expressed as the stretch ratio and the peak values of the intracellular calcium (*Ca*) concentrations. (Courtesy of Torg JS, Thibault L, Sennett B, et al: The pathomechanics and pathophysiology of cervical spinal cord injury. *Clin Orthop* 321:259–269, 1995.)

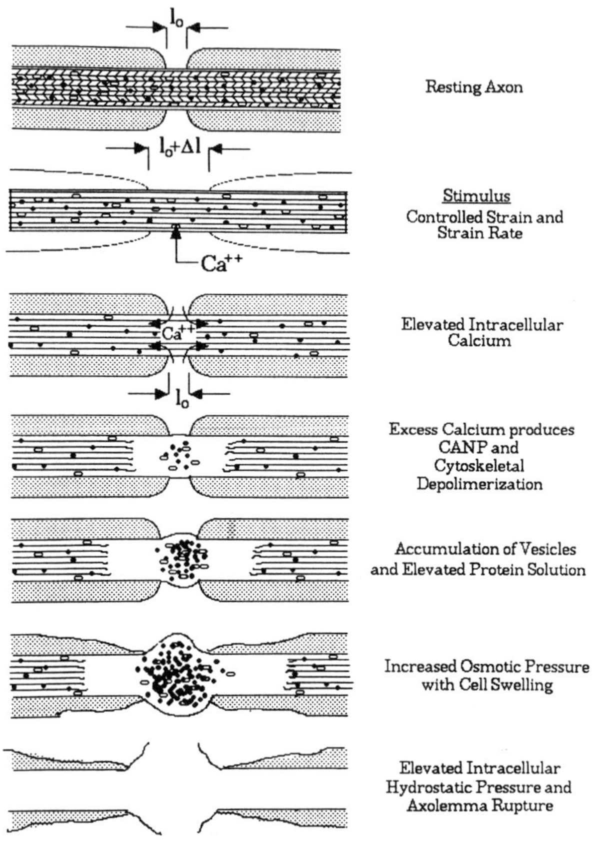

FIGURE 10.—Schematic representation of the effects of elevated intracellular calcium (*Ca*) concentration on cell viability. Specifically, elevated cytosolic free calcium in excess of 50 µmol/L will result in calcium-activated neutral protease (*CANP*) that can damage protein structures of the cell. (Courtesy of Torg JS, Thibault L, Sennett B, et al: The pathomechanics and pathophysiology of cervical spinal cord injury. *Clin Orthop* 321:259–269, 1995.)

reversible, or irreversible in nature. A study of the histochemical response of a squid axon injury model has provided an explanation for these different injury responses.

Methods.—A system designed to apply uni-axial tension at high strain rates was developed and used on the giant axon of the squid, which served as the isolated tissue model. The system's actuator was programmed to deform the axons to various stretch ratios at specific strain rates. Membrane potential, axon deformation, developed tension, and cytosolic free calcium ion concentration as a function of time were determined. Data for the dynamic stretch were recorded over a 100-msec interval. The calcium response was presented over a 30-second time course.

Results.—Axon recovery or failure to recover was found to be directly proportional to the intracellular calcium concentration. This, in turn, was directly proportional to the amount and rate of tension applied to the axon. A curve demonstrating the functional relationship between the magnitude of the mechanical strain and the peak value of the intracellular calcium changes after injury was generated and divided into 5 regions (Fig 9). In range A, the axon will spontaneously recover quickly, with no residual deficit. In range B, the axon will recover, although time to recovery will be extended, and no residual deficit will occur. In range C, the axon will attempt to recover, but a residual deficit will occur, and outcome will depend largely on the cell's ability to pump calcium. Metabolic factors will have a strong effect on this outcome. In range D, the axon will be irreversibly damaged by the initial calcium insult and eventually will die (Fig 10). In range E, the mechanical deformation will lead to structural failure.

Conclusions.—Disruption of cord function results from the effects of local cord anoxia and elevated levels of intracellular calcium in most acute spinal injuries. Initiation of treatment aimed at restoring blood flow and reducing cytosolic calcium may facilitate neurologic recovery in patients with cervical cord injuries.

► These 2 articles (Abstracts 2–18 and 2–19) clearly demonstrate the relationship of the rate, degree, and duration of neuron deformation to reversible and irreversible injury. Both have profound clinical relevance. Specifically, Delamarter et al., by demonstrating the recovery response to prompt decompression of the cord, support the concept of prompt reduction of spinal fractures and dislocation with neurologic involvement.

With regard to the Torg article, this study demonstrates the pathophysiology of cord injury in terms of the specific histochemical responses to neuron deformation. Thus, potential therapeutic measures to reverse both cell membrane permeability failure and increases in cytosolic calcium ion portend a bright future for the potentials of spinal cord resuscitation. The Torg et al. manuscript was awarded the Nicolas Andry Award by the Association of Bone and Joint Surgeons in 1994.

J.S. Torg, M.D.

Cervical Spinal Fractures in Alpine Skiers

Kip P, Hunter RE (Orthopedic Associates of Aspen and Glenwood, Aspen, Colo)

Orthopedics 18:737–741, 1995 2–20

Introduction.—As many as 10 million Americans may engage in alpine skiing, spending 2 weeks on average on the slopes. Past surveys of skiing injuries have focused on extremity trauma. A 5-year review of skiing injuries seen at a hospital and clinic in the Aspen area revealed 18 cases of cervical spine fracture. Two to 5 such injuries were encountered each year.

Observations.—The 16 men and 2 women had an average age of 41 years. Eleven patients were injured in a fall, whereas 7 were involved in a collision—in 2 cases with another skier. Ten patients had posterior column fractures, half of which were at the C7 level. Five patients had neurologic involvement initially. Two of them remained quadriplegic. One of the 7 deaths related to skiing accidents during the review period was caused by a fracture dislocation at C3–C4. Four patients required surgical stabilization of their injuries. Four of the 7 patients involved in collisions either had significant neurologic involvement or died. The 3 oldest patients tended to have relatively serious injuries.

Conclusions.—Cervical spine fracture is a rare but possibly catastrophic injury in alpine skiers. Older skiers, those injured in a collision, and those with facial or head injuries require special attention.

► As the authors have observed, "a collision with an immovable object forces all the kinetic energy that a skier has obtained to dissipate with morbid abruptness." This is particularly true if the energy input occurs through the crown of the head with axial loading of the cervical spine.

J.S. Torg, M.D.

Central Nervous System Lesions and Cervical Disc Herniations in Amateur Divers

Reul J, Weis J, Jung A, Willmes K, Thron A (Technical Univ, Aachen, Germany)

Lancet 345:1403–1405, 1995 2–21

Introduction.—Professional divers and caisson workers, even those who have never experienced decompression sickness, are known to be at risk of long-term neuropsychiatric disorders such as behavioral and memory disturbances, intellectual impairment, and depression. Repeated focal ischemia caused by intravascular gas bubbles and hyalinosis of the walls of small blood vessels may be the source of these symptoms. Amateur divers could have small CNS lesions that cause no acute symptoms, yet could lead to a cumulative effect over time. To investigate this theory, MRI studies of 52 amateur divers and 50 individuals engaged in other athletic activities were performed.

Findings.—Amateur divers had participated in at least 40 dives per year in the past 4 years with self-contained underwater breathing apparatuses. Divers and controls showed no significant differences in medical history. A total of 86 focal hyperintensities were identified with MRI in 27 of 52 divers; a total of 14 such lesions were identified in 10 of 50 controls. A significant difference was noted between groups in terms of both the number of individuals with lesions and the average lesion size. Divers showed a significantly higher incidence of hyperintense lesions of the subcortical cerebral white matter and degenerative changes of the cervical disks. All lesions except 1 were supratentorial and located in the subcortical and central white matter and basal ganglia (Fig 1A). Neither years of diving experience nor total number of dives was significantly correlated

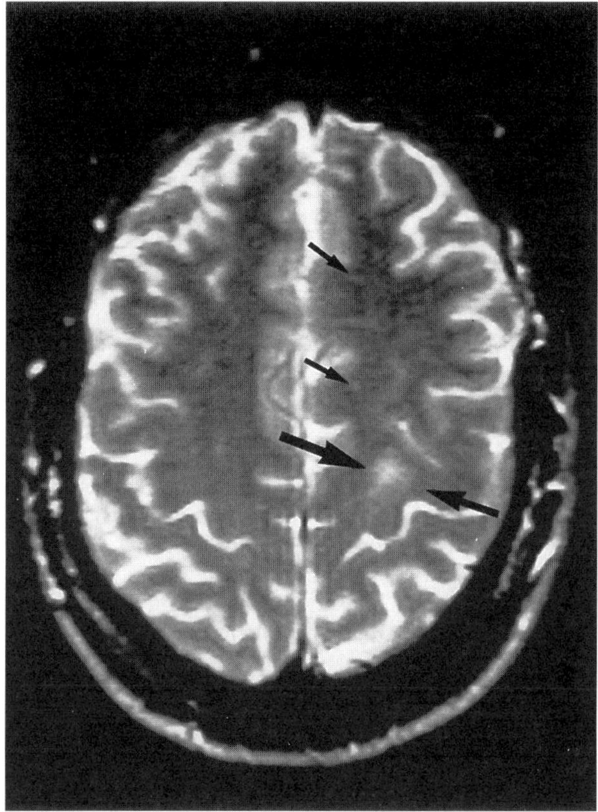

FIGURE 1A.—Large subcortical lesion in the parietal region (*large arrow*) and small symptomless lesions in the frontal lobe (*small arrows*). (Courtesy of Reul J, Weis J, Jung A, et al: Central nervous system lesions and cervical disc herniations in amateur divers. *Lancet* 345:1403–1405, copyright by The Lancet Ltd., 1995.)

with the presence or absence of lesions. Only 9 controls, compared with 32 divers, showed at least 1 degenerated intervertebral disk.

Conclusions.—Amateur divers showed significantly more small hyperintense lesions in the brain and spinal cord than did control participants matched for age and sex. A vascular pathogenesis is suggested by the predominant location of the lesions. Occlusion of small blood vessels by gas bubbles could result in these hyperintense lesions and degenerative cervical disk changes. Comparison with studies of professional divers is complex because of differences in diving technique and medical and technical surveillance. However, even if decompression sickness has not occurred, long-term amateur diving appears to cause increased risk of CNS and vertebral disk degeneration.

▶ This interesting study certainly raises concerns as to the effect of diving on the CNS and intervertebral disks. However, it must be kept in mind that this was primarily an imaging study without pathologic or cognitive function correlation. Neuropsychiatric evaluation and cognitive function studies of the divers and the control group would have been an important addition to the study.

J.S. Torg, M.D.

Airway Preparation Techniques for the Cervical Spine-injured Football Player

Ray R, Luchies C, Bazuin D, Farrell RN (Hope College, Holland, Mich)
J Athletic Train 30:217–221, 1995 2–22

Introduction.—When a football player incurs a cervical spine injury, the problem arises of how best to expose, prepare, and manage the airway while limiting motion of the head and neck. Use of a barrier mask is recommended when performing rescue breathing. A pocket mask having a 1-way air valve is frequently carried by athletic trainers for this purpose. Mannequin studies have shown that rescue breathing may be done in the presence of a football helmet using a modified jaw thrust and a pocket mask that protrudes through the bars of the face mask.

Objective.—Experiments were done on 12 young adult football players to determine whether inserting a pocket mask allows rescue breathing to start sooner, and causes less cervical spine motion, than when the face mask is removed using a manual or power screwdriver or the Trainer's Angel cutting device.

Methods.—Helmet motion was quantified using an opto-electronic motion analysis system, and cervical spine motion was inferred from measured helmet motion. The participants wore a helmet bearing a lineman-type face mask and a hard-shelled chin strap.

Results.—The pocket mask technique of initiating rescue breathing was more expeditious than any method entailing removal of the face mask. Use of the Trainer's Angel caused more rotation, anteroposterior and lateral translation, and peak displacement than any of the other airway preparation methods.

Recommendations.—The helmet should be left undisturbed until spinal injury is confirmed radiographically, and in-line stabilization should be maintained throughout. If the athlete is not breathing, the airway should be opened using a modified jaw thrust. If the athlete still is not breathing, the pocket mask is inserted and rescue breathing or cardiopulmonary resuscitation initiated. A third rescuer may attempt to remove the screws attaching the face mask clips to the helmet, but cut through the clips if necessary. The mask should be cautiously rotated out of position, making every attempt not to move the head or neck.

▶ The authors have made some very important recommendations to follow in these emergencies:

1. Maintain in-line stabilization at all times.

2. Leave the helmet on with the chin strap fastened until radiographs are done.
3. If the athlete is breathing, do not remove or reposition the face mask.
4. If the athlete is not breathing, logroll into position and open the airway using the modified jaw thrust.
5. If the athlete does not begin breathing after step 4, insert the pocket mask and begin rescue breathing or CPR.
6. The third rescuer removes the screws from the face mask.
7. Carefully rotate the face mask.
8. Resume rescue breathing or CPR.
9. Transport the athlete to the emergency room.

In the 1994 YEAR BOOK OF SPORTS MEDICINE, I commented on 2 studies closely related to this one.[1, 2] Certain face masks do not have to be removed before some types of airways can be used. There are tools that make face mask removal a safe and fairly easy procedure. These emergency procedures must be practiced and reviewed annually.

K.L. Knight, Ph.D., A.T.C., and R.I. Moss, Ph.D., A.T.C., have made excellent comments on this study in *Athletic Training Sports Health Care Perspectives.*[3]

F.J. George, A.T.C., P.T.

References

1. Segan RD, Cassidy C, Bentkowski J: A discussion of the issue of football helmet removal in suspected cervical spine injuries. *J Athletic Train* 28:294–305, 1993.
2. Feld F: Management of the critically injured football player. *J Athletic Train* 28:206–212, 1993.
3. Knight KL, Moss RI: *Athletic Training: Sports Health Care Perspectives* 2:140–141, 1996.

3 Shoulder and Upper Extremity

Muscular Synergy in the Shoulder During a Fatiguing Static Contraction

Nieminen H, Takala E-P, Niemi J, Viikari-Juntura E (Tampere Univ, Finland; Inst of Occupational Health, Helsinki)

Clin Biomech 10:309–317, 1995 3–1

Introduction.—Because the shoulder is a complex, tightly connected biomechanical system, it has been difficult to use electromyographic (EMG) measurements from a few muscles to generalize about the operation of the musculature as a whole. Using both a biomechanical 3-dimensional shoulder model and EMG recordings, the synergic operation of shoulder muscles during a fatiguing submaximal arm flexion task was studied.

Methods.—Ten men (median age, 30 years) who volunteered for the study sat on a stool and maintained the extended right arm at 90 degrees of flexion. They were then asked to hold until exhaustion a 4-kg weight suspended on the wrist. Fine wire electrodes were used to obtain IM recordings of muscles of the right shoulder: the pectoralis major, anterior deltoid, middle deltoid, middle trapezius, lower trapezius, and upper trapezius. The biomechanical shoulder model included 30 muscles or muscle parts. Muscles were modeled as stretched strings and bones as rigid bodies. A new optimization method designed to maximize the task endurance time by constantly regulating the force output of each muscle was used in the model. Model predictions on the fatigue order of the shoulder muscles were compared with EMG findings.

Results.—The median endurance time for the 10 study participants was 82 seconds. The first muscles to show EMG signs of fatigue were the deltoid and infraspinatus, demonstrating fatigue during the first 20% of the endurance time. Signs of fatigue appeared rapidly as well in the supraspinatus, pectoralis major, and trapezius muscles. Statistically significant differences in fatigue time were observed between the middle deltoid and the anterior deltoid and between the middle deltoid and the supraspinatus muscles. At a qualitative level, the predictions of the biomechanical model of the order of fatigue corresponded to the EMG results.

However, in contrast to model results, the middle part of the deltoid and the clavicular part of the pectoralis major rapidly showed EMG signs of fatigue.

Discussion.—A correspondence was found between EMG results and the predictions of the biomechanical model regarding the order of fatigue of the shoulder muscles. However, because EMG recordings were limited to 9 muscles or muscle parts and the model used 30, the accuracy of the comparison was decreased. Individual anatomy and learned patterns of muscle activation appeared to influence EMG signs of fatigue, and no clear order for the development of muscle fatigue was found.

▶ This is another study of the very complex human shoulder using a 3-dimensional biomechanical model and EMG recordings. Because of the complexity of the shoulder, it is difficult to use EMG to generalize about the loading of the shoulder. Therefore, biomechanical modeling may be our best bet. Of course there is much to be done, but these authors and others are trying to show us the way.

Col. J.L. Anderson, PE.D.

Kinematics of Shoulder Abduction in the Scapular Plane: On the Influence of Abduction Velocity and External Load

Michiels I, Grevenstein J (Orthopädische Klinik der Johannes Gutenberg-Universität, Mainz, Germany)

Clin Biomech 10:137–143, 1995 3–2

Background.—Previous research on the kinematics of the shoulder complex has been flawed methodologically and yielded uncertain results. To determine how the glenohumeral and scapulothoracic components of shoulder abduction in the scapular plane behave during a continuous movement, the scapular plane was investigated in a kinematic analysis. Whether the "scapulohumeral rhythm" depends on the speed of abduction or an external mechanical load also was investigated.

Methods.—Thirty-eight healthy individuals performed 1 slow and 1 fast abduction in a sitting position (Fig 1). The ratio of the glenohumeral and the scapulothoracic components of the motion was assessed, as was the effect of abduction speed and the external load on it.

Findings.—Although the differences among individuals were great, the abduction process was essentially reproducible for any 1 individual. A strong linear relationship between glenohumeral and scapulothoracic rotation was evident in any individual. The slope of the regression of the glenohumeral component on total arm abduction ranged from 0.75 to 0.5, indicating that only two thirds of arm abduction occurs in the glenohumeral joint. The remaining third occurs through scapular rotation. The slope of the regression was significantly higher in abduction performed slowly than in the high-speed movements. However, differences were small. Statistical analysis of the effect of external load indicated that the

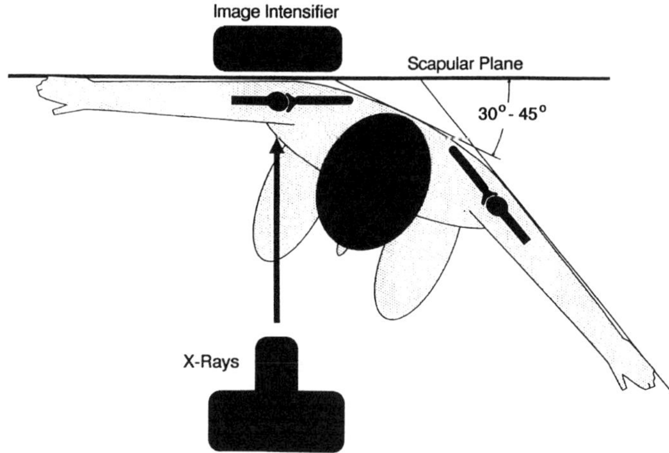

FIGURE 1.—Positioning of the experimental research subject. (Reprinted from *Clinical Biomechanics*, vol. 10, Michiels I, Grevenstein J: Kinematics of shoulder abduction in the scapular plane: On the influence of abduction velocity and external load, pp 137–143, Copyright 1995, with kind permission from Elsevier Science Ltd, The Boulevard, Langford Lane, Kidlington OX5 1GB UK.)

slope of the intra-individual regression is mostly independent of the load. The standard deviation of the abduction parameters determined by different observers varied from 6% to 10% of that between different individuals.

Conclusions.—Knowledge of shoulder joint kinematics is needed to understand subacromial abnormalities, especially impingement problems. The scapulohumeral rhythm depends on the balanced, coordinated function of the involved muscles. The abductor muscle activation pattern appears to be individual and stored as an engram.

► The shoulder joints appear to have replaced the knees as the most prevalent and the most time-loss significant injury within the 17- to 23-year-old age group here at West Point. I believe that most people involved in sports medicine will agree that these shoulder injuries also are much more complex to repair. However, when the entire sports medicine community gets together and begins to study the shoulders in the same way that the knees have been studied for the past 25 years, maybe we will see significant improvement in the prevention and treatment of shoulder injuries. These authors have made a significant contribution to the effort.

Col. J.L. Anderson, PE.D.

Shoulder Kinesthesia in Healthy Unilateral Athletes Participating in Upper Extremity Sports

Allegrucci M, Whitney SL, Lephart SM, Irrgang JJ, Fu FH (Univ of Pittsburgh, Pa)

J Orthop Sports Phys Ther 21:220–226, 1995 3–3

Background.—Kinesthesia—the ability to detect movement—has, along with proprioception, been called the "sixth sense" of bodily function. Kinesthetic deficits have been identified in the lower extremity, including anterior cruciate ligament–deficient and anterior cruciate ligament–reconstructed knees. However, there are relatively few data on shoulder kinesthetic function in athletes whose sports involve the upper extremity. Whether kinesthetic deficits exist in individuals with nonpathologic laxity has been debated. Shoulder kinesthesia, i.e., the threshold to detection of passive motion, was studied in healthy athletes who participated in unilateral overhead sports.

Methods.—Twenty collegiate male athletes who participated in unilateral upper extremity sports—including baseball players, football quarterbacks, and tennis players—were studied. All underwent kinesthetic testing of the dominant and nondominant shoulders using a proprioception testing device, which passively moved the shoulder through an arc of internal and external rotation. The data were analyzed to seek any differences in the threshold of detection of passive motion between shoulders at 0 and 75 degrees of external rotation. Also, possible links between the range of external and internal rotation and the values for threshold to detection of passive motion were assessed.

Results.—At both angles of external rotation, the threshold to detection of motion was significantly higher in the dominant shoulder than in the nondominant shoulder. Kinesthetic acuity was significantly better—that is, the threshold to detection of passive motion scores was lower—at 75 degrees vs. 0 degrees of external rotation in both the dominant and nondominant shoulders. The threshold to detection of passive motion appeared to decrease as the range of internal rotation increased. The range of external rotation was not significantly correlated with the threshold to detection of passive motion.

Conclusions.—Healthy athletes in upper extremity sports may have significant kinesthetic deficits in their throwing shoulder compared with their nondominant shoulder. These deficits may be a possible mechanism for shoulder instability. In both shoulders, kinesthesia is enhanced at 75 degrees of external rotation vs. 0 degrees, at which point the glenohumeral joint capsule is relatively taut.

▶ This study focused primarily on healthy athletes in upper extremity sports such as baseball, football (quarterbacks), and tennis players. Our experience here at West Point, where we have a very physically active population of about 4,000 students from 18 to 23 years of age, is that shoulder injuries have become our biggest sports medicine problem. It has little to do with the type of physical activity they participate in. Although these authors found significant kinesthetic deficits in the throwing shoulder, it has not been my experience that the dominant shoulder is the one most often injured when our entire population is considered. However, that might be an interesting study.

Col. J.L. Anderson, PE.D.

Anterior Shoulder Dislocations: Easing Reduction by Using Linear Traction Techniques

Aronen JG, Chronister RD (Marine Corps Recruit Depot, San Diego; United States Naval Academy, Annapolis, Md)

Physician Sportsmed 23:65–69, 1995 3–4

Background.—Anterior shoulder dislocation is the most common major joint dislocation in athletes. A gentle, linear reduction just after injury—before muscle spasm begins—almost always results in reduction. Delaying treatment for radiographic results is often undesirable. Immediate relief, minimal discomfort, and a decreased risk of re-injury can be achieved through expedient diagnosis and treatment.

Diagnosis and Treatment of Anterior Shoulder Dislocations.—Anterior shoulder dislocations can be diagnosed by assessing the mechanism of injury and taking note of limited arm adduction and shoulder rotation.

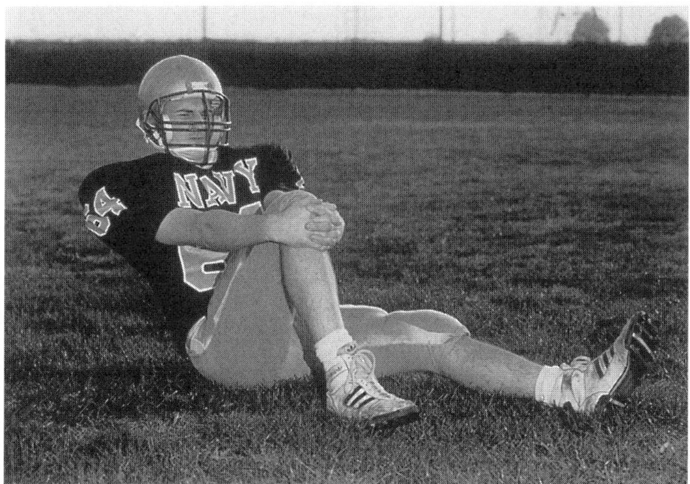

FIGURE 5.—To perform the Aronen self-reduction technique for an anterior shoulder dislocation, the patient sits on the ground and firmly interlocks all fingers in front of the knee on the same side as the dislocated shoulder. The patient then applies steady traction by leaning backward and extending the hip. The patient must maintain full elbow extension and relax the shoulder muscles for this technique to result in a successful reduction. (From Aronen JG, Chronister RD: Anterior shoulder dislocations: Easing reduction by using linear traction techniques. *Physician Sportsmed* 23:65–69, 1995, reprinted with permission of McGraw-Hill, Inc.)

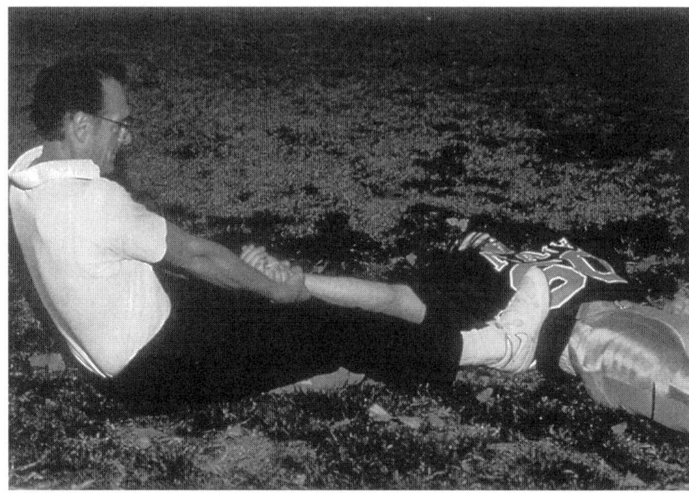

FIGURE 6.—To gently reduce an anterior shoulder dislocation, the physician sits on the ground and places a foot against the supine patient's superior lateral chest wall (not in the axilla) while grasping the patient's wrist with both hands. The practitioner applies gentle, steady traction with the patient's arm in approximately 60 degrees of abduction. The physician's knee is fully extended, and this leg serves as the source of countertraction. (From Aronen JG, Chronister RD: Anterior shoulder dislocations: Easing reduction by using linear traction techniques. *Physician Sportsmed* 23:65–69, 1995, reprinted with permission of McGraw-Hill, Inc.)

The dislocated shoulder loses its normal rounded contour. In addition, the acromion is unusually prominent.

Early reduction reduces discomfort and the risk of further injury by minimizing the amount of muscle spasm that must be overcome. To ensure gentle, safe reduction, all maneuvers performed are limited to those producing linear traction. Inferior and anterior displacement alone will enable the dislocated humeral head to clear the anterior inferior part of the glenoid fossa and result in successful reduction. Gentle, linear reduction will probably not worsen a proximal humerus fracture. Successful methods for reducing dislocations include self-reduction (Fig 5) and the passive traction technique (Fig 6).

Conclusions.—Reduction of anterior shoulder dislocations should be performed as quickly, gently, and safely as possible. In most patients, reduction can be achieved by linear force through a self-reduction technique or a simple, passive traction method.

▶ The authors have described a safe and relatively easy method of reducing anterior shoulder dislocations. Included are pictures and a description of how an individual may safely reduce his own shoulder dislocation. The author stresses the importance of using these procedures within 10–15 minutes of the injury, before the development of severe muscle spasms. Reduction of this injury should always be followed up with an x-ray examination.

F.J. George, A.T.C., P.T.

Physical Therapy Management of Isolated Serratus Anterior Muscle Paralysis

Watson CJ, Schenkman M (Duke Univ Med Ctr, Durham, NC)

Phys Ther 75:194–202, 1995 3–5

Case Report.—Man, 35, who was right hand dominant, had pain "deep inside" the dorsal aspect of his right arm of 2 weeks' duration. The pain was worse when the patient was lying supine. The patient's part-time job in a bakery required him to lift 9- to 14-kg loads, and he had started a weight-lifting program 2- to 3-weeks before the onset of pain. Over-the-counter anti-inflammatory agents and Relafen did not relieve his symptoms. Four days into the 10-day course of Relafen, he received an injection of a nonsteroidal anti-inflammatory agent for pain control, in the emergency department. Pain gradually resolved and disappeared in 6 weeks. The patient then noticed arm weakness. After 5 months, he was referred to physical therapy because of an inability to use his right arm.

Evaluation and Treatment.—Manual muscle testing indicated that the strength of his serratus anterior was 0. Electromyography indicated a long thoracic nerve injury. The patient's complaint was an inability to use his right arm overhead. His scapula would wing when he flexed his shoulder (Fig 1).

Because the patient was already into an intermediate stage of recovery, a home program with regular follow-up was designed.The goals were to prevent loss of range of motion and return the function of the patient's arm. Exercises to strengthen his lower trapezius, serratus anterior, and rotator were performed daily. To strengthening the lower trapezius—which is indicated in cases of paralysis of the serratus anterior muscle—the patient lay prone, laterally rotated the shoulder, and flexed through the pain-free range of motion. Training of the serratus anterior muscle was accomplished by having the patient lie supine and place his arm in the scapular plane. The arm was then projected anterolaterally. As the patient's strength improved, the exercise was performed with elastic bands. A second exercise involved having the patient lie supine with his arm lying on a pillow over his head. He then pressed down on the pillow. He was instructed to bring the inferior angle of the scapula forward and palpate the serratus anterior muscle with the opposite hand. The medial and lateral rotators also were strengthened.

Outcome.—After 5 months, the patient regained full passive range of motion. The strength of his serratus anterior was improved to "poor plus." The strength of the other shoulder muscles was unchanged. His active range of motion increased to 145 degrees of abduction and 155 degrees of flexion. One year after the onset of pain, the strength of his serratus anterior muscle was "good plus," scapular winging, but full active range

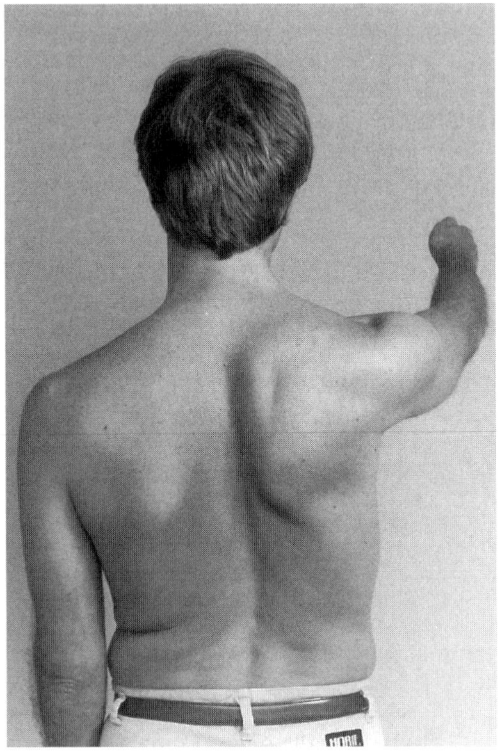

FIGURE 1.—Patient flexing his right shoulder, illustrating the scapular winging. (Courtesy of Watson CJ, Schenkman M: Physical therapy management of isolated serratus anterior muscle paralysis. *Phys Ther* 75:194–202, 1995. Reprinted from *Physical Therapy* with the permission of the American Physical Therapy Association.)

of motion. Seventeen months after the onset of pain, he reported "90% improvement" with a pain-free, but easily fatigued, arm.

Conclusions.—Electromyography revealed an isolated long thoracic nerve injury. With modification of his activity and a home exercise program with regular outpatient follow-up, the patient regained the use of his arm over 17 months.

▶ The authors state that the intermediate stage of this injury begins when pain subsides, and it is during this stage that the nerve is in the process of healing. The treatment goal in this stage is to maintain free range of motion. The authors warn that stretching denervated paralyzed muscles delays, and may even prevent, functional recovery once the involved muscles are reinnervated. They state that "stretching of the denervated muscle should be avoided." However, passive stretching of the antagonist muscles should be done to maintain muscle length. The patient should be instructed in activity modification to protect the serratus anterior and to prevent shoulder impingement.

F.J. George, A.T.C., P.T.

Specificity and Sensitivity of the Anterior Slide Test in Throwing Athletes With Superior Glenoid Labral Tears
Kibler WB (Lexington Clinic Sports Medicine Ctr, Ky)
Arthroscopy 11:296–300, 1995 3–6

Background.—Clinical diagnosis of glenoid labral tears confined to the superior aspect of the glenoid rim is difficult. Several tests have been developed, but none are definitively diagnostic. The sensitivity and specificity of a new test, called the anterior slide test, were assessed by evaluating its accuracy in several populations of athletes.

Methods.—Five groups of athletes were studied, including patients with arthroscopically proven isolated superior glenoid labral tears (group A), with arthroscopically proven partial-thickness articular or bursal side rotator cuff pathology with or without superior glenoid labral tears (group B), with anterior or anterior inferior glenohumeral instability with or without superior labral injuries (group C), with no overt injuries but an internal rotation deficit of the dominant glenohumeral joint (group D), and with no injuries and no involvement with overhead throwing activities.

The patients were examined with their hands on their hips. The examiner stabilized the top of the shoulder with 1 hand with a finger over the anterior aspect of the acromion at the glenohumeral joint and applied a forward and slightly superior force to the elbow and upper arm while the patient resisted this force (Fig 2). Pain, a pop localized at the front of the shoulder, or both was a positive finding.

Results.—There was a positive anterior slide test in 80.4% of group A patients, in 80.5% of group B patients with superior glenoid labral pathology and 18.8% of group B patients without that pathology, in 50% of group C patients with superior labral pathology and 18.2% in group C

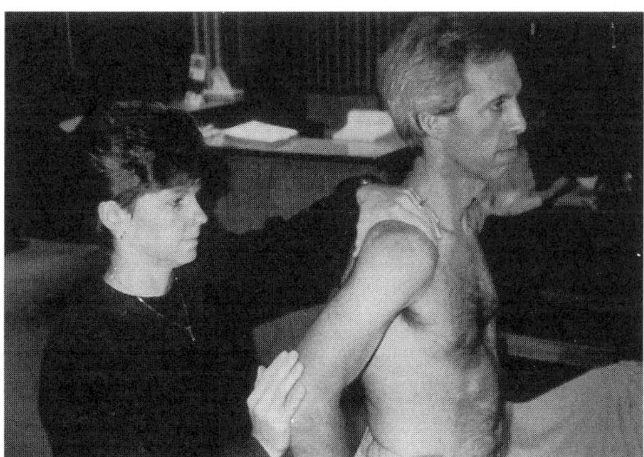

FIGURE 2.—Application of force for anterior slide test. (Courtesy of Kibler WB: Specificity and sensitivity of the anterior slide test in throwing athletes with superior glenoid labral tears. *Arthroscopy* 11:296–300, 1995.)

patients without that pathology, in 11% of group D patients, and in none of the group E patients. The anterior slide test had a sensitivity of 78.4% and a specificity of 91.5%.

Conclusions.—The anterior slide test has a high specificity for superior labral lesions but only a modest sensitivity. Therefore, it should be included in the evaluation of suspected lesions but is not definitively diagnostic in itself.

▶ Although I have had no experience with this clinical test, because it is more sensitive than MRI and is noninvasive compared with arthroscopy it appears to have a place in the evaluation of the shoulder in the throwing athlete.

J.S. Torg, M.D.

Magnetic Resonance Imaging Evaluation of the Rotator Cuff Tendons in the Asymptomatic Shoulder

Miniaci A, Dowdy PA, Willits KR, Vellet AD (Univ of Western Ontario, London, Canada)

Am J Sports Med 23:142–145, 1995 3–7

Objective.—Twenty volunteers who had no shoulder symptoms and no history of shoulder injury had 30 of their shoulders examined by MRI. Most were recreational athletes. The average age was 29 years; only 1 individual was older than 40 years of age.

Findings.—All supraspinatus tendons had areas of intermediate signal intensity that generally were diffuse, but in 2 instances they were focal. About one fourth of the tendons had diffuse, linear, or focal areas of high signal intensity, but this never involved the full thickness of the rotator cuff. Low-grade changes also were consistently found in the infraspinatus tendon, but none of the tendons had areas of high signal intensity. Four subscapularis tendons (13%) had low-grade changes, but all teres minor tendons were normal.

Implication.—Unenhanced MRI may be limited in its ability to demonstrate rotator cuff injury in patients with shoulder pain.

▶ This study substantiates clinical experience that indicates that one must be extremely careful of what is defined as a rotator cuff injury on an MRI scan. However, the number of shoulders in the study was small, and none of the findings were confirmed or refuted surgically or by arthrogram.

J.S. Torg, M.D.

Suprascapular Nerve Entrapment by Ganglion Cysts: A Report of Six Cases With Arthroscopic Findings and Review of the Literature

Fehrman DA, Orwin JF, Jennings RM (Univ of Wisconsin, Madison)
Arthroscopy 11:727–734, 1995 3–8

Introduction.—Suprascapular nerve entrapment is an increasingly recognized form of shoulder pain/dysfunction. The addition of 6 cases of entrapment by a ganglion cyst make a total of 70 reported instances.

Mechanisms.—The suprascapular nerve, a mixed nerve arising from the upper trunk of the brachial plexus, passes posterior to the plexus and deep to the trapezius, where it traverses the suprascapular notch. The notch is roofed by the transverse scapular ligament (Fig 1). The nerve supplies the

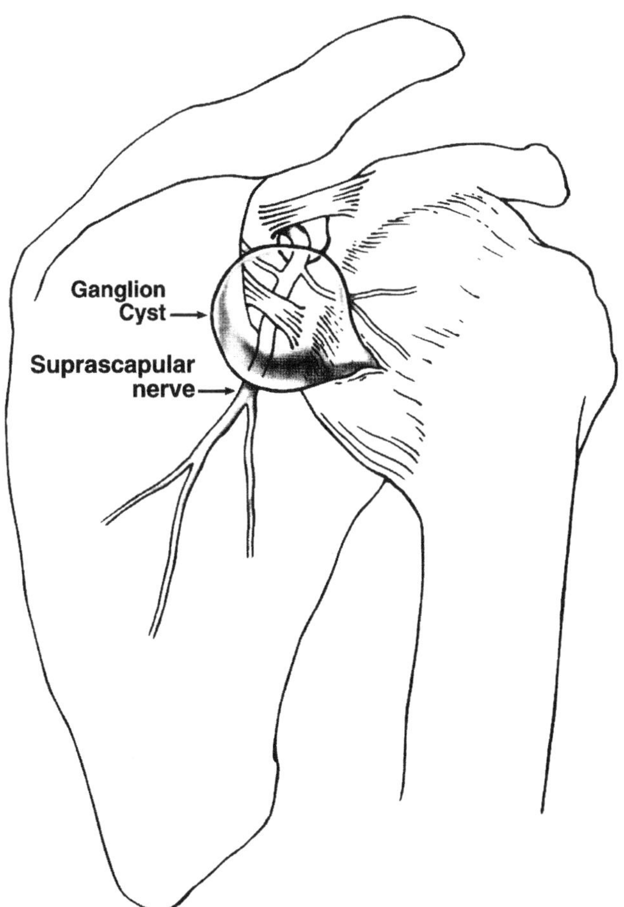

FIGURE 1.—Anatomy of the region showing a ganglion cyst at the spinoglenoid notch. (Courtesy of Fehrman DA, Orwin JF, Jennings RM: Suprascapular nerve entrapment by ganglion cysts: A report of six cases with arthroscopic findings and review of the literature. *Arthroscopy* 11:727–734, 1995.)

supraspinatus muscle and receives sensory branches from many neighboring structures, including the rotator cuff. The spinoglenoid ligament, or inferior transverse scapular ligament, is variably present. Compression or dysfunction of the suprascapular nerve may result from trauma, including scapular fracture and shoulder dislocation; overuse; or a mass lesion such as a tumor, ganglion, or hematoma.

Clinical Picture.—Typically, patients describe deep, diffuse pain of long duration in the posterolateral shoulder. Often they report trouble sleeping. Usually external rotation is weak, and the range of motion may be limited. Chronic dysfunction may lead to wasting of the infraspinatus muscle. Radiographs may demonstrate callus or a bony tumor at the suprascapular or spinoglenoid notch. The best means of diagnosing entrapment is electromyography combined with nerve conduction studies.

Management.—Dysfunction unrelated to an apparent mass lesion calls for rest followed by physical therapy, nonsteroidal drugs, and possibly modification of activities. In patients who remain symptomatic after 4–6 months, operative release of the suprascapular ligament usually solves the problem. Most agree that excision is the best approach to a ganglion causing symptomatic compression of the suprascapular nerve. Ten of 14 reported patients did very well after having a ganglion excised. Aspiration of a ganglion under ultrasonic or CT guidance has been described.

▶ It is important to understand that extrinsic compression of the suprascapular nerve at the spinoglenoid notch by a ganglion cyst should be considered in those patients with subscapular nerve entrapment. As pointed out by the authors, it is necessary to evaluate and treat the intra-articular pathology as well as the ganglion cyst to successfully manage this subset of patients.

J.S. Torg, M.D.

The Arthroscopic Mumford Procedure: An Analysis of Results

Snyder SJ, Banas MP, Karzel RP (Southern California Orthopedic Inst, Van Nuys)

Arthroscopy 11:157–164, 1995 3–9

Background.—Although many patients with injury to the acromioclavicular joint can be successfully treated with physical therapy, oral anti-inflammatory drugs, and corticosteroid injections, some will require surgery. The Mumford procedure involves resection of the distal clavicle and has been used to treat posttraumatic, degenerative disease of the acromioclavicular joint associated with osteoarthritis, distal clavicle osteolysis, fractures, and other conditions. Traditionally performed as an open surgical procedure, it can result in significant morbidity. Arthroscopic shoulder surgery avoids many of the problems associated with open procedures. Forty-six patients who underwent 50 arthroscopic distal clavicle excisions from 1990 through 1993 were retrospectively reviewed.

Methods.—The 46 patients (average age, 42 years) received a diagnosis of acromioclavicular degeneration based on evidence from physical examination, radiography, acromioclavicular joint injection, bone scan, and MRI. All patients had pain and tenderness to palpation over the acromioclavicular joint, and a positive adduction test eliciting pain was obtained for 40 shoulders. Patients underwent distal clavicle resection using the Claviculizer, a specially designed burr with a short sheath to prevent excessive penetration into the clavicle. All procedures were performed on an outpatient basis. Immediately after surgery, passive range of motion and pendulum exercises were started, and exercises for the forearm, wrist, and hand were added soon thereafter. After 1–2 weeks, overhead lifting was allowed. Patients were evaluated using the University of California at Los Angeles Shoulder Rating Scale and completed questionnaires about the surgical outcome.

Results.—All patients were noted during surgery to have acromioclavicular joint degeneration with destruction of the articular cartilage. Forty-one patients had an intrascalene block as a supplement to general anesthesia. Follow-up radiography showed that the average distal clavicle resection was 14.8 mm, with a range of 7–20.5 mm. No intraoperative complications occurred. The outcome for 47 shoulders (94%) was good to excellent according to the University of California at Los Angeles shoulder scoring system; for 3 shoulders, it was fair. No patient had a poor result. Twenty-six patients said they had an excellent result; 11, a very good result; 10, a good result; and 3, a poor result. Forty-five said they would recommend the procedure. On average, patients returned to work within 43 days, although 4 returned to work on the day of surgery. Twenty-five patients who considered themselves athletes returned to their pre-injury level of competition.

Discussion.—Arthroscopic resection of the clavicle does not violate the deltoid and trapezius muscular fascia, helping avoid postoperative shoulder weakness and painful scars. The arthroscopic Mumford procedure using the Claviculizer appears to be effective in treating acromioclavicular joint pathology.

► The observations and conclusions of the authors are in keeping with my own clinical experience.

J.S. Torg, M.D.

Arthroscopic Subacromial Decompression: Two-to-Seven-Year Follow-up

Roye RP, Grana WA, Yates CK (Univ of Oklahoma, Oklahoma City)
Arthroscopy 11:301–306, 1995 3–10

Introduction.—Impingement of the rotator cuff beneath the coracoacromial arch is a common cause of shoulder pain in athletes or workers who engage in repetitive overhead activities. For 88 patients who underwent arthroscopic subacromial decompression for stage II or early stage III impingement syndrome of the shoulder, results compared were in different categories of patients.

Patients and Methods.—Follow-up data were available retrospectively for 88 of 102 patients who underwent shoulder arthroscopic procedures at the study institution from March 1985 through May 1990. In 2 cases both shoulders were injured. Patients were interviewed by telephone to confirm and supplement clinical and rehabilitation records. Clinical outcome was evaluated according to results of Neer's criteria, the University of California at Los Angeles Shoulder Rating Scale, and the Shoulder and Elbow Surgeons Rating Scale. The group was divided among patients with partial rotator cuff tears (43 shoulders) and those without (47 shoulders). Other subgroups identified were athletes (56 shoulders) and throwers (34 shoulders).

Results.—Most of the patients with impingement syndrome of the shoulder were men (71%), and the injuries were primarily in the dominant shoulder (74%). Sixty-eight shoulders had rotator cuff weakness preoperatively; 32 had a history of trauma. The groups with and without partial rotator cuffs did not differ in age, male:female ratio, status as athlete vs. nonathlete, the presence of night pain, functional outcome, or other variables. At follow-up, 80% of patients met Neer's criteria for satisfactory results, 94% met the University of California at Los Angeles Shoulder Rating Scale criteria, and 95% had a satisfactory outcome by the Shoulder and Elbow Surgeons Rating Scale. Responses to the questionnaire expressed satisfaction in 93% of cases. By the Neer rating, 90% of nonthrowing athletes but only 68% of throwing athletes obtained satisfactory results. Only half of the competitive baseball and softball pitchers had satisfactory results. The only complications were keloid scar formation at portal sites in 2 patients.

Conclusions.—Arthroscopic subacromial decompression in patients with stage II or early stage III impingement syndrome of the shoulder yielded satisfactory results overall. Few complications occurred, and patients were soon able to return to normal activities. Patients with and without rotator cuff tears fared equally well, although throwing athletes, especially pitchers, had a poorer prognosis than other patients.

▶ The author's statement that "our impression is that arthroscopic subacromial decompression is an acceptable alternative to open anterior acromioplasty with comparable results for the treatment of the impingement lesion" is not supported by the data. Specifically, there is no randomly selected open acromioplasty group with which to make a comparison. The important point of this article is that throwing athletes do not have as good a prognosis with regard to maintaining high-caliber, pain-free shoulder activities as do non-throwing athletes after arthroscopic subacromial decompression.

J.S. Torg, M.D.

Titanium Anchors for the Repair of Rotator Cuff Tears: Preliminary Report of a Surgical Technique

Caniggia M, Maniscalco P, Pagliantini L, Bocchi L (Università degli Studi di Siena, Italy)

J Orthop Trauma 9:312–317, 1995 3–11

Introduction.—Transbone suturing is now the most commonly used and most effective means of repairing a ruptured rotator cuff, but it is a lengthy

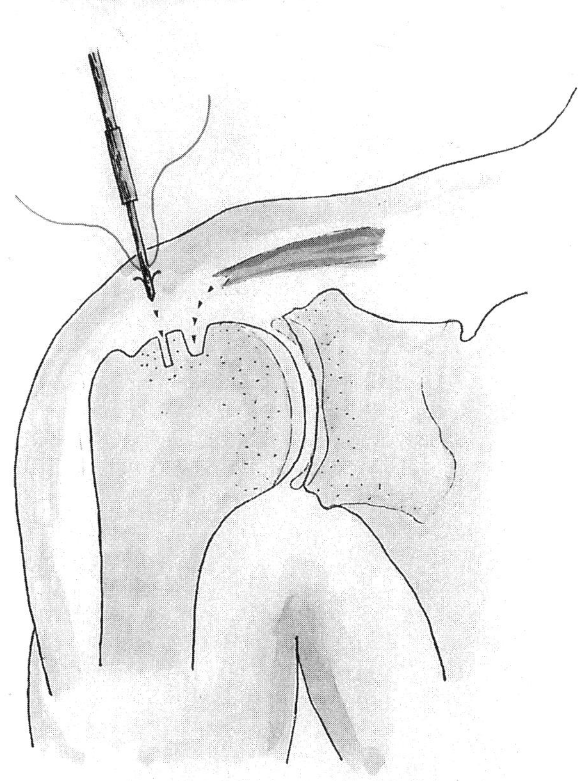

FIGURE 3.—The anchors are inserted into the holes. (Courtesy of Caniggia M, Maniscalco P, Pagliantini L, et al: Titanium anchors for the repair of rotator cuff tears: Preliminary report of a surgical technique. *J Orthop Trauma* 9:312–317, 1995.)

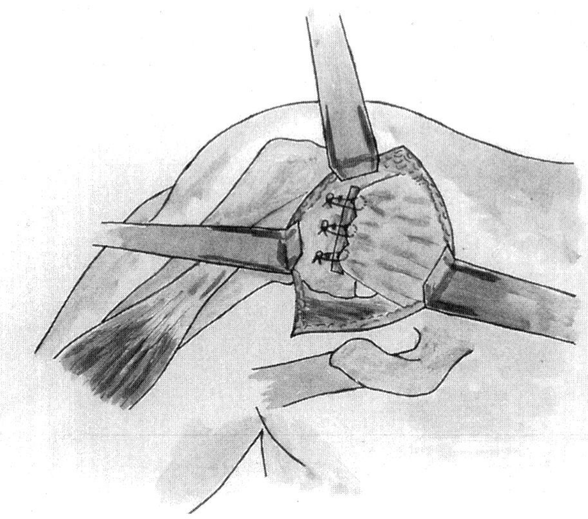

FIGURE 4.—The rotator cuff has been sutured. (Courtesy of Caniggia M, Maniscalco P, Pagliantini L, et al: Titanium anchors for the repair of rotator cuff tears: Preliminary report of a surgical technique. *J Orthop Trauma* 9:312–317, 1995.)

and laborious operation. As an alternative, titanium anchors were used to repair rotator cuff tears in 34 patients younger than 60 years of age who had good-quality bone and no known metabolic bone disease. Ten tears had been present for a year or longer before repair. Ten small, 15 medium-sized, and 9 large tears were repaired.

> *Technique.*—With the patient in the so-called astronaut's (semi-reclining) position, an incision is made down the superior part of the anterolateral side of the acromion, and the deltoid muscle is split distally and freed. The subacromial bursa is removed and an acromioplasty done with resection of the coracoacromial ligament. From 6 to 9 mm of the inferior acromial edge is excised. The rotator cuff is extensively detached so that it may be re-inserted at the desired point after cutting the margins. A shallow trough 3–4 cm long is carved in the humeral cortex to facilitate re-attachment of the rotator cuff. Three holes then are drilled about 1.5 cm apart, 0.5 cm distal to the trough, and anchors threaded with non–re-absorbable sutures are inserted (Fig 3). After engaging the anchors, the rotator cuff is repaired (Fig 4) and its terminal part re-inserted into the trough. The repair is tested by rotating the arm before re-inserting the deltoid into the acromion by trans-bone suturing. The arm is immobilized in adduction and splinted.

Results.—Thirty of the 34 patients were satisfactorily relieved of pain and had adequate active forward flexion and muscle strength after 6 months to 2 years of follow-up. Eighteen had excellent results and 12 had good results based on University of California at Los Angeles scores. No implant failures occurred. Two patients had inadequate function despite good pain relief, and 2 others were dissatisfied with the overall outcome.

Conclusion.—Titanium anchors are useful in repairing rotator cuff tears that are not too old or large, as long as there is bone of adequate quality and patient compliance is likely.

► I fully agree with the authors that the use of titanium anchors facilitates the task of the surgeon in rotator cuff tears requiring approximation of the cuff to bone. This particular innovation has simplified the technical task, reduced operative time, and produced results comparable with traditional transbone suturing.

J.S. Torg, M.D.

Treatment of Calcifying Tendinitis of Rotator Cuff by Extracorporeal Shock Waves: A Preliminary Report

Loew M, Jurgowski W, Mau HC, Thomsen M (Univ of Heidelberg, Germany)

J Shoulder Elbow Surg 4:101–106, 1995 3–12

Introduction.—Rotator cuff calcification may occur in up to half of patients with shoulder pain. These calcifications can lead to impaired function and pain in many cases; the problem can become chronic, with constant pain both at rest and with movement. Extracorporeal shock wave application (ESWA) has been useful in patients with multilocalized enthesiopathies and calcifying tendinitis. Its value for the treatment of calcifying tendinitis of the shoulder was systematically assessed.

Methods.—The prospective study included 20 patients with chronic, symptomatic, calcifying shoulder tendinitis. All had had symptoms for at least 1 year and rotator cuff calcifications measuring greater than 10 mm in diameter on anteroposterior radiographs. All patients underwent application of high-energy shock waves, 18–22 kV, in a lithotripter. The patients received 2 sessions of ESWA therapy at 2,000 pulses each. The subjective and functional results were assessed at 6 and 12 weeks after treatment using the Constant score. Radiographs and MRI scans were obtained as well.

Results.—By 12 weeks, 15 patients showed a marked reduction of symptoms. The Constant score improved by an average of 30% in this group. The calcifications were completely eliminated on radiographic evaluation in 7 patients and partially disintegrated in 5 patients. A transient subcutaneous hematoma was observed in 14 patients, although overall morbidity was low. No enduring damage to the bone or soft tissue was seen on MRI scans.

Conclusions.—In the short term, ESWA can eliminate calcium deposits in the rotator cuff in some patients. The mechanism of their elimination is unclear, but a change in consistency does occur. This allows the calcific structure either to break into the subacromial bursa or to be resorbed in the tendon tissue. A long-term, controlled study is under way.

▶ This article certainly presents an innovative approach to an old problem. One question is whether it is the tendon or the juxtaposition bursal tissue that actually calcifies. The authors do point out reports of 100% spontaneous healing of these lesions. Another question is whether a well-placed injection of a corticosteroid solution might not give more prompt and effective therapeutic results. Of course, this would require a prospective study with random selection.

J.S. Torg, M.D.

Effect of Lesions of the Superior Portion of the Glenoid Labrum on Glenohumeral Translation

Pagnani MJ, Deng X-H, Warren RF, Torzilli PA, Altchek DW (Hosp for Special Surgery, New York; Lipscomb Clinic, Nashville)

J Bone Joint Surg (Am) 77–A:1003–1010, 1995 3–13

Objective.—Clinical indications that lesions of the superior part of the glenoid labrum lead to increased glenohumeral translation prompted a biomechanical study of the effects of labral detachment in cadavers.

Methods.—The superior part of the glenoid labrum anterior to the biceps was stripped, disrupting the superior and middle glenohumeral ligaments. The shoulders were mounted on a special apparatus so that 50-newton anterior, posterior, superior, and inferior forces and a 22-newton joint-compressing load could be applied. A 55-newton force was applied to the tendon of the long head of the biceps brachii. Shoulders were tested in 7 positions of glenohumeral elevation and rotation. The labral lesion then was extended posteriorly to include the part connected to the biceps tendon as well as that associated with glenoid attachments of the posterosuperior aspect of the capsule, and tests were repeated.

Results.—Takings lesions from only the anterosuperior part of the glenoid labrum did not significantly alter anteroposterior or superoinferior glenohumeral translation, even when force was applied to the biceps brachii tendon. The more extensive lesion, however, destabilized the biceps insertion and significantly increased glenohumeral translation in both planes. Anterior translation increased about 6 mm at 45 degrees of glenohumeral elevation, and inferior translation increased by about 2 mm.

Conclusion.—Lesions of the superior glenoid labrum that involve the biceps insertion increase glenohumeral translation in multiple directions.

▶ As the authors point out, lesions of the superior portion of the labrum detaching the insertion of the biceps are not usually associated with overt instability. However, the patient may have subtle increases in humeral head translation on physical examination and may relate subjective sensation of the shoulder being loose or slipping. This is an excellent study in which the relatively small increases in translation may explain the symptoms associated with an isolated lesion of the superior portion of the labrum.

J.S. Torg, M.D.

Arthroscopic Fixation of Superior Labral Lesions Using a Biodegradable Implant: A Preliminary Report

Pagnani MJ, Speer KP, Altchek DW, Warren RF, Dines DM (Vanderbilt Univ, Nashville, Tenn; Duke Univ, Durham, NC; Hosp for Special Surgery, New York)

Arthroscopy 11:194–198, 1995 3–14

Background.—Arthroscopy now allows more detailed examination of intra-articular pathology in patients with shoulder pain and dysfunction. One cause of such pain is a lesion of the superior glenoid labrum that also involves the long head of the biceps brachii. Lesions that destabilize the biceps "anchor" result in increased translation of the glenohumeral joint, which causes symptoms as the unstable labrum is caught within the shoulder joint. The experience of several years was reviewed in treating SLAP lesions, which involve "an injury to the superior aspect of the labrum which begins posteriorly and extends anteriorly...including the 'anchor' of the biceps tendon to the glenoid."

Patients and Methods.—Twenty-two patients underwent arthroscopic fixation of a superior labral lesion and were followed up for an average of 2 years. All had undergone conservative treatment, which had not been effective. Injury was related to overhead sports in 13 patients, to contact injury in 5 others, and to traction injury in 1; the other patients could not recall a precipitating event.

Using arthroscopy, a biodegradable implant was used to fix the labrum to the glenoid. The drill bit was advanced to an approximate depth of 12 mm into the bony glenoid (Fig 2). After the drill bit was removed, leaving a wire in place, a tack was placed over the wire and set into place using a cannulated pusher (Fig 3). This procedure was performed only if the lesion resulted in pathologic instability of the biceps insertion; lesions that did not involve the insertion were not stabilized with the implant.

Patients underwent examination and completed a detailed questionnaire about shoulder stability and function 1 year or longer after surgery. In addition, shoulder function was evaluated with the system of the American Shoulder and Elbow Surgeons.

Results.—On the basis of the American Shoulder and Elbow Surgeons scores before and after surgery, significant improvements were seen in pain, stability, and function after insertion of the implant. Nineteen of the patients (86%) were satisfied with the procedure, including 14 of 16 patients with type II lesions and 5 of 6 patients with type IV lesions. Full shoulder function was regained for 12 of 13 overhead-activity athletes and 2 of 3 contact-activity athletes. No patient had instability or looseness of the shoulder. Two patients continued to experience pain after surgery, and

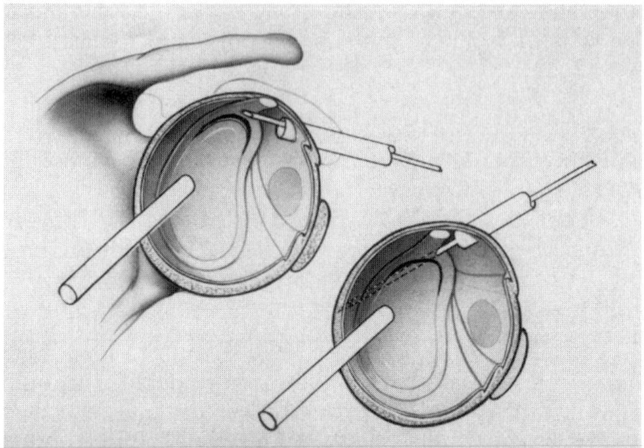

FIGURE 2.—**Left,** a cannulated drill bit with a guide wire is introduced through the anterosuperior arthroscopic portal. **Right,** the guide wire is used to pierce the labrum. The labrum is then repositioned on the superior portion of the glenoid. The drill bit and guide wire are then advanced into the bony glenoid with a motorized drill. (Courtesy of Pagnani MJ, Speer KP, Altchek DW, et al: Arthroscopic fixation of superior labral lesions using a biodegradable implant: A preliminary report. *Arthroscopy* 11:194–198, 1995.)

3 had restricted motion, lacking 10 degrees to 20 degrees of rotation. Two of these 3 were dissatisfied with their result, but 20 patients reported a significant improvement in pain.

Discussion.—Simple débridement of unstable superior labral lesions is not generally successful, although it may be considered for some types of lesions. The arthroscopic stabilization procedure is not recommended for patients older than 40 years of age in whom lesions are found incidentally.

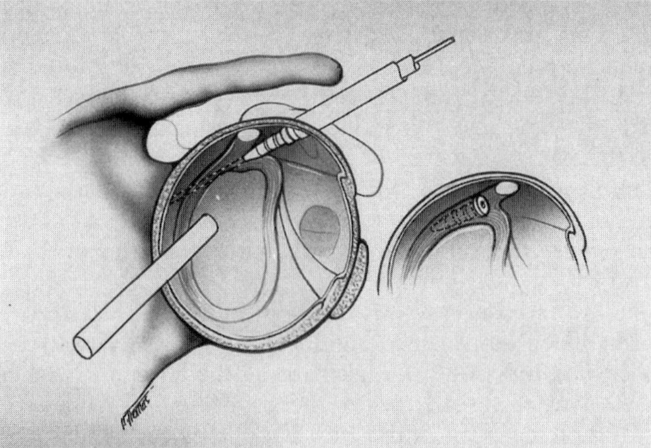

FIGURE 3.—**Left,** the drill bit is removed leaving the wire in place. The tack is placed over the wire and placed using a cannulated pusher. **Right,** seated tack after removal of the guide wire. (Courtesy of Pagnani MJ, Speer KP, Altchek DW, et al: Arthroscopic fixation of superior labral lesions using a biodegradable implant: A preliminary report. *Arthroscopy* 11:194–198, 1995.)

It is, however, justified in young, athletic individuals who experience shoulder pain with overhead activity.

An Analysis of 140 Injuries to the Superior Glenoid Labrum

Snyder SJ, Banas MP, Karzel RP (Southern California Orthopedic Inst, Van Nuys)

J Shoulder Elbow Surg 4:243–248, 1995 3–15

Introduction.—Shoulder arthroscopy has allowed the recognition of a specific injury to the superior glenoid labrum known as a superior labrum anterior and posterior (SLAP) lesion. This lesion begins posterior to the biceps tendon and extends anterior to the biceps tendon to a point at or above the midglenoid notch. Because of the variable disruption of the insertion of the biceps tendon, the SLAP lesion can cause disability. The clinical experience with SLAP lesions at 1 institution during an 8-year period was reviewed.

Methods.—The findings of 2,375 shoulder arthroscopies performed between 1985 and 1993 were reviewed to identify 140 patients (6%) with superior labral injuries. The symptoms and mechanisms of injury were examined. Intraoperative findings, treatment, and outcome were reviewed.

Results.—All of the patients had shoulder pain and 49% had mechanical symptoms, including locking, catching, popping, or snapping. Falling or a direct blow to the shoulder was the most common mechanism of injury. Other mechanisms included glenohumeral subluxation or dislocation, lifting a heavy object, participating in overhead racquet sports, and throwing. Neither the mechanism of injury nor physical examination findings were significantly predictive of the type of labral lesion. Preoperative radiographs did not indicate superior labral injury.

Intraoperative findings indicated that the lesions were type I in 21%, type II in 55%, type III in 9%, type IV in 10%, and complex in 5%. The superior labral lesions were isolated in 28% and were associated with partial tearing of the rotator cuff in 29%, with full-thickness tearing of the rotator cuff in 11%, with Bankart labral detachments in 22%, with acromioclavicular joint spurring or degeneration in 16%, and with glenohumeral chondromalacia in 10%.

Treatment depended on the type of lesion and involved either débridement alone or with glenoid abrasion, suture anchor, or suture repair. Eighteen patients underwent repeat arthroscopies. Healing occurred in 3 of 5 type II lesions treated with débridement and glenoid abrasion, in 4 of 5 type II lesions treated with tack fixation, in the 3 type III lesions and 1 type IV lesion treated with débridement, in 2 type IV lesions treated with suture repair, and in 2 complex type II and III lesions treated with débridement and suture anchor fixation.

Conclusions.—Superior glenoid labral injuries are not common, but they should be suspected in patients with pain and mechanical catching. These lesions are most commonly type II and can be reliably treated with suture anchor fixation. Suture repair of the superior labrum and the split biceps tendon can have good results with type IV lesions.

▶ These 2 articles (Abstracts 3–14 and 3–15) must be considered technique reports. Although Pagnani et al. stated that 86% of the patients were "satisfied with the procedure," they reported an average follow-up of 2 years, with a range of 12 to 24 months. Somehow this does not compute. With regard to Snyder et al., they essentially concluded that "suture anchor fixation of type II lesions can reliably reconstruct the normal anatomic attachment of the superior labrum to the glenoid." There is no mention of the length or results of follow-up.

J.S. Torg, M.D.

Results of Arthroscopic Debridement of Glenoid Labral Tears
Martin DR, Garth WP Jr (Univ of Alabama, Birmingham)
Am J Sports Med 23:447–451, 1995 3–16

Objective.—The results of arthroscopic débridement of labral flap tears were reviewed in 23 athletes having 24 affected shoulders.

Patients.—Twelve anteroinferior and 12 posterior glenoid labral lesions were treated. All the patients were functionally unstable, but none had ligament detachment. All but 1 of the 23 athletes were male. Their average age at the time of treatment was 19 years. Throwing was implicated in 14 injuries and a blow to the arm or shoulder in 9 instances. All individuals were symptomatic during activity with the arm overhead. Rotator cuff rehabilitation had been tried for at least 6 weeks. Three patients had a history of documented anterior shoulder dislocation.

Treatment.—Patients were managed on an outpatient basis by standard arthroscopic techniques while they were under general endotracheal anesthesia. All lesions were débrided back to a stable rim; associated injuries also were débrided. Patients engaged in throwing sports were restricted until full external rotator strength returned, as documented by isokinetic testing. The average follow-up was 4 years.

Results.—Good-to-excellent clinical results were achieved in 21 shoulders. Sixteen patients, including 5 of 8 baseball pitchers, were able to return to their customary level of activity. Excellent results were obtained in 5 of 9 shoulders with positive impingement signs. Two patients with persistent anterior instability were considered to have failed treatment; they subsequently required capsular shift because of recurrent painful subluxation. Isokinetic testing demonstrated some increase in concentric external rotation strength but trace weakness in eccentric external rotation.

Conclusions.—Persistently good-to-excellent results were achieved in nearly 90% of cases, warranting an initial attempt at arthroscopic débridement of anteroinferior and posterior labral flap tears. Capsulorrhaphy is not necessary as a first measure if gross instability and a Bankart lesion are ruled out.

► The observations and conclusions of the authors are in keeping with my own clinical experience. We have previously reported on arthroscopic resection of glenoid labral tears in the athlete.[1] In reports on 29 cases, our experience indicated that a history of the inability to engage in overhead throwing and striking activities associated with the presence of a "click" on physical examination identifies a subgroup of patients with possible longitudinal tears of the anterior glenoid labrum. Arthroscopic resection of these lesions in a stable joint can relieve a patient's discomfort and allow a return to athletic competition. However, in patients with anterior instability, labral débridement was not a successful alternative to formal stabilization.

J.S. Torg, M.D.

Reference

1. Glasgow SG, Bruce RA, Yacobucci GN, et al: Arthroscopic resection of glenoid labral tears in the athlete. *Arthroscopy* 8:48–54, 1992.

Arthroscopic Debridement of Glenoid Labral Tears in Athletes

Tomlinson RJ Jr, Glousman RE (Southern California Orthopedic Inst, Van Nuys; Kerlan Jobe Orthopaedic Clinic, Inglewood, Calif)

Arthroscopy 11:42–51, 1995 3–17

Introduction.—Results of arthroscopic treatment of glenoid labral tears have varied widely, from as few as 7% of patients to as many as 91% having acceptable results. The effectiveness of arthroscopic labral débridement in athletes with glenoid labral lesions but without overt shoulder instability was evaluated retrospectively.

Patients and Methods.—Fifty-two patients were treated from June 1988 through June 1990. Six were excluded after undergoing shoulder reconstruction during follow-up. The other 46 patients had an average age of 24 years at the time of arthroscopic treatment of glenoid labral lesions. The average duration of symptoms was 18 months, and the mean follow-up was 30 months. The 43 men and 3 women in the group were all involved in athletics that required overhead use of the affected shoulder. All had pain with athletic movement; 30 had pain with daily activities. Conservative treatment had been tried for 1 to 6 months without a positive response. Outcome was graded subjectively and objectively according to postoperative level of pain and level of competition attained after surgery.

Results.—Results after arthroscopic débridement were judged excellent in 18 patients, good in 7, fair in 17, and poor in 4. Thus, only slightly more than half of the patients (54%) had a good or excellent result. Patients with or without shoulder laxity did not differ significantly in outcome. Similarly, outcome did not appear to be affected by mechanism of injury, the presence of rotator cuff lesions, or labral lesion location. A statistically significant difference in outcome was found for professional baseball players, 75% of whom had an excellent or good outcome. In contrast, only 43% of the remaining nonprofessional group had outcomes classified as good to excellent.

Conclusions.—The long-term results of arthroscopic débridement were not consistent in this group of young athletes with glenoid labral lesions in the absence of overt shoulder instability. A consistent, aggressive rehabilitation program offers the greatest chance for early recovery; however, later reconstructive surgery may be needed.

▶ Because Tomlinson and Glousman reported that 54% of patients had good or excellent results and Martin and Garth (Abstract 3–16) reported that 90% had good or excellent results, this indicates to me that there is a place for arthroscopic débridement of glenoid labral tears. In all likelihood, patient selection is the key to success.

We previously reported on 28 overhead throwing and striking athletes who underwent partial glenoid labral resection, with the indications for the procedure being a sudden inability to perform because of pain and presence of a palpable "click" on clinical examination.[1] In those with stable joints, there was 91% chance of good or excellent functional outcome, whereas for those with unstable joints there was a 25% chance of good functional outcome. It appears that arthroscopic resection of an anterior longitudinal labral tear in a stable shoulder can relieve a patient's discomfort and allow a return to athletic competition. On the other hand, in patients with anterior instability and labral tears, labral débridement was not a successful alternative to formal stabilization.

J.S. Torg, M.D.

Reference

1. Glasgow SG, Bruce RA, Yacobucci GN, et al: Arthroscopic resection of glenoid labral tears in the athlete. *Arthroscopy* 8:48–54, 1992.

Arthroscopic Bankart Procedure: Two- to Five-Year Followup With Clinical Correlation to Severity of Glenoid Labral Lesion

Green MR, Christensen KP (Tripler Army Med Ctr, Hawaii)

Am J Sports Med 23:276–281, 1995 3–18

Introduction.—Morgan and Bodenstab described an arthroscopic procedure for anterior shoulder instability in which sutures are passed through drill holes in the scapular neck. This method eliminates the need for anterior dissection of the shoulder and the resultant scarring and loss of external rotation.

Objective.—The results of the transglenoid suture procedure were assessed in 60 consecutive patients (average age, 25 years). All but 3 of the

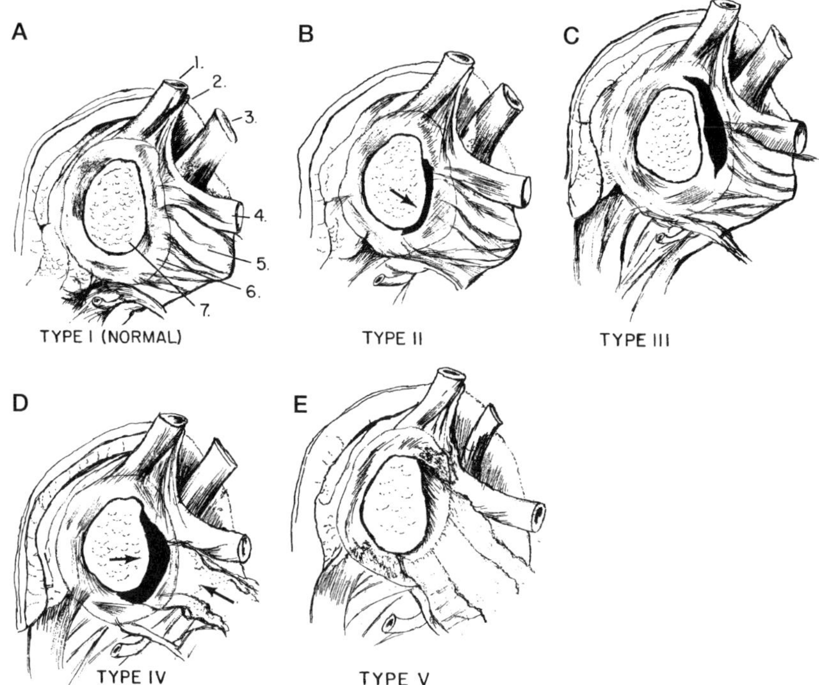

FIGURE 1.—Classification of labral lesions. **A,** type I is a normal labrum (*1,* long head of the biceps; *2,* superior glenohumeral ligament; *3,* subscapularis; *4,* middle glenohumeral ligament; *5,* inferior glenohumeral ligament; *6,* glenoid labrum; and *7,* glenoid). **B,** type II is a simple detachment of the labrum from the glenoid. Clinically, there is associated instability, and this type is usually repairable by arthroscopic or open techniques. **C,** type III is a disturbance tear of the glenoid labrum. Clinically, there may be pain, clicking, or mechanical symptoms, and this type is amenable to open or arthroscopic débridement. **D,** type IV is a detachment of the labrum with significant fraying or degeneration. Clinically, there is associated instability, but this type is usually not amenable to arthroscopic reattachment. **E,** type V is a complete degeneration or absence of the glenoid labrum. Clinically, there is associated instability, but this type is not amenable to arthroscopic re-attachment. (Courtesy of Green MR, Christensen KP: Arthroscopic Bankart procedure: Two- to five-year followup with clinical correlation to severity of glenoid labral lesion. *Am J Sports Med* 23:276–281, 1995.)

patients had had at least 1 episode of frank dislocation and all were found to have a detached glenoid labrum (Fig 1).

Results.—Forty-seven patients were available for evaluation an average of 41 months after arthroscopic surgery. Eighteen patients had recurrent dislocation during follow-up, and 3 had episodes of subluxation. The overall failure rate was 42%. Among 37 evaluable patients, surgery failed in only 1 of 22 who had simple labral detachment and no other significant lesion (type II labrum). In contrast, surgery failed in 13 of 15 patients with a type IV or type V labrum in whom the labrum-inferior glenohumeral ligament complex was significantly compromised. The patients without recurrent instability regained an average of 94% of their preoperative function. Strength in abduction and external rotation was normal, and the loss of external rotation averaged only 1.5 degrees. Few complications occurred.

Conclusion.—The outcome of this procedure relates directly to the degree of disruption of the glenoid labrum-inferior glenohumeral ligament complex. Arthroscopic Bankart repair is recommended only for patients in whom injury is limited to detachment of the glenoid labrum.

Arthroscopic Stabilization for Recurrent Anterior Shoulder Dislocation: Results of 59 Cases

Walch G, Boileau P, Levigne C, Mandrino A, Neyret P, Donell S (Centre Hospitalier Lyon-Sud, Pierre-Bénite, France)

Arthroscopy 11:173–179, 1995 3–19

Objective.—The development of shoulder arthroscopy has made it possible to repair chronic anterior shoulder disability using Morgan's technique, which uses transglenoidal suture of the inferior glenohumeral ligament. Recent reports of a significant recurrence rate have prompted a review of patients who have had surgery that used this technique.

Methods.—Morgan's technique, using 2 sutures from anterior to posterior taking the inferior glenohumeral ligament–labrum complex, was used in 48 patients with recurrent anterior dislocation of the shoulder. A variation also was used, with the superior suture including the middle glenohumeral ligament (6 patients) or the superior part of the tendon of the subscapularis (5 patients). After 4 weeks of immobilization, rehabilitation was begun, and return to sports was allowed beginning 4 months postoperatively. Patients were followed up for an average of 49 months.

Results.—Results were excellent in 20 patients, good in 5, fair in 5, and poor in 29. In patients with poor results, 26 had another anterior dislocation, and 3 had recurrent subluxation an average of 13 months after surgery. Only 18 patients were able to return to their pre-injury level of sports activity. Recurrence rates were associated with preoperative findings of inferior hyperlaxity, a Bankart lesion, and extended ligamentous lesions.

Conclusion.—Because the successful outcome for this procedure is only 50%, the technique, until perfected, should be limited to clinical trials.

Arthroscopic Bankart Suture Repair for Recurrent Traumatic Unidirectional Anterior Shoulder Dislocations

Youssef JA, Carr CF, Walther CE, Murphy JM (Dartmouth-Hitchcock Med Ctr, Lebanon, NH)

Arthroscopy 11:561–563, 1995 3–20

Objective.—The results of arthroscopic repair were reviewed in 30 consecutive patients treated for a Bankart lesion after traumatic anterior shoulder dislocation. Patients were followed for at least 2 years after repair and for an average of 38 months.

Patients.—Twenty-three men and 7 women with an average age of 26½ years were operated on. All of them had a "pure" dislocation; patients with instability resulting from subluxation or multidirectional instability were excluded. The patients had had an initial frank dislocation that was documented radiographically or required help to reduce. All but 4 patients had multiple dislocations. Nine patients regularly took part in collision-type sports activities. All but 2 of 15 double-contrast CT arthrograms demonstrated a Bankart lesion.

Outcome.—A transglenoid Bankart suture repair was performed by 3-portal arthroscopy. Eleven patients had an excellent functional outcome based on the Rowe grading system and 8 had a good outcome by these criteria. Three patients had fair results, and 8 (27%) had a poor outcome. Six of the latter 8 patients had frank redislocation after repair, 5 as a result of sports-related trauma. Three patients had degenerative changes in the glenohumeral joint.

Conclusion.—Arthroscopic transglenoid suture repair failed in more than one fourth of patients in this series with unidirectional anterior shoulder dislocations. This procedure no longer is performed in athletic patients younger than 30 years of age who have recurrent traumatic unidirectional shoulder instability.

► Morgan and Bodenstab[1] described the arthroscopic procedure to reattach the Bankart lesion to the anterior glenoid rim and scapular neck with a transglenoid suture. Reporting on 25 cases, they claimed 100% excellent results, with all patients achieving full active range of motion and return to pre-injury activity level, including contact and throwing sports, without symptoms of pain or instability.

The results of these 3 reports—a 42% recurrent dislocation/subluxation rate by Green and Christensen (Abstract 3–18), a 49% recurrent dislocation/subluxation rate by Walch et al. (Abstract 3–19), and a 27% failure rate by Youssef et al. (Abstract 3–20)—are most disconcerting. These articles suggest that patient selection is most important—specifically, that the procedure not be performed on patients who are younger than 30 years old who participate in collision or competitive sports. Furthermore, the procedure is recommended only for patients with isolated detachment of the glenoid labrum. It is also recommended that this particular arthroscopic technique only be performed as part of a prospective controlled trial until the technique is perfected.

J.S. Torg, M.D.

Reference

1. Morgan CD, Bodenstab AB: Arthroscopic Bankart suture repair: Technique and early results. *Arthroscopy* 3:111–122, 1987.

Arthroscopic Bankart Repair With the Suretac Device: Part I. Clinical Observations

Warner JJP, Miller MD, Marks PM, Fu FH (Univ of Pittsburgh, Pa)

Arthroscopy 11:2–13, 1995 3–21

Introduction.—Arthroscopic Bankart repair has been touted as more anatomical, faster, and less inclined to produce patient morbidity than are the open techniques and has become an accepted method of surgical stabilization for anterior shoulder instability. However, the failure rate of this procedure is still unacceptably high. A cannulated, absorbable fixation device made of polyglyconate was devised to avoid iatrogenic injury and the risks that metal implants pose around joint surfaces and to remove the requirement for an accessory posterior incision. This device (Suretac: Acufex Microsurgical, Mansfield, Mass) enjoyed initial favor but has since been attributed a long-term follow-up failure rate similar to that of other arthroscopic repair techniques. Healing after arthroscopic Bankart repair with the Suretac device was investigated through observation of 15 patients so treated who underwent "second-look" arthroscopic evaluation.

Methods and Findings.—Patients underwent the "second-look" procedure an average of 9 months after the original surgery to address the complications of recurrent instability (7 patients), pain (6 patients), or pain with stiffness (2 patients). Of the 8 patients with stable shoulders, the Bankart repair had healed completely in 5 and partially in 3. However, the Bankart repair was completely healed only in 3 and partially healed only in 1 of the 7 patients with recurrent instability. Lax capsular tissue was present in 6 of these patients; technical errors during the original repair were retrospectively detected in 4. Biopsy of the repair sites of 2 patients performed 6–8 months after the original surgery showed residual polyglyconate polymer debris surrounded by a histiocytic infiltrate.

Conclusions.—High failure rates among arthroscopic repair techniques are probably attributable to patient selection and technical pitfalls. These procedures do offer some advantages, however, and their success rate should improve with more rigid patient selection criteria. For example, arthroscopic repair is well suited to a patient with a unidirectional, posttraumatic anterior dislocation or subluxation and a discrete Bankart lesion with well-developed, thick-appearing glenohumeral ligaments. The healing strength of the Bankart repair is still in question, although complete healing does not appear necessary for shoulder stability.

Arthroscopic Bankart Repair With the Suretac Device: Part II. Experimental Observations

Warner JJP, Miller MD, Marks P (Univ of Pittsburgh, Pa)

Arthroscopy 11:14–20, 1995 3–22

Introduction.—Arthroscopic Bankart repair has been performed using a variety of techniques. The Suretac device (Acufex Microsurgical, Mans-

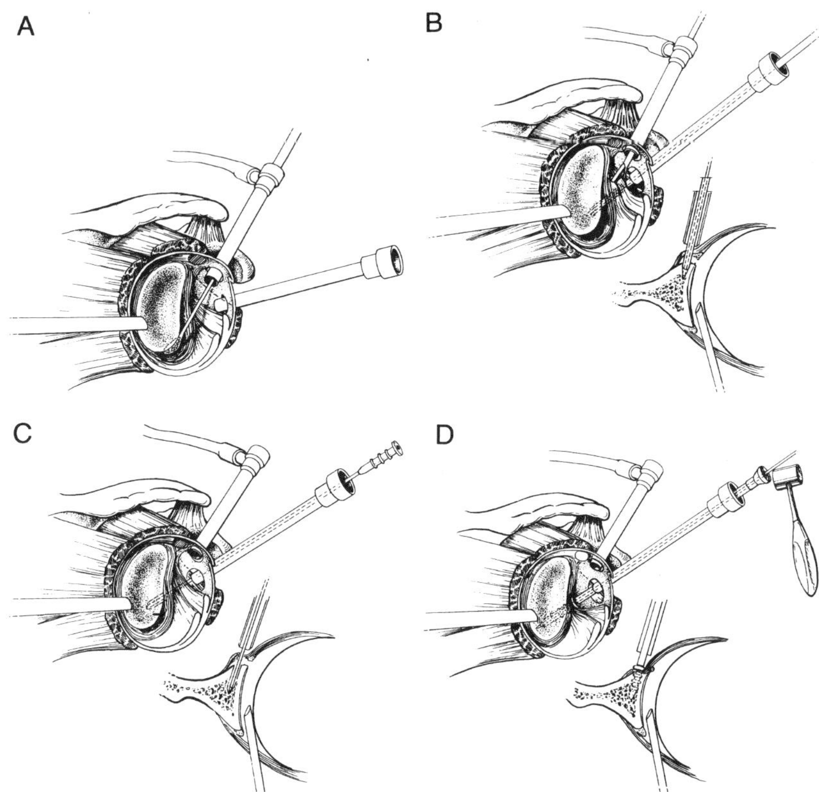

FIGURE 1.—Arthroscopic Bankart repair technique using the Suretac device. **A**, diagrammatic representation of mobilization of the labrum and inferior glenohumeral ligament (*IGHL*) off the scapular neck. **B**, diagrammatic representation of superior shift of the IGHL before drilling. **C**, diagrammatic representation of the guide wire through the IGHL. **D**, diagrammatic representation of the Suretac repair. The IGHL has been pulled up and compressed against the anterior and inferior juxta-articular scapular neck after repair with the Suretac device. (From Warner JJP, Miller MD, Marks P: Arthroscopic Bankart repair with the Suretac device: Part II. Experimental observations. *Arthroscopy* 11:14–20, 1995. Adapted from Warner JJP, Warren RF: Arthroscopic Bankart repair using a cannulated, absorbable, fixation device. *Op Tech Orthop* 1:192–198, 1991.)

field, Mass) was developed to avoid the technical limitations of the stable repair technique and the suture repair technique. The technical limitations and pitfalls of this absorbable, cannulated fixation device composed of polyglyconate polymer were investigated using a cadaver model.

Methods.—Bankart lesions were created arthroscopically in 8 cadaver shoulders. These lesions were then repaired with arthroscopic Bankart repair using the Suretac device (Fig 1). Placement of the Suretac devices and adequacy of repair were evaluated by dissection. To evaluate placement of the Suretac device relative to the articular surface, the glenoids were transected in the transverse plane and embedded in clear methylmethacrylate.

Results.—Several technical errors were identified, including inadequate abrasion of the anterior and inferior juxta-articular neck of the scapula and inadequate superior and medial shift of the inferior glenohumeral ligament (before placement of the lowest Suretac device). Other errors noted regarding the Suretac device were inappropriate medial placement relative to the articular margin and insufficient capture and compression of capsular tissue.

Discussion.—Several technical steps in arthroscopic repair using the Suretac device require meticulous attention to detail. These include: (1) extensive mobilization of the inferior glenohumeral ligament down to the 6-o'clock position of the glenoid rim, (2) creation of a shallow bony trough by thorough débridement and burring of the juxta-articular neck of the scapula down to the 6-o'clock position, (3) shift of the inferior glenohumeral ligament superior-medially, (4) positioning of the lowest Suretac device below the 4-o'clock position, and (5) good capture and compression of capsuloligamentous tissue against the scapular neck via use of 3 Suretac devices placed close to the glenoid rim. If any of these goals cannot be achieved, the surgeon is best advised to switch to an open repair technique.

Arthroscopic Bioabsorbable Tack Stabilization of Initial Anterior Shoulder Dislocations: A Preliminary Report

Arciero RA, Taylor DC, Snyder RJ, Uhorchak JM (Keller Army Hosp, West Point, NY)

Arthroscopy 11:410–417, 1995 3–23

Purpose.—Patients with an acute, initial anterior shoulder dislocation have traditionally been treated by conservative means, with reduction, immobilization, and rehabilitation. Age continues to be the main prognostic factor influencing recurrence. In initial studies comparing conservative therapy with arthroscopic surgery, the recurrence rate of instability was reduced from 80% to 14%. Since then, the arthroscopic technique has been changed, including the addition of a bioabsorbable fixation device to eliminate the need for transglenoid drilling and tying of suture over the posterior soft tissues. The early results of this technique were evaluated.

Patients.—The patients were 26 consecutive Army cadet athletes who had an acute, initial anterior shoulder dislocation. Manual reduction was required for initial treatment in all cases. The patients underwent arthroscopic surgery within 10 days; these procedures were performed with use of the Beach chair position and interscalene anesthesia. The arthroscopic findings were avulsion of the anteroinferior capsulolabral complex from the glenoid rim—or Bankart lesion—in 25 patients and lateral detachment of the inferior glenohumeral ligament from the humeral neck in 1. A Hill-Sachs lesion was noted in 23 patients and a SLAP tear in 3. For all patients with Bankart lesions, repair was performed using a cannulated bioabsorbable fixation device.

Outcomes.—Preliminary results in 19 patients, all with more than 1 year of follow-up, are reported. The patients' average age was 19.5 years. At an average of 19 months' follow-up, they had lost an average of 3 degrees of external rotation. None of the patients experienced recurrent dislocation, although 1 had a single episode of resubluxation. According to the Rowe point score, the results were excellent in 16 patients, good in 2, and fair in 1. All the cadets returned to their previous level of athletic performance.

Conclusions.—In young athletes with an acute, initial anterior shoulder dislocation, arthroscopic bioabsorbable tack stabilization appears to be an effective treatment alternative. It should be used only for initial, traumatic dislocations that require manual reduction. The technique described provides an anatomical repair with low morbidity that, in early experience, appears to reverse the natural history of frequent recurrence.

► These 3 articles (Abstracts 3–21, 3–22, and 3–23) clearly define the current laboratory and clinical status of the Suretac device in dealing with anterior glenohumeral dislocation. As pointed out by Warner et al., high failure rates seem to be a result of patient selection as well as technical pitfalls. They believe the patients with unidirectional posttraumatic anterior dislocation or subluxation are ideally suited for this approach when they have a discrete Bankart lesion with well-developed, thick-appearing glenohumeral ligaments. Patients with significant ligamentous injury, on the other hand, should be treated with open techniques. Arciero et al. conclude that the procedure should be reserved for young athletes with initial traumatic dislocation requiring reduction. It should be pointed out that Warner et al. did not state the length of follow-up and Arciero stated his to be "over 1 year" without giving a range. Should the technical problems be resolved, will the technique withstand the test of time?

J.S. Torg, M.D.

Clinical Anatomy and Pathomechanics of the Elbow in Sports

Guerra JJ, Timmerman LA (American Sports Medicine Inst, Birmingham, Ala; Univ of California, Davis)

Sports Med Arthro Rev 3:160–169, 1995 3–24

Elbow Injuries.—The baseball pitch is the best studied and understood athletic motion. Throwing in baseball and other sports involves tremendous forces and torques above the elbow, which can result in tension, lateral compression, and posterior impaction elbow injuries. Valgus stress on the medial elbow can occur during arm cocking, arm acceleration, and to a lesser extent, arm deceleration in the throwing motion. Most athletes can tolerate these forces with proper warm-up, conditioning, and mechanics. Microscopic tears and subsequent laxity are most likely to occur to the ulnar collateral ligament if the athlete has poor flexibility or is fatigued. A concomitant flexor-pronator tendinitis may develop in the presence of valgus instability. Etiologic factors for ulnar nerve symptoms are traction, compression, and friction. It is likely that more than one of these factors is in effect with ulnar nerve symptoms. In young athletes with open growth plates, the valgus force on the medial side of the elbow can result in "little leaguer's" elbow. Injuries may include medial epicondylar apophyseal inflammation, fragmentation, delayed ephiphyseal closure, and growth plate separation. Lateral elbow compression injuries are most likely to occur at the end of the throw when a compressive shearing force is focused on the inferior and medial aspect of the capitellum. The result can be damage to the articular cartilage with fibrillation and fraying. Traumatic osteochondritis dissecans may occur in adolescent athletes as an expression of lateral overload from repetitive throwing. Posterior impaction injuries are most likely to occur during arm acceleration and arm deceleration throwing phases. The most likely posterior impaction injuries are osteophyte buildup, stress fractures of the olecranon, and disturbances in the olecranon epiphysis in immature athletes.

Conclusion.—An understanding of the anatomy and mechanics of the elbow will help develop a rational approach to evaluation, treatment, and rehabilitation of sports-related injuries.

▶ This article is a comprehensive review of the clinical anatomy and pathomechanics of the elbow. The original paper is recommended reading for those interested in the subject matter.

J.S. Torg, M.D.

Arthroscopic Assessment of the Medial Collateral Ligament Complex of the Elbow

Field LD, Callaway GH, O'Brien SJ, Altchek DW (Mississippi Sports Medicine and Orthopaedic Ctr, Jackson; Hosp for Special Surgery, New York)

Am J Sports Med 23:396–400, 1995 3–25

Objective.—Elbow arthroscopy is increasingly performed to diagnose and treat various disorders, but the extent to which the medial collateral ligament (MCL) complex, the chief stabilizer of the elbow, can be visualized remains uncertain.

Methods.—Ten fresh cadaveric elbows from different individuals were examined. The MCL complex was exposed by a muscle-splitting incision, and the anterior and posterior bundles were marked with nylon sutures. Two experienced surgeons then examined the joints arthroscopically using a 30-degree 4-mm instrument.

Observations.—In only 1 of the 10 elbows was part of the anterior bundle of the MCL visualized, even when the elbow was moved through 130 degrees. In no case was the ulnar or humeral insertion of the anterior bundle seen. In contrast, the entire posterior bundle of the MCL complex was visualized in all elbows, most readily through a posterocentral portal 4 cm proximal to the olecranon process. During examination of the posteromedial gutter, the arthroscope pushed directly against the nerve and was separated from it only by a thin capsule and the posterior bundle.

Conclusion.—Unless the MCL complex is completely disrupted, the inability to visualize the anterior bundle arthroscopically may limit the diagnostic value of this procedure.

▶ In addition to pointing out the problem associated with visualization of the anterior bundle of the partially torn MCL arthroscopically, the authors recommend that "the surgeons should exercise a low threshold for performing an arthrotomy to ensure protection of the ulnar nerve whenever difficulty is encountered in performing any arthroscopic procedure in the posterior medial gutter."

J.S. Torg, M.D.

Painful Olecranon Physeal Nonunion in an Adult Weight Lifter: A Case Report

Walker LG (Univ of California, Los Angeles)

Clin Orthop 311:125–128, 1995 3–26

Background.—Persistent olecranon physes is an uncommonly reported condition, with only 3 cases described to date. In each of these 3 patients, the physeal nonunion was bilateral, and either unilateral, bipartite, or tripartite patellae were noted. In the present case, an adult weight lifter had a painful unilateral physeal nonunion.

Case Report.—Man, 20, who had been involved in competitive weight lifting since 14 years of age, was evaluated for intermittent pain about the dominant elbow. The pain had begun 18 months previously, was localized over the olecranon, and was aggravated by weight lifting. Although pain was substantially reduced when decreasing the amount of weight lifted, increasing the poundage reportedly led to recurrent pain.

Full range of elbow motion was noted on physical examination, although joint swelling and tenderness over the olecranon were observed. On radiographic evaluation, a chronic epiphysis with smooth sclerotic borders was observed in the affected elbow, whereas all physes were closed in the contralateral elbow. Radiographs of the knees were unremarkable.

Conservative treatment was initiated, but after 6 months, no improvement was noted. Curettage of the physis, together with tension bone wiring augmented by iliac crest bone graft, was subsequently undertaken. On histologic assessment, columnar organization of hyaline cartilage, indicative of a persistent epiphyseal plate, was noted.

After an uneventful postoperative course and 4 weeks of long arm casting, a rehabilitation program was initiated. Normal elbow motion and evidence of radiographic union were observed 2 years after surgery, and the patient remained symptom-free after returning to competitive weight lifting. No further treatment was undertaken.

Conclusions.—The growth centers of the elbow are well-established problem areas in active preadolescent and adolescent patients. At present, the association between weight lifting and epiphyseal damage in the adolescent remains controversial; studies aimed at evaluating the safety of weight lifting among individuals in this age group therefore are encouraged. The development of guidelines for preadolescent and adolescent weight lifters, as well as other athletes, may help prevent stress-related injuries in young individuals.

Fractures of Unfused Olecranon Physis: A Re-evaluation of This Injury in Three Athletes

Turtel AH, Andrews JR, Schob CJ, Kupferman SP, Gross AE (Am Sports Medicine Inst, Birmingham, Ala; Univ of Toronto; New York, NY)

Orthopedics 18:390–394, 1995 3–27

Objective.—Acute fracture separations or stress fractures of the incompletely fused physis of the olecranon can occur in athletes. These injuries are thought to result from violent and repetitive forces generated by the triceps as the arm goes through the acceleration phase of throwing. The mechanism of fracture of the unfused olecranon is reconsidered in a report of 3 such injuries, 2 of which occurred in professional baseball players.

Case 2.—Man, 26, fell directly on his right elbow while it was in flexion. The patient was a right-handed major league shortstop who had previously been noted to have an asymptomatic, unfused olecranon apophysis. Radiographs showed a displaced fracture through the synchondrosis. The patient underwent open reduction and internal fixation without bone grafting. A stable fibrous union was achieved, and the patient had full range of motion and no symptoms at 3½ years' follow-up.

Discussion.—The cases described in this article, along with previous biomechanical data, suggest that persistent physis of the olecranon does not result from tensile forces through the olecranon enthesis of the triceps during active extension. Because more eccentric type triceps contractions appear to occur during throwing, it might be best to emphasize this type of training for throwing athletes. Acute, displaced fractures of the unfused olecranon physis can be managed by anatomical stable fixation without grafting; bone grafting of the synchondrosis is needed in patients with the atraumatic chronic condition.

▶ We have previously reported 2 cases of nonunion of a stress fracture to the olecranon physeal plate occurring in adolescent baseball pitchers.[1, 2] Both patients were successfully treated with inlaid bone grafts. The question has been raised as to whether these lesions in adolescents will heal without surgery. Walker's report as well as that by Kovach et al.[3] substantiates that the acute lesion can go on to either a disruption of the olecranon or a painful olecranon physeal nonunion. Unless there is complete healing with closure of the physeal line after conservative management, open reduction and either bone grafting or internal fixation is recommended.

J.S. Torg, M.D.

References

1. Torg JS, Moyer RA: Non-union of a stress fracture through the olecranon epiphyseal plate observed in an adolescent baseball pitcher: A case report. *J Bone Joint Surg (Am)* 59A:264–265, 1977.
2. Pavlov H, Torg JS, Jacobs B, et al: Nonunion of olecranon epiphysis: Two cases in adolescent baseball pitchers. *Am J Roentgenol* 136:819–820, 1981.
3. Kovach J II, Baker BE, Mosher JE: Fracture separation of the olecranon ossification center in adults. *Am J Sports Med* 13:105–111, 1985.

Wrist Kinematics Differ in Expert and Novice Tennis Players Performing the Backhand Stroke: Implications for Tennis Elbow

Blackwell JR, Cole KJ (Univ of Iowa, Iowa City)
J Biomech 27:509–516, 1994 3–28

Background.—Novice tennis players experience a greater incidence of lateral humeral epicondylitis (tennis elbow) than do expert players. Investigators suggest that this may reflect the novice players' use of faulty mechanics for the backhand stroke. Wrist kinematics, including flexion and extension, grip pressures, and wrist muscle electromyographic activity were examined in novice and expert tennis players performing the backhand stroke.

Participants and Methods.—Eight novice and 8 expert tennis players aged 18–30 years were investigated. History of injury or elbow and forearm pain was not noted in any player. Skill levels were evaluated using the National Tennis Rating Program scale, which ranges from 0 to 7 with 7 designating a world-class player. All novices had scores of less than 2, whereas experts achieved scores greater than 5. After preliminary flexor and extensor muscle electromyelograms (EMGs) and maximum grip pressure data were obtained, participants were instructed to return tennis balls projected from a machine using a flat backhand ground stroke. No instructions with respect to grip, body orientation, or stroke were issued.

Results.—All participants moved their wrists in the flexion direction before ball-racket collision. However, expert players reversed their initial wrist motion and performed the backhand stroke with wrists extended (i.e., neutral alignment of the forearm and hand dorsum). In expert players, ball-racket impact occurred with the wrist extended at an average of

0.41 rad, approximately 23 degrees from neutral alignment. In addition, their wrists moved further into extension at impact. In comparison, novice players hit the ball with the wrist flexed 0.22 rad, at about 13 degrees from neutral alignment. Moreover, novice players moved their wrist further into flexion on impact. Similar levels of activity were observed on wrist extensor EMGs during the 500-msec interval before ball-racket collision. However, expert players had greater electromyographic levels after contact, consistent with the accompanying wrist extension. The combined wrist kinematic and electromyographic data showed that novice players eccentrically contracted their wrist extensor muscles while performing the backhand stroke.

Conclusions.—It is suggested that conditions facilitating stretch of wrist extensor muscles during ball-racket impact are present in novice players. The subsequent eccentric contraction of wrist extensor muscles may play a role in the development of lateral tennis elbow in novice players. Emphasis on proper body position for the background stroke may reduce the severity or incidence of injury in tennis players.

▶ The purpose of this study was to determine whether novice and expert tennis players performing the backhand stroke differ in wrist kinematics. This goal has been accomplished. However, to my knowledge, there are no hard data substantiating the premise that there is a greater prevalence of lateral humeral epicondylitis in novice tennis players than in expert players. Also, even if this were so, the data as presented do not support the conclusion that wrist kinematics correlate with the occurrence of tennis elbow.

J.S. Torg, M.D.

The Results of Operative Treatment of Medial Epicondylitis

Kurvers H, Verhaar J (Univ Hosp Maastricht, The Netherlands; Univ Hosp Rotterdam, The Netherlands)

J Bone Joint Surg (Am) 77–A:1374–1379, 1995 3–29

Background.—Although medial epicondylitis is common, it is incompletely understood. It may be related to an isolated traumatic event or to overuse, and sometimes coexists with ulnar neuritis. Nonoperative treatment is recommended, but when it is insufficient, use of various operative procedures has been described. Results of operative forms of treatment have not been well documented. The results of operative treatment for medial epicondylitis in 38 patients (40 elbows) were assessed, with emphasis on the influence of certain preoperative variables on outcome.

Methods.—Patients ranged in age from 22 to 56 years (mean, 42 years); 24 elbows showed coexistent ulnar neuritis. All patients underwent an operative procedure in which the attachment of the common flexor muscle of the forearm to the medial epicondyle was released. In 17 of the 24 elbows with coexistent ulnar neuritis, the retinaculum over the cubital tunnel was also released. Follow-up continued for a mean of 44 months. Results of treatment were assessed retrospectively based on subjective outcome, pain during resisted palmar flexion of the hand and wrist, patient satisfaction, and grip strength.

Results.—Overall subjective outcome was considered good for 25 elbows. Twenty-eight elbows experienced resolution of preoperative pain. Elbows with coexistent ulnar neuritis were less likely to experience a good overall subjective outcome than were those without. At follow-up, 11 of 16 elbows with isolated medial epicondylitis, but only 3 of 24 elbows with coexistent ulnar neuritis, were symptom-free. Symptoms of ulnar neuritis persisted in 15 elbows. Grip strengths did not differ between affected elbows and their normal contralateral counterparts.

Discussion.—The operative treatment is intended to reduce the tensile forces of the flexor muscles. The outcome of this procedure for isolated medial epicondylitis is comparable to that of other published reports on this technique and to reports of extensor release for lateral epicondylitis. However, when ulnar neuritis is coexistent neither flexor release alone nor combined with retinacular release provides satisfactory results. This may be because the degenerative changes of medial epicondylitis in these patients are not limited to the origin of the flexor muscles but also involve peritendinous tissue. Increased pressure in the cubital tunnel or direct irritation of the ulnar nerve may be related to the ulnar neuritis. Additional anterior transposition of the ulnar nerve could have more beneficial results. Grip strength does not appear to be a valid measure of outcome for patients with ulnar neuritis.

Resection and Repair for Medial Tennis Elbow: A Prospective Analysis

Ollivierre CO, Nirschl RP, Pettrone FA (Virginia Sports Medicine and Rehabilitation Inst, Arlington)

Am J Sports Med 23:214–221, 1995 3–30

Background.—Medial tennis elbow tendinosis may develop in the overhead repetitive-action athlete as a result of injury to the tendinous origin of the flexor-pronator muscle mass. Such injury can result from repetitive activities requiring valgus or flexion forces about the elbow, such as occur in improperly hit forearm shots in racket sports. Patients must be evaluated to distinguish primary ulnar nerve neuropathy and medial collateral ligament abnormalities from true tendinosis. Nonoperative management using PRICEMM (preventive education, rest, immobilization, compression, elevation, medications, and modalities) is attempted first but is ineffective in some patients. Fifty elbows with tennis elbow tendinosis in 48 patients were refractory to nonoperative management, necessitating surgical intervention. The outcomes of these procedures were evaluated.

Methods.—Racket sports were implicated in 21 cases, with golf and swimming the next most common initiating activities. Twelve patients had associated ulnar nerve symptoms at the time of surgery. Symptoms had

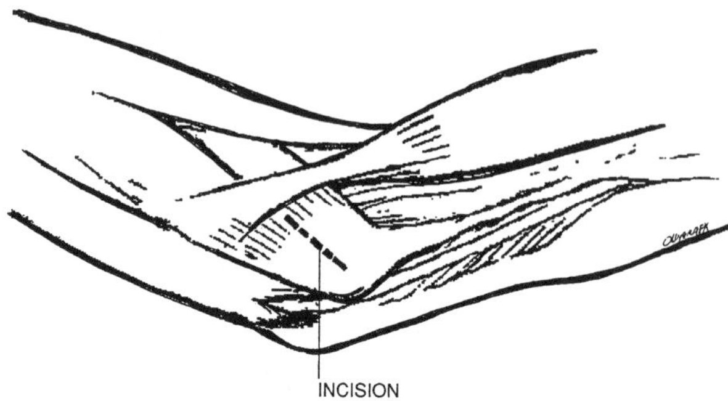

FIGURE 3.—Incision along the flexor carpi radialis-pronator teres interval. (Courtesy of Ollivierre CO, Nirschl RP, Pettrone FA: Resection and repair for medial tennis elbow: A prospective analysis. *Am J Sports Med* 23:214–221, 1995.)

been present for an average of 2.5 years before surgery and the patients had received a total of 130 injections of a local anesthetic and/or cortisone. Pain occurrence and intensity were rated before and after surgery at rest, during activities of daily living, and during the activity that aggravated the symptoms. The surgical procedure involved excision of the diseased tendon, usually through the flexor carpi radialis-pronator teres interval (Figs 3, 4, 5). A rehabilitation program was started on the first day after surgery involving finger, wrist, and shoulder motion.

Results.—The injured tendon was located at the flexor carpi radialis-pronator teres interval in 28 cases, whereas the flexor carpi ulnaris was involved in 6 cases and the common flexor origin in 16. All patients with ulnar nerve symptoms had ulnar nerve compression. Pain reduction on follow-up (average, 37 months) was reported by all patients. None of 14 patients with preoperative pain at rest continued to have such pain after surgery, and only 2 of 32 who had pain with activities of daily living continued to have residual discomfort. Eight patients who related their

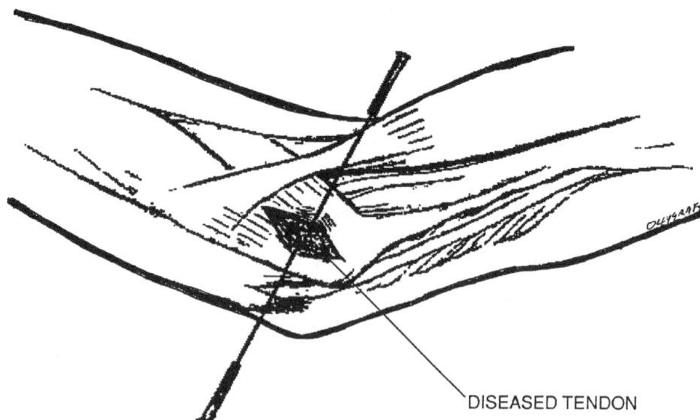

FIGURE 4.—Flexor carpi radialis-pronator teres interval exposed, revealing diseased tendon tissue. (Courtesy of Ollivierre CO, Nirschl RP, Pettrone FA: Resection and repair for medial tennis elbow: A prospective analysis. *Am J Sports Med* 23:214–221, 1995.)

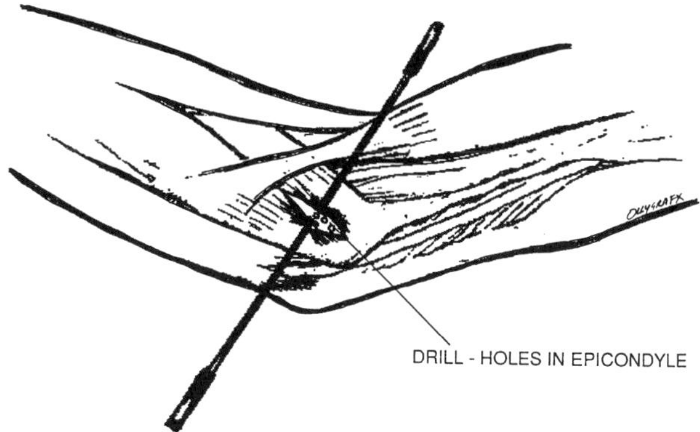

FIGURE 5.—Drill holes are made into the cortical bone of the medial epicondyle at the site of the excised tendon. (Courtesy of Ollivierre CO, Nirschl RP, Pettrone FA: Resection and repair for medial tennis elbow: A prospective analysis. *Am J Sports Med* 23:214–221, 1995.)

symptoms to sports did not return to the preinjury level of participation, and 2 occupational athletes were also unable to return to preinjury levels of involvement. These patients did report a decrease in pain intensity, however. Histologic analysis showed an absence of acute inflammation with angiofibroblastic hyperplasia tendinosis and the fibrillary degeneration of collagen. Dynamometer strength testing showed that all patients improved significantly after surgery.

Discussion.—Medial tennis elbow is an uncommon occurrence, and few reports on this subject are found in the medical literature. Most cases will resolve with nonoperative management and a good rehabilitation program. Intractable pain, however, requires surgery, followed by a quality rehabilitation program. Most patients treated in this way will be able to return to their previous activities and will experience significant pain relief.

Operative Treatment of Medial Epicondylitis: Influence of Concomitant Ulnar Neuropathy at the Elbow

Gabel GT, Morrey BF (Mayo Clinic, Rochester, Minn; Baylor College of Medicine, Houston)

J Bone Joint Surg (Am) 77–A:1065–1069, 1995 3–31

Objective.—The results of surgery for medial epicondylitis were reviewed in 26 patients with 30 affected elbows, 16 of which exhibited ulnar neuropathy. The patients had an average age of 43 years at the time of surgery and were followed for at least 2 years.

Clinical Aspects.—Symptoms began acutely in a setting of trauma in 8 patients. The average time of symptoms before surgery was 31 months. Tenderness over the medial epicondyle was a constant finding. The most sensitive means of eliciting pain was resisted pronation of the forearm. Ulnar neuropathy was mild in 11 elbows, moderate in 4, and severe in 1.

Operative Findings and Management.—Exploration revealed a focus of inflammation in 17 elbows and focal ulnar nerve compression in 9 elbows. The nidus of inflammation most often was in the middle-to-lateral portion of the tendon mass, involving the pronator teres and flexor carpi radialis tendons. Thirteen elbows underwent elevation of the flexor-pronator origin with débridement, epicondylar shaving, and reattachment of the flexor pronator origin. Four other elbows had the same operation but without reattachment. Medial epicondylectomy was done in 2 cases. Submuscular transposition of the ulnar nerve was the usual procedure when decompression was necessary.

Results.—Follow-up an average of 7 years after surgery revealed 11 excellent, 15 good, 2 fair, and 2 poor results. All but 1 of 25 elbows with no more than mild ulnar neuropathy had a good or excellent outcome, compared with only 2 of 5 elbows with moderate or severe ulnar neuropathy. Several patients did not achieve maximal improvement until more than 6 months had elapsed.

Discussion.—The only factor consistently associated with the outcome of repair was the degree of involvement of the ulnar nerve. If only mild neuropathy is present and there is no focal compression, it is enough to treat the epicondylitis. Cubital tunnel release is preferred if decompression is necessary.

▶ These 3 reports (Abstracts 3–29, 3–30, 3–31) present operative management of medial epicondylitis by 2 different techniques. Kurvers and Verhaar expose the flexion origin and completely divide it transversely close to its attachment to the medial epicondyle. In those patients with preoperative symptoms of ulnar neuritis, the retinaculum of the cubital tunnel was left undisturbed. In this latter group of patients, they report that "the results of release of flexor muscle alone without release of the retinaculum of the cubital tunnel were not satisfactory." On the other hand, Ollivierre et al. selectively debrided the injured tendon located in the flexor carpi radialis-pronator teres interval, the flexor carpi ulnar being involved in 6 cases and the common flexor origin in 16. In those cases with signs and symptoms with referral to the ulnar nerve, the nerve was explored concurrently. When necessary, the nerve was decompressed. In those patients with nerve subluxation or dislocation it was transferred subcutaneously anterior to the medial epicondyle. Unfortunately, the authors did not report the specific response to surgery in the subgroup that had ulnar nerve transpositions. Although Gabel et al. included either release of the cubital tunnel retinaculum or ulnar nerve transposition depending on the degree of nerve involvement, their results depended on the degree of preoperative nerve compression. Thus, the results of surgery, in all likelihood, depend on the initial condition of the ulnar nerve.

J.S. Torg, M.D.

Sports Fractures of the Distal Radius: Epidemiology and Outcome
Lawson GM, Hajducka C, McQueen MM (Royal Infirmary of Edinburgh, Scotland)
Injury 26:33–36, 1995 3–32

Background.—During the past 20 years, the number of people participating in recreational or sporting activities has increased, yet little is known about sports-related fractures of the distal radius. To address this deficiency, the epidemiology, management, and outcome of sports-related fractures of the distal radius seen during a 5-year period were reviewed.

Patients.—Between 1988 and 1993, 2,774 patients were seen at a trauma unit in Edinburgh with fractures of the distal radius. Of those, 221 (8%) sustained 225 fractures during a sporting or recreational activity. Follow-up consisted of radiographic examination at 6 weeks and questionnaires at an average of 27 months after treatment.

Treatment.—All but 4 fractures were treated by closed manipulation and/or cast application. Twelve percent required further extensive treatment, including closed reduction and external fixation in 16, open reduction with bone grafting and K-wire fixation in 7, open reduction and internal fixation with buttress plate in 1, and remanipulation in 2.

Results.—The majority of the fractures occurred in young men aged 20–29 years. Half of the fractures occurred during soccer, 12% during skiing, 9% during dancing, and 7% during rugby. The majority of the fractures sustained during soccer, football, and skiing occurred during play on synthetic surfaces. High energy sports, such as skiing and horse riding, and increasing age were associated with more severe and complex fractures, whereas football and rugby were associated with more benign, extra-articular fractures. Complications occurred in 14%, mainly malunion. Of the 131 participants who completed the questionnaires, 72.5% returned to their original sport, and this was influenced primarily by the preinjury standard of competition and the patient's age.

Summary.—The epidemiology of fractures of the distal radius that occur during sports or recreational activities reflects the epidemiology of other sports injuries as a whole. High energy sports and increasing age result in more complex and severe fractures, and playing on synthetic turf increases the risk of wrist fractures. The rate of complication is low. Return to sports is affected largely by preinjury standard of competition and commitment and not fracture severity.

▶ Although not specifically analyzed, this report indicates a correlation between playing surfaces and the occurrence and severity of wrist fractures. Specifically, in those fractures resulting from soccer, 54% were sustained on synthetic turf, 28% on grass, and 18% on other surfaces.

J.S. Torg, M.D.

Delayed Onset of Forearm Compartment Syndrome: A Complication of Distal Radius Fracture in Young Adults

Simpson NS, Jupiter JB (Massachusetts Gen Hosp, Boston)

J Orthop Trauma 9:411–418, 1995 3–33

Objective.—The outcome was reviewed in 5 patients having a total of 8 isolated intra-articular fractures of the distal radius in whom features of elevated pressure developed in the volar compartment of the forearm 18–54 hours after injury.

Clinical Aspects.—All 5 patients, 4 men and a woman, were younger than 45 years of age and were engaged in manual work when injured. All fractures were closed high-energy injuries, 7 caused by a fall and 1 by a motorcycle accident. All fractures were manipulated with the use of local anesthesia. A local hematoma block was performed in 5 cases and a Bier's block in 3. The fracture was better aligned after manipulation in all instances but, after 18–54 hours, the patients experienced increased pain and paresthesias in conjunction with tense swelling of the forearm. Pressures in the flexor forearm compartment ranged from 65 mm Hg to 90 mm Hg.

Management and Outcome.—The superficial and deep flexor compartments were decompressed along with the carpal tunnel via an anterior approach, without using a tourniquet. One patient also had the ulnar nerve and artery released bilaterally. In 5 of 8 extremities the flexor muscles appeared dark, edematous, and contused but regained a normal appearance after decompression. In most cases alignment was restored using the AO minidistractor attached to Schanz screws in the radius and second metacarpal. A volar buttress T plate was applied in 4 cases, and Kirschner wires were used to secure bony fragment in 7 cases. Evidence of compartment syndrome was eliminated within several hours in 6 instances. One patient required a second fasciotomy. Split-skin grafting was required for closure in 3 cases. Three of the 5 patients were able to resume their previous work. Bony union was achieved an average of 8 weeks after injury. Objective ratings of the wrist indicated a good outcome in 4 cases and a fair result in 3.

Conclusions.—There is a risk of delayed compartment syndrome developing after a high-energy fracture of the distal radius. When surgery is indicated, it is necessary to do a complete volar decompression.

► The authors call attention to the fact that selective recording of forearm intercompartmental pressures may be advised in patients at risk.

J.S. Torg, M.D.

Gymnast's Wrist (Pseudorickets Growth Plate Abnormality) in Adolescent Athletes: Findings on Plain Films and MR Imaging

Liebling MS, Berdon WE, Ruzal-Shapiro C, Levin TL, Roye D Jr, Wilkinson R (Columbia Presbyterian Med Center, New York)

AJR 164:157–159, 1995 3–34

Introduction.—Adolescents are engaging more and more in competitive sports in general, and in gymnastics in particular, making the so-called gymnast's wrist a matter of increasing interest.

Case Report.—Boy, 13½ years, was a competitive gymnast who sometimes worked out several hours a day, and who had pain in both wrists, chiefly in a dorsal and radial distribution. The pain was worsened by hanging from the rings or high bar. On examination, the patient described pain on full-forced dorsiflexion and

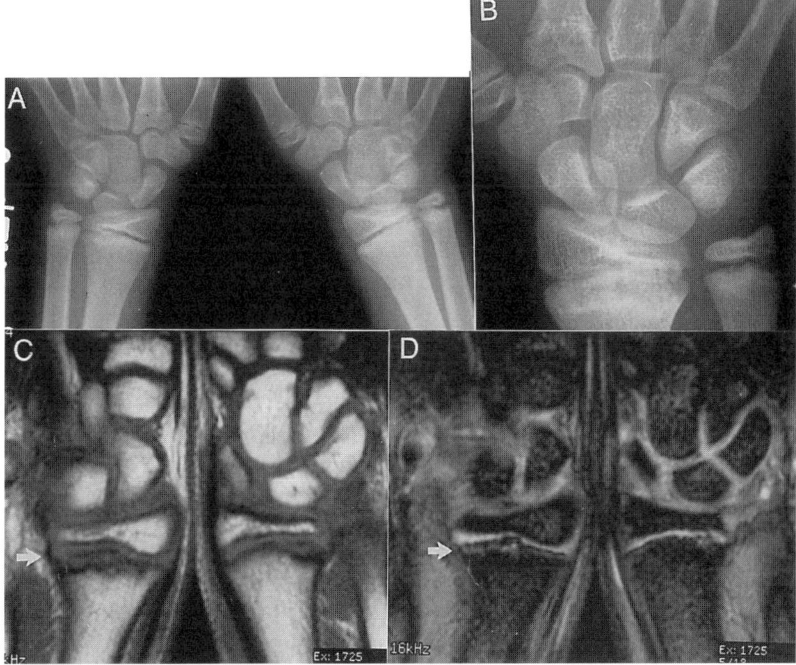

FIGURE 1.—Gymnast's wrist in a 13½-year-old boy. **A,** radiograph of the wrists shows slight widening of distal radial and—to a lesser extent—ulnar physes, and mild irregularity of bordering metaphyses. **B,** magnification radiograph of left wrist obtained 3 months after (**A**) because of continued pain shows interval progression of growth plate changes, which resemble those seen in rickets. Similar changes were seen on right side (not shown). **C,** coronal, 4-mm section T1-weight (600/17) MR image of 4-mm section of wrists shows line of intermediate signal intensity (*arrow*) proximal to and isointense with physis and irregularity of bordering high marrow signal of distal radial metaphysis. **D,** coronal gradient echo (600/22, 35 flip angle) MR image of 4-mm section of wrists shows a fine irregular line of high signal intensity (*arrow*) just proximal to normal high signal intensity of physis. (Courtesy of Liebling MS, Berdon WE, Ruzal-Shapiro C, et al: Gymnast's wrist [pseudorickets growth plate abnormality] in adolescent athletes: Findings on plain films and MR imaging. *AJR* 164:157–159, 1995.)

palmar flexion, and there was slight tenderness over the radial part of the wrist. Pain persisted 3 months later despite the use of splints and nonsteroidal anti-inflammatory drugs. Radiographs at this time demonstrated widened, irregular distal radial physes, especially on the left where pain was worse. Similar but less prominent changes were noted in the distal ulnar physes. Magnetic resonance images confirmed widened growth plates and irregular metaphyses, and demonstrated a fine, irregular line of high signal intensity near the open growth plate (Fig 1). The growth plates appeared radiographically more normal 6 months after the patient ceased activities that stressed the wrist.

Discussion.—The fact that the ligaments and joint capsule are substantially stronger than the open growth plate makes this site vulnerable to injury by compressive loading and shearing forces. Repeated microtrauma may produce temporary ischemia in the zone of provisional calcification, impairing calcification of the growth plate and resulting in physeal widening and metaphyseal irregularity. Stopping gymnastics is curative but may not be acceptable to the patient.

► This report includes useful photographs of the classic radiographic "pseudorickets" signs and the classic MRI signs of the growth plate injuries of "gymnast's wrist." Because the ligaments and joint capsule are 2–5 times stronger than the open growth plate, the latter takes the brunt of the injury, with ischemia, inhibited calcification, physeal widening, and metaphyseal irregularity. Similar changes can be seen in "catcher's knee." Gymnasts are prone to wrist injury because this joint bears much stress during the pommel horse, uneven parallel bars, and floor exercises. The use of dowel grips on the uneven parallel bars can worsen the injury.[1] In 1 survey, radiographic changes of gymnast's wrist were seen in 84% of top-flight adolescent gymnasts. The onset of wrist pain is gradual and usually worse with weight-bearing and dorsiflexion. Focal tenderness over the radial condyle may occur. With cessation of the causative stress, pain will subside and radiographic abnormalities will resolve without impairment of growth. These authors recommend pretraining and annual follow-up wrist radiographs to monitor injury in gymnasts who are skeletally immature.

E.R. Eichner, M.D.

Reference

1. 1992 Year Book of Sports Medicine, p 84.

Arthrography of the Wrist: Assessment of the Integrity of the Ligaments in Young Asymptomatic Adults

Kirschenbaum D, Sieler S, Solonick D, Loeb DM, Cody RP (Robert Wood Johnson Univ Hosp, New Brunswick, NJ)

J Bone Joint Surg (Am) 77–A:1207–1209, 1995 3–35

Introduction.—The value of wrist arthrography is limited because the prevalence of asymptomatic ligament perforations is unknown. Degenerative perforations of wrist ligaments are common after age 49 years. The prevalence of perforations of wrist ligaments of asymptomatic young and middle-aged adults was analyzed.

Methods.—Arthrography of the wrist was performed in 52 asymptomatic volunteers. The mean age of 38 men and 14 women was 28 years. All but 4 were right-hand dominant. The right wrists of 23 research subjects and the left wrists of 29 were randomly chosen for arthrography. Medical history was obtained and physical examination of both upper extremities was conducted. Measurements were taken of active motion with a goniometer, strength testing with a dynamometer, ballottement testing for impingement, and palpation for wrist tenderness.

Results.—In 14 (27%) of 52 wrists, communication of the contrast material was observed. Multiple communications were observed in 4 wrists with positive findings on the arthrogram. The most common positive finding in 6 of 14 wrists was a perforation of the triangular fibrocartilage alone. Other perforations were: 2 wrists—scapholunate ligament alone; 2 wrists—lunotriquetral ligament alone; 2 wrists—triangular fibrocartilage and the scapholunate and lunotriquetral ligaments; 1 wrist—triangular fibrocartilage and the scapholunate ligament; and 1 wrist—triangular fibrocartilage and the lunotriquetral ligament. There were no significant differences in range of motion or grip strength between wrists that were examined arthrographically and the contralateral wrists. No ballottement or tenderness was noted in any wrists. There were no significant differences in range of motion, grip strength, hand dominance, or sex between wrists with perforation and those with no perforation. Those wrists with perforation had a slightly larger positive ulnar variance, compared to those with no perforation.

Conclusion.—The usefulness of arthrography of the wrist may be limited. Ligament perforation is a common finding in young asymptomatic adults. A positive result on arthrography should be correlated with other clinical parameters.

► The clinical relevance of this study is that the arthrogram should not be considered a definitive study for diagnosis of a clinically important injury involving a wrist ligament.

J.S. Torg, M.D.

Factors Associated With Wrist Pain in the Young Gymnast

DiFiori JP, Puffer JC, Mandelbaum BR, Mar S (Univ of California, Los Angeles; Santa Monica Orthopaedics and Sports Medicine Group, Calif; Pacific Athletic Club, Pacific Palisades, Calif)

Am J Sports Med 24:9–14, 1996 3–36

Introduction.—Gymnastics is growing rapidly in popularity. The gymnast's upper extremities often are used to bear weight, subjecting the wrist in particular to compression, rotation, and distraction forces of considerable magnitude. Improper techniques and previous injury may render the gymnast at risk of wrist pain syndrome.

Objective.—Mechanisms of wrist pain were studied in 52 gymnasts aged 5–16 years. The participants, with an average age of 12 years, trained for 12 hours per week on average and had started at age 6½ years.

Findings.—Nearly three fourths of the gymnasts (73%) had had wrist pain in the past 6 months, a majority of them in both wrists. Pain was mainly present dorsally and most often was described as aching. Floor exercises were likeliest to have produced pain, but many subjects also associated pain with use of the pommel horse. Older and heavier subjects and those who had trained longer and more intensively were relatively likely to experience wrist pain. Those with pain had started training at a relatively late age.

Conclusion.—Whether a gymnast will experience wrist pain depends in part on the age at onset of training in relation to current age and the intensity of training.

▶ The stated purpose of this study was "to determine the prevalence of wrist pain in a group of nonelite young gymnasts, and determine the training factors associated with the pain." This has been accomplished with appropriate statistical substantiation. Unfortunately, the design of the study did not deal with several important points. Although the age of the individual was significantly correlated with wrist pain, the factor of skeletal maturity was not assessed. Most important, no explanation was forthcoming with regard to the cause of the pain. Also, the issue of whether modifying training loads will decrease the prevalence of the injury was not addressed.

J.S. Torg, M.D.

Acute Gamekeeper's Thumb: Quantitative Outcome of Surgical Repair

Downey DJ, Moneim MS, Omer GE Jr (Univ of New Mexico, Albuquerque)

Am J Sports Med 23:222–226, 1995 3–37

Background.—Chronic laxity affecting the thumb metacarpophalangeal joint, sometimes known as "gamekeeper's thumb," is most often the result of sporting injuries and falls on the thumb. Partial tears of the ulnar collateral ligament have been treated by plaster immobilization and complete tears either by this method or by operative repair. Diagnosis of a complete tear is required before operative treatment is undertaken. Ten consecutive patients with complete tears who had early surgical repair were followed for long-term outcome.

Methods.—The 10 patients had 11 complete ulnar collateral ligament tears, 9 of which resulted from athletic activities and 2 from domestic injuries. Patients had an average age of 35 years and underwent surgery an average of 6 days after injury. Diagnosis was based on clinical stress testing, with the contralateral thumb used to determine degree of laxity for the given patient. A complete tear was diagnosed by the absence of an end point in full extension and slight flexion. Complete tears were confirmed at surgery and repaired.

Results.—With an average follow-up of 42 months, patients subjectively reported pain as only an occasional mild ache. On a scale of 1–10, the mean level of pain was 1.6, the mean degree of strength was 9.3, and the mean functional score was 9.2. Range of motion in the involved joint was significantly decreased compared to that of the uninjured thumb (mean 50.9 degrees vs. 73.7 degrees). There was a trend toward decreased ulnar laxity in the affected thumbs, but the affected and contralateral thumbs were similar in grip, pulp pinch, key pinch, and radial laxity.

Conclusion.—Forceful radial deviation of the proximal phalanx results in acute instability of the ulnar side of the metacarpophalangeal joint of the thumb. A complete tear of the ulnar collateral ligament can be diagnosed accurately by stress testing. Partial tears are treated successfully with a cast but complete tears should be repaired surgically soon after the injury. Overall, repair achieved good long-term stability and strength with only slight loss of motion and occasional mild pain.

▶ The conclusions of the authors are in keeping with current orthopedic thinking. However, it should be pointed out that the study group was quite small and that there were no nonsurgically treated controls.

J.S. Torg, M.D.

4 Hips, Thighs, Knees, Foot, and Ankle

When Groin Pain Signals an Adductor Strain

Hasselman CT, Best TM, Garrett WE Jr (Univ of Pittsburgh, Pa; Univ of Wisconsin, Madison; Duke Univ, Durham, NC)

Physician Sportsmed 23:53–60, 1995 4–1

Introduction.—Thigh adductor strains most commonly occur in soccer players, although they have also been associated with hockey, football, tennis, horseback riding, bowling, and running. The adductor longus is the most frequently injured muscle. Patients usually report a groin "twinge" or "pull," indicating soft-tissue injury with severe groin pain that may render them unable to walk. When adductor injuries become chronic, patients may have either persistent groin pain that does not respond to conservative treatment or a painless mass in the groin. The diagnosis, treatment, and prevention of adductor strains were reviewed.

Diagnosis.—The diagnosis of adductor strains should emphasize history and physical examination. Most strains occur with forceful abduction of the thigh during adduction or with hyperabduction. The patient should be asked about the location, duration, severity, and quality of pain, together with any aggravating or alleviating factors. Most strains do not result in a palpable defect, although ecchymosis in the medial midthigh is a common finding. Inspection and palpation of the groin, the scrotum, and the abdominal musculature are performed, and active and passive range of motion are evaluated. Having the patient perform sit-ups against minimal resistance can help to differentiate between abdominal and adductor strains.

Imaging studies provide an important adjunct to the history and physical examination. Hip radiographs can be used to rule out fracture or joint disease. Herniography may detect hernias not found on physical examination. Computed tomography may be used for patients with persistent symptoms that are unexplained by history and physical examination. Magnetic resonance imaging can accurately localize the injury, but it cannot distinguish between acute injuries, chronic injuries, and delayed-onset muscle soreness.

Treatment.—Conservative management is used for acute strains and should be tried for chronic injuries. Immediate treatment includes ice, elevation, rest, and compression, followed in several days by heat, passive stretching, support bandages, and isometric strengthening. Nonsteroidal anti-inflammatory drugs, steroids, analgesics, and muscle relaxants may be useful. The authors recommend primary surgical repair for acute complete muscle ruptures, although this is controversial. Patients with chronic injury may need surgery if they have persistent pain that resists rehabilitation efforts.

Prevention.—Adductor strains may be avoided by proper warm-up techniques such as stretching. Static and proprioceptive neuromuscular facilitation stretches are thought to be more effective than ballistic stretching or bouncing. Strength training has also been recommended for the prevention of muscle strain.

Summary.—Muscle strain injury, usually of the adductor muscles, is a common cause of groin pain in athletes. Diagnosis is by history and physical examination, with CT or MRI reserved for uncertain cases. Management seeks to relieve pain and swelling and to restore early range of motion. Patients with acute complete muscle rupture or with chronic muscle rupture and persistent pain may require surgical repair. Research is needed to identify the best preventive measures.

► Groin pain in athletes may be very disabling and is usually caused by an injury to the adductor muscles. A related study, entitled Abdominal wall muscle tears in hockey players,[1] was abstracted and commented on in *Athletic Training Sports Health Care Perspectives.* G.A. Thibodeau in his comment states, "The authors confirm earlier speculation that sportsman's hernia is directly related to weakness of abdominal muscles in the floor of the inguinal ring. In addition they extend the diagnosis to hockey players and present evidence for the first time to show that actual thinning or tears in the floor of the inguinal ring (internal oblique muscles) are the causative factors."[2]

The authors of this study describe an excellent technique for making a differential diagnosis. They recommend using a minimally resisted sit-up to recreate the pain. If there is pain in the groin during this test, an injury of the abdominals should be suspected.

F.J. George, A.T.C., P.T.

References

1. Simonet WT, Saylor HL III, Sim L: Abdominal wall muscle tears in hockey players. *Int J Sports Med* 16:126–128, 1995.
2. Thibodeau GA: *Athletic Training Sports Health Care Perspectives.* Vol. 1, pp 393–394, 1995.

Surgical Release of the 'Snapping Iliopsoas Tendon'

Taylor GR, Clarke NMP (Southampton Univ Hosps NHS Trust, England)

J Bone Joint Surg (Br) 77-B:881–883, 1995 4–2

Purpose.—Pain snapping in the groin with an ache that radiates to the thigh may result from abnormal subluxation of the iliopsoas muscle at the iliopectineal eminence. This is a sporadically reported cause of hip pain that occurs mainly in young, active patients, such as dancers. Although surgical treatment has been reported, it is not widely known. Some cases of snapping iliopsoas tendon fail to respond to conservative treatment. The results of iliopsoas tendon release in 14 patients with "snapping psoas" were reported.

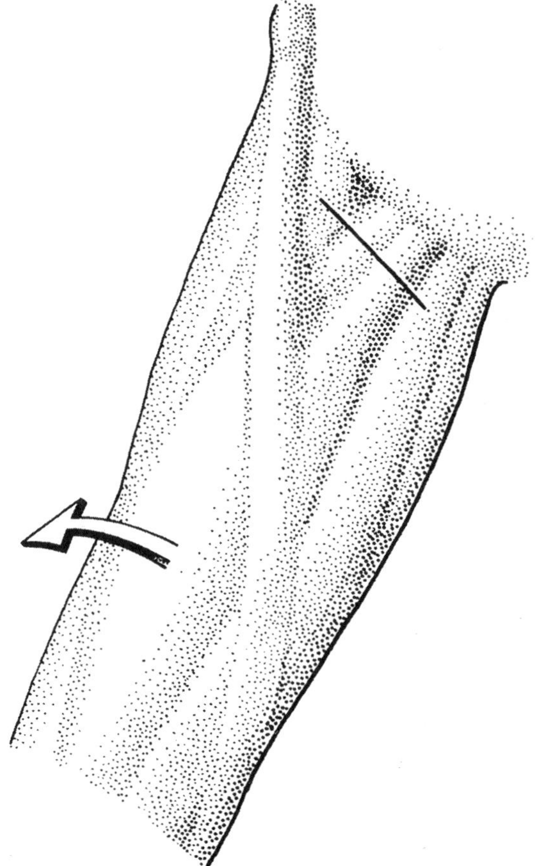

FIGURE 1.—Surface landmarks of the incision. The 5-cm incision straddles the palpable tendons of the adductors approximately 2.5 cm below and parallel to the inguinal skin crease. (Courtesy of Taylor GR, Clarke NMP: Surgical release of the 'snapping iliopsoas tendon.' *J Bone Joint Surg (Br)* 77-B: 881–883, 1995.)

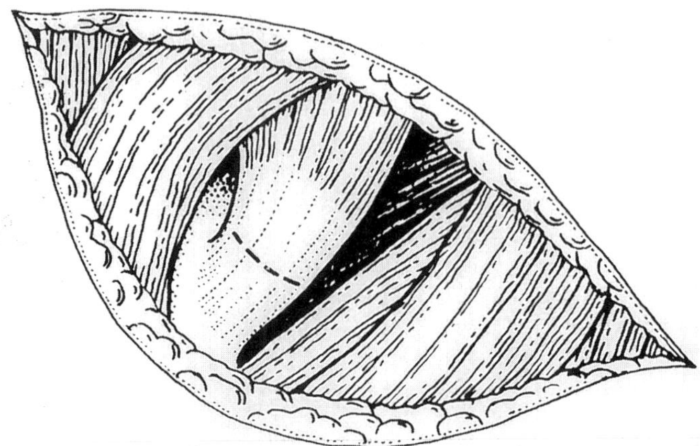

FIGURE 2.—Development of the incision. The fascia is divided and blunt dissection develops a plane between pectineus, medially, and adductor longus and the deeper brevis, laterally. External rotation of the leg delivers the lesser trochanter and the iliopsoas tendon into the wound. The tendinous part is cleared of areolar tissue, lifted, and divided (*dotted line*). (Courtesy of Taylor GR, Clarke NMP: Surgical release of the 'snapping iliopsoas tendon.' *J Bone Joint Surg (Br)* 77-B:881–883, 1995.)

Patients.—The patients were 19 women and 3 men (mean age, 21 years). All had painful snapping of the groin, followed by a dull ache that often radiated to the thigh and lasted for minutes to hours. In most patients, extension of the affected hip from a flexed, abducted, and externally rotated position reproduced the click. Most patients had tenderness in the adductor triangle. The results of plain radiography and arthrography were normal. Each patient received a clinical diagnosis of subluxation of the iliopsoas tendon.

Treatment and Outcomes.—Fourteen patients failed to respond to conservative management, which consisted of avoidance of provoking activities for at least 6 weeks and treatment with physiotherapy, including assisted extension and ultrasound. The 14 patients who still had symptoms underwent surgical release of the iliopsoas tendon. Two patients in this group had bilateral pain. The release was performed by a medial approach through a 5-cm horizontal incision over the palpable border of the adductors (Fig 1). The incision was developed to identify the iliopsoas tendon, the true tendinous portion of which was divided under direct vision (Fig 2). The associated muscle fibers were left intact.

At a mean follow-up of 17 months, the click had resolved in 10 of 16 hips. Five hips still had an occasional, painless click, and 1 hip was unchanged. There were no early complications, although 2 patients had some persistent flexion weakness of the hip.

Discussion.—The "snapping psoas" is a painful condition that may produce disproportionately disabling symptoms in a small number of patients. In cases that fail to respond to conservative measures, surgical release of the iliopsoas tendon can provide relief. The diagnosis can be made clinically using the "extension test" described in this report.

► This particular problem, although rare, may result in disproportionately disabling symptoms. The "extension test" described by the authors involves reproducing the click by extending the affected hip from a flexed, abducted, and externally rotated position. It should be noted that although the operation is generally successful in modifying the "iliopsoas snap" and relieving the pain, it does not always abolish it.

J.S. Torg, M.D.

Drop Leg Lachman Test: A New Test of Anterior Knee Laxity

Adler GG, Hoekman RA, Beach DM (Saint Mary's Hosp, Grand Rapids, Mich)

Am J Sports Med 23:320–323, 1995 4–3

Background.—For the determination of anterior cruciate ligament (ACL) laxity, the Lachman test has 85% accuracy with conscious patients and 100% accuracy with anesthetized patients. However, a large limb, control of flexion and contraction, lack of patient relaxation, and other difficulties all may confound the Lachman test. A modification, called the drop leg Lachman (DLL) test was developed and tested.

Methods.—To perform the DLL test, the patient is positioned supine with the leg abducted off the side of the table and flexed approximately 25 degrees. The examiner holds the patient's foot between his/her legs, stabilizes the thigh to the table with 1 hand, and applies the anteriorly directed force of the Lachman test with the other hand (Fig 1). Fifty-two patients having unilateral ACL deficiency were studied prospectively. The patients were examined with the DLL test either while conscious, under anesthesia, or both. A KT-1000 arthrometer was used to measure trans-

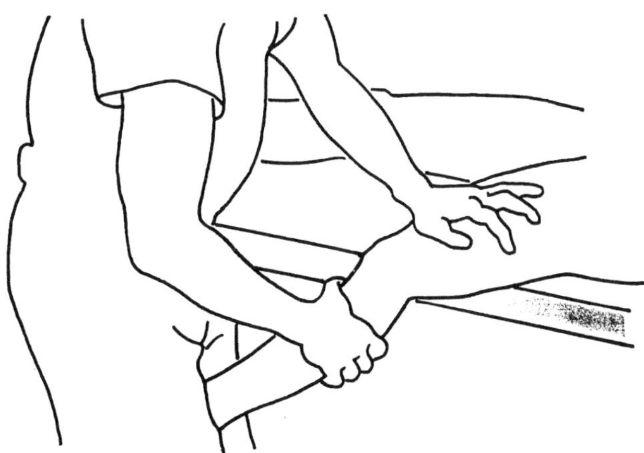

FIGURE 1.—The drop leg Lachman test is performed with the patient supine and the involved extremity abducted so that the knee can be flexed 25 degrees. (Courtesy of Adler GG, Hoekman RA, Beach DM: Drop leg Lachman test: A new test of anterior knee laxity. *Am J Sports Med* 23:320–323, 1995.)

lation with both the DLL and the traditional Lachman test in both injured and contralateral legs. The differences in results between the 2 tests were analyzed.

Results.—In conscious patients, the average displacement in intact knees was 4.3 mm with the Lachman test and 4.8 mm with the DLL test, whereas in injured knees, the average displacement was 8.1 mm with the Lachman test and 10.4 mm with the DLL test. In anesthetized patients, the average displacement in intact knees was 5.4 mm with the Lachman test and 5.3 mm with the DLL test; in injured knees, the average displacement was 10.5 mm with the Lachman test and 12.8 mm with the DLL test. There was no correlation between the magnitude of the difference between the 2 tests and previous surgery, previous injury, age, sex, weight, or the time since injury.

Conclusion.—Significantly greater anterior translation was measured in the majority of the ACL-deficient knees with the DLL test than with the Lachman test in both conscious and anesthetized patients. In addition, the DLL test is easier to perform than the traditional Lachman test.

▶ Lachman created the Lachman test, and Torg described it in 1976.[1] Feagin and Cooke proposed the prone examination for anterior cruciate ligament insufficiency.[2] Wroble and Lindenfeld described the stabilized Lachman test.[3] Now Adler, Hoekman and Beach have described the "drop leg Lachman test." Clearly, a rose by any other name would smell the same.

J.S. Torg, M.D.

References

1. Torg JS, Conrad W, Kalen V: Clinical diagnosis of anterior cruciate ligament instability in the athlete. *Am J Sports Med* 4:84–93, 1976.
2. Feagin JA, Cooke TDV: Prone examination for anterior cruciate ligament insufficiency. *J Bone Joint Surg* 71B:863, 1989.
3. Wroble RR, Lindenfeld TN: The stabilized Lachman test. *Clin Orthop* 237:209–212, 1988.

Derivation of a Decision Rule for the Use of Radiography in Acute Knee Injuries

Stiell IG, Greenberg GH, Wells GA, McKnight RD, Cwinn AA, Cacciotti T, McDowell I, Smith NA (Univ of Ottawa, Ont, Canada)
Ann Emerg Med 26:405–413, 1995 4–4

Objective.—In response to the need for more efficient use of radiography in the emergency department, an attempt was made to develop a decision rule for examining acute knee injuries. Such a guideline should identify all fractures and should be reliable and easily applied.

Methods.—To derive such a rule, a study was initiated including adult patients seen at 2 teaching hospital emergency departments who had acute blunt knee injuries occurring in the previous week. Twenty-three standardized clinical variables derived from clinical experience, the literature, and a pilot study were applied. Emergency physicians were trained to assess these variables in a standardized manner. The goal was to identify all fractures of the knee or patella, excluding avulsion fragments less than 5 mm wide that were not associated with a complete tendon or ligament disruption. Radiographs were interpreted by staff radiologists having no knowledge of the clinical findings.

Series.—All but 13% of 1,212 eligible patients were enrolled in the study during a 14-month period. Sixty-eight of the 1,047 study patients (6%) had a fracture, and 66 had clinically significant injuries. Radiography was done in the emergency department in 707 patients.

Results.—The final decision rule included 5 variables: age 55 years and older; tenderness over the head of the fibula; isolated patellar tenderness; inability to flex the knee to 90 degrees; and inability to bear weight. The presence of 1 or more of these findings would have identified all fractures with a specificity of 0.54. Radiographs would have been obtained from 49% of patients, rather than 69% as actually occurred.

Conclusion.—This clinically based decision rule is a practical, reliable, and very sensitive means of deciding when to obtain radiographs in patients seen in the emergency department with acute blunt knee injuries.

▶ The presence of 1 or more of the 5 cited findings identified fractures in the study population with the sensitivity of 1.0 (95% confidence interval) and specificity of 0.54 (95% confidence interval). Several modifiers were mentioned. Importantly, clinical application of the proposed decision rule should await prospective validation. Also, the rule is not applicable at this point to patients younger than 18 years of age. The authors believe that the most important benefit of their findings is the potential for more cost-effective patient management. They cite, on the basis of data, a potential for a 28% reduction in the use of radiography. Considering the recent position of the American Academy of Orthopaedic Surgeons that orthopedic surgeons are qualified to read plain radiographs, perhaps the radiologist is on his way to becoming a vestigial organism.

J.S. Torg, M.D.

Magnetic Resonance Imaging of Knee Disorders: Clinical Value and Cost-effectiveness in a Sports Medicine Practice

Gelb HJ, Glasgow SG, Sapega AA, Torg JS (Univ of Pennsylvania, Philadelphia)

Am J Sports Med 24:99–103, 1996 4–5

Background.—An increasing number of patients with knee injuries are undergoing MRI. The clinical value of MRI in such patients was investigated in a 3-part study.

Methods.—In the first part of the study, 72 consecutive patients were interviewed regarding the ordering of their MRI scan. Next, the treating physicians at 1 center were asked whether the MRI findings affected diagnosis or treatment. Finally, clinical assessments were compared with MRI findings in 37 patients who had diagnoses confirmed arthroscopically.

Findings.—The physicians believed that MRI results would have affected the diagnosis in 3 patients. Magnetic resonance findings were thought to contribute to patient treatment in only 14 of the 72 patients. When compared with arthroscopic findings, clinical assessment had a sensitivity and specificity of 100% for the diagnosis of anterior cruciate ligament injuries, and MRI had a sensitivity of 95% and a specificity of 88%. For isolated meniscal lesions, the sensitivity and specificity were 91% for clinical assessment and 82% and 87%, respectively, for MRI. Clinical assessment and MRI had a positive predictive value of 100% and 33%, respectively, for articular surface damage.

Conclusion.—Magnetic resonance imaging appears to be overused in the assessment of knee disorders. Compared with the assessment of a skilled examiner, MRI is not an accurate, cost-effective method for evaluating such injuries.

▶ The data presented support the concept that in many, if not most, instances, MRI of sports-related musculoskeletal problems is overutilized, overpriced, and over-read. Clearly, an adequate history and competent physical examination remain paramount in the orthopedist's diagnostic armamentarium.

J.S. Torg, M.D.

The Diagnosis of Acute Complete Tears of the Anterior Cruciate Ligament: Comparison of MRI, Arthrometry and Clinical Examination

Liu SH, Osti L, Henry M, Bocchi L (Univ of California, Los Angeles; Univ of Siena, Italy)

J Bone Joint Surg (Br) 77–B:586–588, 1995 4–6

Objective.—The usefulness of a number of clinical maneuvers for detecting complete tears of the anterior cruciate ligament (ACL) was determined in 38 patients who underwent arthrometry as well as MRI. The patients, 27 males and 11 females 16 to 43 years of age, were all operated on within 3 weeks after injury. All had sports-related injuries.

Methods.—All patients were first examined within a week of injury, the average interval being 3 days. The same examiner performed a Lachman test, an anterior-drawer test at 90 degrees of knee flexion, and a pivot-shift test. The patients then were tested with a KT-1000 arthrometer at 15 and 20 lb of active displacement. A side-to-side difference exceeding 3 mm was considered a positive result. Magnetic resonance imaging was performed using a surface coil with the leg extended and externally rotated up to 20 degrees.

Results.—Magnetic resonance imaging detected all but 3% of ACL injuries, but it was only 82% sensitive for complete ruptures. The best clinical results were obtained using the Lachman test and arthrometry. Arthrometry was 97% sensitive using a displacement criterion of 3 mm and 100% sensitive at 2 mm. The Lachman test detected 95% of injuries. The drawer and pivot-shift tests were the least sensitive methods.

Conclusion.—Magnetic resonance imaging is not necessary before deciding to reconstruct a completely ruptured ACL.

▶ The findings and conclusions of the authors are in keeping with our recently published report on the clinical value and cost-effectiveness of MRI of knee disorders in the sports medicine practice.[1]

J.S. Torg, M.D.

Reference

1. Gelb HJ, Glasgow SG, Sapega AA, et al: Magnetic resonance imaging of knee disorders: Clinical value and cost-effectiveness in a sports medicine practice. *Am J Sports Med* 24:99–103, 1996.

Partial ACL Rupture: An MR Diagnosis?

Yao L, Gentili A, Petrus L, Lee JK (Univ of California, Los Angeles; Samaritan Hosp, Troy, NY)

Skeletal Radiol 24:247–251, 1995 4–7

Background.—The ability of MRI to distinguish between partial and complete anterior cruciate ligament (ACL) ruptures has not been established. Such a distinction may have an effect on prognosis and management. A study to clarify the ability to make such a distinction was undertaken.

Methods.—Eighty-eight patients underwent arthroscopy and MRI. Thirty-six of these patients had normal ACLs, 21 had partial ACL ruptures, and 31 had complete ACL ruptures. Scans were interpreted by an experienced clinician unaware of other findings. The scans were scored for 4 primary and 7 secondary signs.

Findings.—The sensitivity of MRI was lower for partial than for complete ACL ruptures. On MRI, most detected partial ACL ruptures looked like complete ruptures. Although secondary signs did not significantly improve the detection of partial ACL ruptures, they did help distinguish partial from complete ACL ruptures. Complete ACL rupture was indicated by displacement of the posterior horn of the lateral meniscus and popliteus muscle injury.

Conclusion.—Magnetic resonance imaging shows most partial ACL ruptures. However, MRI is less sensitive for partial than for complete ACL ruptures. Distinguishing between partial and complete ACL ruptures on MR assessment can be improved slightly by the use of secondary signs.

Diagnosis of Partial Tears of the Anterior Cruciate Ligament of the Knee: Value of MR Imaging

Umans H, Wimpfheimer O, Haramati N, Applbaum YH, Adler M, Bosco J (Albert Einstein College, Bronx, NY)
AJR 165:893–897, 1995 4–8

Background.—Magnetic resonance imaging is sensitive and specific in the diagnosis of complete anterior cruciate ligament (ACL) rupture. In this case-control study, MR findings in patients with arthroscopically proven partial ACL tears were compared with findings in patients with complete ACL tears or no evidence of injury.

Methods.—All reports of arthroscopy performed at 2 institutions during 1990–1992 and 1992–1993, respectively, revealed 13 patients with partial ACL tears. Thirteen patients with intact ACLs and 13 with completely ruptured ACLs were selected randomly from the same period to serve as controls. Diagnostic criteria included the absence of findings of complete ACL tear together with abnormal intrasubstance signal, bowing of the ACL, or nonvisualization of the ACL on 1 MRI sequence with visualization of intact fibers on other sequences.

Findings.—Magnetic resonance imaging had a sensitivity of 40% to 75% and a specificity of 62% to 89% for detecting partial ACL tears. Variability in both interobserver and intraobserver interpretations was greater than 0.7 kappa in all combinations but 1 when comparing the diagnostic consistency of each of 3 readers with himself, using 2 readings on separate days, and with each separate interpretation by the other 2 radiologists.

Conclusion.—Magnetic resonance imaging is not sensitive enough to establish the diagnosis of partial ACL tears without arthroscopy. However, this study had certain limitations, such as a small sample size and the heterogeneity of the MRI technique.

► Clearly, diagnosis of complete disruption of the ACL is predicted on clinical examination, i.e., a positive Lachman test. The unacceptable sensitivity and specificity of MRI in diagnosing partial ACL tears further negates the use of this imaging technique in evaluating trauma to the knee joint. To be noted: Umans et al. conclude that "Our results show that MR evaluation of partial ACL tears is not sufficiently sensitive to establish the diagnosis without arthroscopy". If that be the case, who needs MRI?

J.S. Torg, M.D.

Open Versus Closed Chain Kinetic Exercises After Anterior Cruciate Ligament Reconstruction: A Prospective Randomized Study

Bynum EB, Barrack RL, Alexander AH (Naval Med Ctr, Oakland, Calif)
Am J Sports Med 23:401–406, 1995 4–9

Objective.—Opinions differ regarding the optimum strength training protocol after anterior cruciate ligament (ACL) reconstruction. Closed kinetic chain exercises performed at full flexion are thought to add joint stability. Open chain exercises, on the other hand, performed at 30 degrees to 90 degrees, create shearing forces across the joint. The results of a prospective, randomized study of open and closed kinetic chain exercises during accelerated rehabilitation to determine if closed chain exercises are safe and more effective than conventional rehabilitation were presented.

Methods.—After reconstruction of the ACL, 100 patients (9 women) aged 18–48 years were randomly assigned to 1 of the 2 protocols. Evaluations using the Lysholm knee function scoring scale, a modified Tegner activity rating scale, and patient assessments were performed preoperatively and at 3-month intervals postoperatively for 1 year and then yearly by blinded orthopedic residents. The average follow-up was 19 months.

Results.—Three patients did not complete the study. There were 47 patients in the open kinetic chain protocol and 50 patients in the closed kinetic chain protocol. Surgery restored stability in more than 90% of knees. Severe patellofemoral pain was reported by 42% of patients before surgery and 21% after surgery. Subjective improvement, Lysholm score, and Tegner activity level increased significantly after surgery. In 95% of patients, full range of motion was restored. The closed kinetic chain group had lower mean KT-1000 arthrometer side-to-side differences and less patellofemoral pain in all follow-up periods, rated their results as excellent or good, and believed they returned to their daily activities and sports activities faster than expected.

Conclusion.—The closed chain kinetic exercises are safe and yield better objective and subjective results than do the open chain kinetic exercises in patients with ACL reconstruction.

► This study confirmed the findings of other studies that using closed chain exercises in the early rehabilitation stages of ACL-reconstructed knees is better than using open chain methods. In fact, a closed chain accelerated exercise protocol is now considered conventional in the rehabilitation of ACL reconstruction using patella tendon grafts. The authors confirm a number of advantages to using this type of program. There is less stiffness and patellofemoral pain. The program is safe because it puts less stress on the maturing graft and the patellofemoral joint. According to the authors, it is cost-effective and convenient and has excellent patient acceptance and satisfaction. There is also less chance of residual losses of range of motion in both extension and flexion.

The authors have accepted this type of program for their ACL reconstructions. Please read Abstracts 4–10 and 4–11.

F.J. George, A.T.C., P.T.

Ligament Stability Two to Six Years After Anterior Cruciate Ligament Reconstruction With Autogenous Patellar Tendon Graft and Participation in Accelerated Rehabilitation Program

Shelbourne KD, Klootwyk TE, Wilckens JH, De Carlo MS (Methodist Sports Medicine Ctr, Indianapolis, Ind)

Am J Sports Med 23:575–579, 1995 4–10

Introduction.—Accelerated rehabilitation programs for patients with anterior cruciate ligament (ACL) reconstruction were developed to avoid the stiffness, weakness, and patellofemoral problems associated with traditional restrictive rehabilitation approaches. However, observations in animals have raised concerns about possible graft stretching or graft failure resulting from accelerated rehabilitation after ACL reconstruction. Patients from 1 accelerated rehabilitation program were studied for signs of patellar tendon graft stretching.

Methods.—The study included 209 patients who underwent autogenous central-third patellar tendon graft ACL reconstruction and followed the same postoperative accelerated rehabilitation program. In this program, the emphasis was on early full hyperextension, early weight-bearing as tolerated, and closed-chain functional activities. When patients reached full range of motion and approximately 65% of strength and were able to perform prescribed running and agility drills, they were permitted to return to sports participation. To be eligible for the study, patients had to have KT-1000 arthrometer follow-up at the time they reached full range of motion and at 2 years or longer after surgery. The data were examined for signs of a change in the length of the patellar tendon graft, as indicated by a KT-1000 arthrometer manual maximum difference between the operated and normal knees.

Results.—The patients took an average of 12 weeks to reach full range of motion. The average KT-1000 arthrometer measurement was 2.06 mm at that time and 2.10 mm at an average follow-up of 3 years. The difference was nonsignificant. The difference between the involved and uninvolved knees was 3 mm or less initially in 78% of patients; at follow-up, it was 83%. The patients' responses to modified Noyes questionnaires showed an average stability score of 19.6. Only 3% of patients had any complaints of instability.

Conclusion.—For patients undergoing ACL reconstruction, accelerated rehabilitation does not appear to alter long-term stability, as reflected by KT-1000 arthrometer measurements. In their experience of 2–6 years with a program of early full hyperextension, early introduction of functional activities, and rapid return to sports, the authors have not observed stretching or instability of the patellar tendon graft.

▶ This is another study from Dr. Shelbourne who is considered to be the first to describe the accelerated rehabilitation program for ACL reconstruction.[1] This should be read with the previous study (Abstract 4–9), which confirms the effectiveness of the accelerated closed chain program. This study confirms the fact that the patella tendon grafts maintain their integrity for up to 6 years, with the average of 209 patients being tested at 3 years after repair.

As I stated after the previous study, the closed chain accelerated program has become the conventional rehabilitation program for ACL reconstructed knees using patella tendon grafting. T.A. Blackburn, in commenting on this study, states, "I still find an alarming number of patients that are not allowed to progress in their post-operative programs because of excuses that the graft will stretch out. Patients with this type of surgery may be weight bearing as soon as possible, may move the involved leg through a full range of motion, may use any muscle group they want in open and closed chain positions, and progress their functional activities as they develop the range of motion, strength, power, endurance, proprioception and joint healing necessary to move from one stage to the next at their own speed."[2]

F.J. George, A.T.C., P.T.

References

1. Shelbourne KD, Nitz P: Accelerated rehabilitation after anterior cruciate ligament reconstruction. *Am J Sports Med* 18:292–299, 1990.
2. Blackburn TA: *Athletic Training Sports Health Care Perspectives* Vol. 2, pp 166–167, 1996.

Strength of the Quadriceps Femoris Muscle and Functional Recovery After Reconstruction of the Anterior Cruciate Ligament: A Prospective, Randomized Clinical Trial of Electrical Stimulation

Synder-Mackler L, Delitto A, Bailey SL, Stralka SW (Univ of Delaware, Newark; Univ of Pittsburgh, Pa; Washington Univ, St Louis, et al)

J Bone Joint Surg (Am) 77–A:1166–1173, 1995 4–11

Introduction.—Causes for incomplete recovery of the quadriceps femoris after surgery are still elusive. An earlier study involving few patients demonstrated that judiciously administered regimens of electric stimulation improve the recovery of the quadriceps femoris in the first 6 weeks after surgery. After reconstruction of the anterior cruciate ligament (ACL), the effectiveness of electric stimulation as an adjunct to ongoing intensive rehabilitation in the early postoperative phase was assessed, specifically the strength of the quadriceps femoris muscle and some variables of gait.

Methods.—After reconstruction of the ACL, 110 patients were divided into 4 groups: 31 received treatment with high-intensity neuromuscular electric stimulation; 34 received high-level volitional exercise; 25 received low-intensity neuromuscular electric stimulation; and 20 received combined high- and low-intensity neuromuscular electric stimulation. All of the rehabilitation treatment was isometrically performed with the knee flexed at 65 degrees. All patients performed intensive closed kinetic chain exercises. Measurements were taken of the strength of the quadriceps femoris muscle and kinematics of the knee during stance phase after 4 weeks of treatment.

Results.—In the groups that received high-intensity stimulation, either alone or combined with low-intensity electric stimulation, the quadriceps strength averaged 70% or more of the strength of the uninvolved side. In the group that received high-level volitional exercise, the quadriceps strength averaged 57%, whereas in the group treated with low-intensity electric stimulation, quadriceps strength averaged 51%. The strength of the quadriceps was significantly and directly correlated with the kinematics of the knee joint. The type of operation performed also significantly affected the recovery of the quadriceps and the gait. Patients who had reconstruction of the ACL with the use of an autologous patellar-ligament graft did poorly when compared with the others.

Discussion.—There is a clear advantage to using high-intensity electric stimulation to restore the strength of the quadriceps, and there is no advantage to using low-intensity stimulation. Open kinetic chain exercises for the quadriceps femoris, such as 15 contractions 3 times a week, combined with high-intensity electric stimulation improves the recovery of the quadriceps and the functional outcome after reconstruction of the ACL.

▶ The authors express concern about the persistent weakness of the quadriceps muscle, which is seen in many patients who have undergone ACL reconstruction and are rehabilitated using only closed chain exercises. They report on significant differences in quadriceps strength in those subjects who received high-intensity electric stimulation. They also comment on the significance and correlation between quadriceps strength and kinematics of the knee joint. They state, "First, there is a tendency for patients who have a weak quadriceps femoris muscle to hold the knee in slight flexion at heel-strike and to continue to flex only slightly after heel-strike...Second, they fail to demonstrate a dynamic return to an extended position during mid-stance...; the knee is held in slight flexion throughout the period of single limb support." They also point out that judicious application of open kinetic chain exercises for the quadriceps femoris muscle (with the knee in a position that does not stress the graft) with the use of high-intensity neuromuscular electric stimulation improves the strength of this muscle and the functional outcome after reconstruction of the ACL.

F.J. George, A.T.C., P.T.

Femoral Nerve Block as an Alternative to Parenteral Narcotics for Pain Control After Anterior Cruciate Ligament Reconstruction

Edkin BS, Spindler KP, Flanagan JFK (Vanderbilt Univ, Nashville, Tenn)

Arthroscopy 11:404–409, 1995 4–12

Background.—Significant postoperative pain follows anterior cruciate ligament (ACL) reconstruction. Parenteral narcotics are usually required.

Femoral nerve block (FNB) after arthroscopically assisted ACL reconstruction with autograft patellar tendon was evaluated prospectively. Parenteral narcotic administration was used as an indicator of clinical efficacy.

Methods and Findings.—Twenty-four patients underwent arthroscopically assisted autograft patellar tendon ACL reconstruction using Winnie's "3-in-1" FNB as the main method of postoperative pain control. Ninety-two percent of the patients received no parenteral narcotics after FNB. Ninety-five percent said that FNB was beneficial and that they would request it again. The mean duration of pain control was 29 hours. Seventy-nine percent of the patients believed that they could be discharged within 23 hours. Two patients, or 8%, did not respond to FNBs. No major complications occurred.

Conclusion.—Femoral nerve block is a safe, reliable, effective form of analgesia after ACL reconstruction. When successful, it eliminates the need for parenteral narcotics. In addition, patients tolerate FNB well. Thus, FNB is a valuable adjunct to ACL reconstruction surgery.

► In view of the established efficacy of local anesthesia with IV sedation in the performance of virtually all surgical arthroscopic procedures except those involving ligamentous reconstruction, I question the use of either an FNB or a "3-in-1" nerve block for routine procedures. However, the femoral and 3-in-1 nerve blocks appear to be useful adjuncts in the control of post-ACL reconstruction pain. It would appear that this would be particularly so if the procedure is done on an outpatient basis.

J.S. Torg, M.D.

Functional Knee Bracing

Liu SH, Mirzayan R (Univ of California, Los Angeles)

Clin Orthop 317:273–281, 1995 4–13

Background.—With the development of advanced surgical techniques for reconstruction of the anterior cruciate ligament (ACL), the results of treatment for knee injuries have improved. As the number of functional knee braces prescribed increases, so does the number of commercially available braces. However, studies of the effectiveness of such braces have yielded conflicting results. Current knowledge of the effectiveness of functional knee bracing was reviewed.

Findings.—The review includes the results of static and dynamic studies of knee bracing and a comparison of custom vs. off-the-shelf functional knee braces. The available data suggest that the performance of functional knee braces depends, in large part, on soft-tissue compliance. For example, brace function appears to be enhanced by the presence of a bulky thigh compartment. Studies of design characteristics have found that the optimal hinge design is one that matches the knee joint's kinematic characteristics and axis of rotation. Compared with custom-made braces, off-the-shelf braces offer the advantages of greater accessibility and lower cost. It remains uncertain whether custom braces are any more effective than off-the-shelf braces. Restraint of anterior tibial displacement appears to be greatest with shell, bilateral hinge-type brace designs. In addition, these braces are more durable than strap-type braces.

Discussion.—Along with other advances, functional knee bracing has improved the results of treatment for ACL injuries and permitted injured athletes to return to their previous activity level. The comprehensive rehabilitation protocol for knees with ACL deficiency and ACL reconstruction should include functional knee bracing. Further study is needed to establish the effectiveness of different types of off-the-shelf braces.

▶ Where are we with functional knee bracing for ACL-deficient knees and postsurgical ACL knees? In the 1970s and 1980s, all our ACLs, both the postsurgical and ACL-deficient knees, wore a functional knee brace. In the 1990s, we have seemed to lose confidence in these braces and what we were expecting of them. Perhaps we were expecting too much. It may have taken 20 years, but we have come to realize that there is no brace that will take the place of a normal ACL. We are expecting less from these braces now and understand their limitations better.

Because of these lower expectations, we are, again, becoming more receptive to braces. They are not weightless; they are not completely comfortable; they may not provide complete protection in a stressful situation. However, the athlete may feel better using one, and function may be improved. It has been difficult to prove this improved function because of an increase in proprioceptive feedback, but that may be the case. The authors state, "Functional knee bracing does have a role in the treatment of patients with anterior cruciate ligament deficiency and anterior cruciate ligament reconstruction... [it] should be an integral part of a comprehensive rehabilitation program..."

F.J. George, A.T.C., P.T.

Comparison of Two Regional Anesthetic Techniques for Knee Arthroscopy

Bonicalzi V, Gallino M (Ospedale Molinette, Torino, Italy; Ospedale Gradenigo, Torino, Italy)

Arthroscopy 11:207–212, 1995 4–14

Background.—Regional anesthesia of the lower limb is a rational and effective approach to anesthesia for patients undergoing arthroscopic knee surgery. The "3-in-1" block—in which the femoral, lateral femoral cutaneous, and obturator nerves are blocked with a single injection—has been reported to be useful for this purpose. The 3-in-1 block was compared with femoral nerve block (FNB) for knee arthroscopy.

Methods.—The prospective, randomized study included 280 inpatients admitted for knee arthroscopy. One hundred patients were assigned to receive 3-in-1 block and 180 to receive FNB. All patients were premedicated with atropine and diazepam. Four anesthesiologists experienced in performing lower extremity blocks for orthopedic surgery performed all blocks. The 3-in-1 block was performed using a total of 20 mL of 0.5% bupivacaine without epinephrine. The 2 groups were compared for the success of regional anesthesia, for various pain-related factors, and for side effects.

Results.—The 3-in-1 block successfully provided anesthesia for 75 of 100 patients assigned to it. Twenty required supplemental local anesthesia and 5 required conversion to general anesthesia. Femoral nerve block was successful in 88 of 180 patients. Intravenous flunitrazepam and/or fentanyl was necessary in 90 patients and general anesthesia in 2. Muscle relaxation was better and postoperative analgesia longer lasting with the 3-in-1 block. Neither group experienced any side effects.

Conclusion.—The 3-in-1 block appears to be the most reliable, safe, and effective regional anesthetic technique for knee arthroscopy. The 3-in-1 block provides a deep, profound, and prolonged anesthesia that allows the surgeon to maneuver without difficulty.

Local Anesthesia for Knee Arthroscopy: Efficacy and Cost Benefits

Shapiro MS, Safran MR, Crockett H, Finerman GAM (Univ of California, Los Angeles)

Am J Sports Med 23:50–53, 1995 4–15

Background.—Knee arthroscopy is the most common orthopedic surgical procedure in the United States. Arthroscopic procedures can be performed successfully using local anesthesia, but many orthopedic surgeons do not use it, possibly because of fear that the surgery will take longer, that it is not useful for arthroscopic surgery, or that the anesthesia will be ineffective and patients will be dissatisfied. The efficacy of local, regional, and general anesthesia in knee arthroscopy was evaluated retrospectively.

Methods.—In 123 patients between 16 and 71 years of age, 165 arthroscopic procedures were performed. Of the 165 procedures, 124 were performed using local anesthesia with minimal IV sedation, 35 using general endotracheal anesthesia, and 6 using spinal-epidural blocks or regional anesthesia. Medical records were reviewed for surgical time, efficacy of anesthesia, complications, and recuperation time before discharge. Patient satisfaction was also recorded.

Results.—Local anesthesia did not increase operative time and shortened recovery time; patient satisfaction was also high. Procedures successfully completed using local anesthesia included partial meniscectomy, débridement, abrasion arthroplasty, lysis of adhesions, loose body removal, synovectomy, meniscal repair, lateral release, and plica resection. There were no complications.

Discussion.—These findings show that local anesthesia for outpatient knee arthroscopy is effective and less costly than other anesthetic techniques and results in high patient satisfaction. Some orthopedic surgeons may not be familiar with the local anesthesia technique for knee arthroscopy. It is also believed that expertise is required because more precise portal location and technique are required when using local anesthesia. Local anesthesia is recommended for most patients scheduled for knee arthroscopy on an outpatient basis.

► The findings of the authors confirm our previously published paper entitled "Arthroscopic surgery of the knee under local anesthesia."[1] One major point that I disagree with is the suggestion that midazolam hydrochloride be used as the IV sedative. Our experience has been that use of this agent—which has a central action resulting in nervous system disinhibition and quadriceps spasm—can make the procedure most difficult to perform. Also, propofol predisposes the patient to excessive verbal communication, which can be somewhat distracting for the surgeon. I personally recommend that fentanyl in intravenous doses of 1 to 3 mg be used for sedation.

J.S. Torg, M.D.

Reference

1. Yacobucci: GN, Bruce R, Conahan TJ, et al: Arthroscopic surgery of the knee under local anesthesia. *Arthroscopy* 6:311–314, 1990.

Arthroscopic Posteromedial Visualization of the Knee

Boytim MJ, Smith JP, Fischer DA, Quick DC (Minneapolis Sports Medicine Ctr)

Clin Orthop 310:82–86, 1995 4–16

Introduction.—Arthroscopic posteromedial visualization of the knee is a technique in which the posteromedial compartment is entered and visualized through an anterolateral portal. Although this technique is simple to perform, has some key diagnostic and treatment advantages, and poses little risk of complications, it is not commonly used. The posteromedial compartment is commonly involved in such articular problems as tears of the posterior horn of the medial meniscus and loose bodies. The value of posteromedial visualization was demonstrated in a prospective study.

Methods.—The study included 3 orthopedic surgeons who performed posteromedial visualization in each of 117 consecutive patients undergoing arthroscopy. This was done through a standard anterolateral portal by placing the arthroscope in the medial aspect of the intercondylar notch. With the knee in 40 to 60 degrees of flexion, the arthroscope was moved medially to the posterior cruciate ligament until it entered the posterior compartment. Visualization of the posteromedial compartment was enhanced by changing from a 30-degree to a 70-degree arthroscope. The surgeons rated the value of posteromedial visualization for each patient.

Results.—The study patients were undergoing arthroscopy for diagnosis and/or treatment of 209 pathologic conditions, the most common being tears of the medial meniscus. The surgeons rated posteromedial visualization procedure as easy to perform in 78% of patients. It was more difficult in patients with degenerative joint disease. The surgeons rated posteromedial visualization as helpful for diagnosis or treatment in 13% of cases and essential in another 4% of cases. Its value was greatest for patients with tears of the posterior horn of the medial meniscus, especially for those tears that were undetected by visualization from the anteromedial compartment alone. Eighty-nine percent of patients were rated as having adequate visualization of the posteromedial compartment. The procedure carried no morbidity.

Conclusion.—For most patients undergoing arthroscopy of the knee, posteromedial visualization is easy to perform, entails little risk of morbidity, and allows good visualization of the posteromedial compartment. In some patients, it can detect conditions that might be missed by visualization from the anteromedial compartment alone. Posteromedial visualization should be a routine part of arthroscopic knee examination.

The Posteromedial Portal in Knee Arthroscopy: An Analysis of Diagnostic and Surgical Utility

Gold DL, Schaner PJ, Sapega AA (Univ of Pennsylvania, Philadelphia)

Arthroscopy 11:139–145, 1995 4–17

Introduction.—The gold standard for the diagnosis of intra-articular knee disorders is arthroscopy. This is in spite of the "blind spots" to the arthroscope, including the posterior periphery of the menisci, the posterior cruciate ligament and the posterior capsule, which can lead to false negative findings. If there is going to be a site of diagnostic errors, the posteromedial corner of the knee is the likely site. This is a result of using the anterior portal for diagnosis of posteromedial lesions. Obviously, the scope must be inserted where it is most needed in the joint. Clinical experience with the use of the posteromedial portal was reported.

Methods.—The authors retrospectively reviewed the records of 400 consecutive arthroscopies. Routine anterior and medial portals were used. Supplemental posteromedial portals were used where indicated, in accordance with established indications. If a posteromedial portal was found to have been used, clinical indications, technical information about the surgery and surgical notes and other pertinent records were obtained.

Results.—A total of 400 surgeries were reviewed. A posteromedial portal was not necessary in 73 cases because of the nature of their problem. In 61 of the remaining 327 cases, a posteromedial portal was used for a total of 18.5% of cases. A diagnostic portal alone was used in 42 cases and 2 portals (diagnostic and surgical) were used in 17 cases. The need to examine of the posterior periphery of the medical meniscus was the reason for 92% of the diagnostic portals. Thirteen of the 19 surgical posteromedial portals were for meniscal débridement or meniscectomy. There were a total of 78 posteromedial portals made in the 327 patients. Two thirds of the 59 diagnostic portals yielded treatable lesions. The use of this portal was mostly for the treatment of the medical meniscus. Ten percent of the medical meniscectomies involved using the posteromedial portal. There were 22 patients in whom a medial meniscal tear was seen only by using the posteromedial portal. The only complications involved 1 patient with a partial loss of saphenous nerve sensation, which could have been the result of other surgical work done at the same operation, and a patient who had serous drainage after walking 3 miles on the first postoperative day.

Conclusion.—There appear to be 2 indications for the use of the posteromedial portal: first, when posteromedial lesions are frequent (such as in anterior cruciate ligament–deficient knees) on the basis of preoperative symptoms or prior imaging studies; second, when complete visualization of the full superior meniscosynovial junction cannot be accomplished using normal anterior portals. If a frontal approach is either inefficient or unsuccessful, one should consider using the posteromedial approach.

▶ The position of the authors in Abstracts 4–16 and 4–17—that visualization of the posterior medial compartment should be performed in routine arthroscopic examinations—is well taken. A third technique worth mentioning is a direct posterior medial portal. This portal requires that the knee be fully distended and runs the danger of injury to the saphenous vein.

J.S. Torg, M.D.

Optimizing Arthroscopic Knots

Loutzenheiser TD, Harryman DT, Yung S-W, France MP, Sidles JA (Univ of Washington, Seattle)

Arthroscopy 11:199–206, 1995 4–18

Introduction.—The need to use instruments rather than fingers to secure sutures may be 1 reason why arthroscopic suture repairs may be less secure than the same procedure performed in open fashion. Many of the knots tied during arthroscopy consist of an initial slip knot to remove slack, followed by a series of half-hitches. The latter may be difficult to avoid when asymmetric tension is applied to the strands; thus, the security of arthroscopically tied knots may be less than that of square knots. A series of experiments were performed in an attempt to determine why certain knots are successful and others fail.

Methods.—After extensive practice, 8 different configurations of knots were tied by hand and with a knot pusher (Fig 1). The various knots were compared for security under cyclic and peak loading conditions.

Results.—Knot configurations in which the half-hitch throws were reversed and the posts alternated were the most secure (Fig 6). Knots begun with a simple slip knot failed immediately. Hand-tied knots showed better loop-holding capacity than identical knots tied using a pusher.

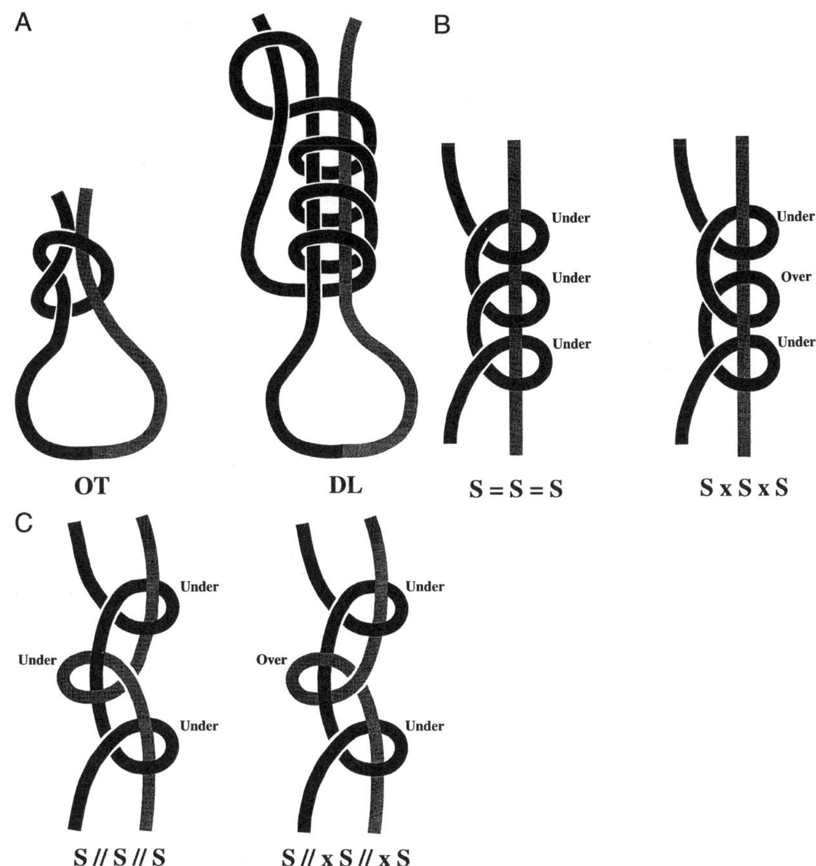

FIGURE 1.—A, the slip knot configurations shown were used initially to remove slack from the suture loop. The overhand throw sliding knot (*OT*) configuration designates the simple overhand throw and the Duncan loop sliding knot (*DL*) configuration designates the complex Duncan loop configuration. **B,** the half-hitch configurations shown represent 2 combinations that do not incorporate post switching. The labels "over" and "under" indicate the direction for the initial pass around the post when making each half-hitch loop. Note that the direction of the half-hitch loops are reversed for the SxSxS configuration. **C,** the half-hitch configurations shown represent 2 combinations that incorporate post switching and reversal of the loop direction. Note that the S//xS//xS configuration combines post switching and loop direction reversal. (Courtesy of Loutzenheiser TD, Harryman DT, Yung S-W, et al: Optimizing arthroscopic knots. *Arthroscopy* 11:199–206, 1995.)

Conclusion.—When tying knots arthroscopically, the surgeon can best control holding capacity and minimize suture loop displacement by properly alternating the tying strands and reversing the loop with placing hitches. The security of arthroscopic knots can be optimized by careful attention to the specific techniques by which knot throws are made. Arthroscopic surgeons should practice and examine pusher-tied knots to optimize consistency before using them clinically.

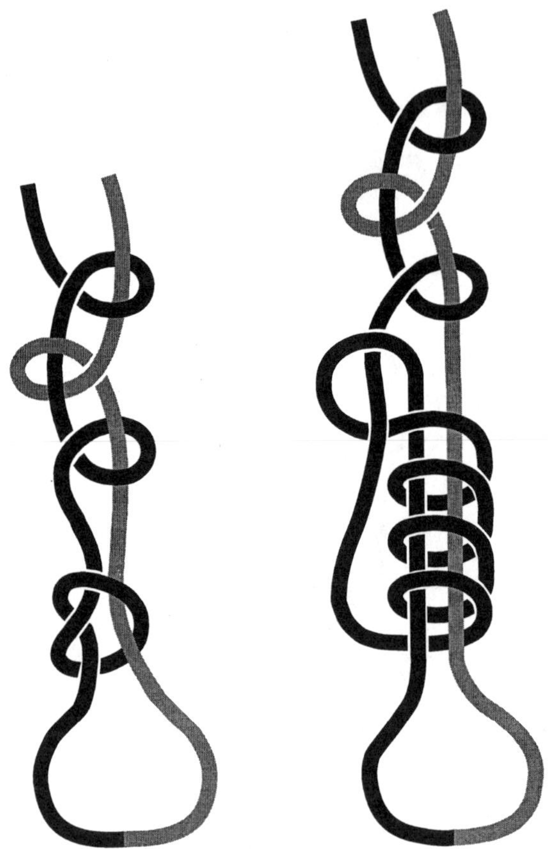

FIGURE 6.—The knot combinations shown exhibited the least loop displacement under load and the best loop holding capacity. The Duncan loop (*DL*) = S//xS//xS knot outperformed all others except the overhand throw (*OT*) = S//xS//xS configuration. (Courtesy of Loutzenheiser TD, Harryman DT, Yung S-W, et al: Optimizing arthroscopic knots. *Arthroscopy* 11:199–206, 1995.)

► This excellent paper is strongly recommended reading for all arthroscopic surgeons. The simple, but excellent, illustrations are most helpful in demonstrating proper knot tying techniques.

J.S. Torg, M.D.

Identification and Treatment of Plica Syndrome: A Chiropractic Approach

Meisenheimer JL, Duermit BH (Wichita, Kan; Loveland, Ohio)

Chiroprac Tech 7:94–97, 1995 4–19

Background.—In up to 60% of the population, a plica in the knee is normal. A plica is a synovial fold present from birth. When patients, especially adolescents, report prepatellar discomfort, examination is indicated to rule out conditions with similar symptoms. Plica syndrome results from the inflammation of the specific knee joint structures. This is caused by chronic overuse, repetitive stress, or repetitive trauma from activities such as jogging, contact sports, and bicycling. A chiropractic approach to the identification and treatment of plica syndrome was discussed.

Plica Syndrome.—Three plicae are located in the knee joint: the suprapatellar, infrapatellar, and medial patellar. Initially, patients usually report a snapping pain or knee stiffness that is like an arthritic condition. Although normal plicae can be palpated, they become more marked when thickened and inflamed, causing a snapping when flexing and extending the leg. Several functional tests can be done to establish the diagnosis of plica syndrome. In one, with the patient supine, the examiner pressures the patella medially with the heel of the hand while palpating the medial femoral condyle with the fingers of the same hand. The knee is then flexed and the tibia slightly medially rotated. A tender fold reproducing the familiar, painful snapping sensation may then be palpable. Other useful tests are the patellar grind, patellar compression, and Apley's distraction tests; pain at the end of passive range of knee flexion; and a false positive McMurray's test.

Chiropractic treatment of plica syndrome is very basic. The practitioner initially applies ice or pulsed ultrasound to relieve inflammation. Transverse friction massage is then performed across the main point of tenderness to realign the developed scar tissue, providing the biological healing response needed to rehabilitate the area. Stretching the hamstrings and strengthening the quadriceps are important, with special consideration given to the vastus medialis.

Conclusion.—The increase in active lifestyles will increase the number of patients seen with plica syndrome. This common knee abnormality can be identified only through a meticulous case history and a comprehensive orthopedic assessment. The conservative treatment afforded by chiropractors is especially useful for providing relief when plica syndrome is the only condition present and initially has a positive prognosis.

▶ The authors recommend reducing inflammation in the plica. After the inflammation has subsided, they recommend the use of transverse friction massage, hamstring stretching, and vastus medialis oblique strengthening to relieve this painful syndrome.

F.J. George, A.T.C., P.T.

Running Injuries to the Knee

James SL (Univ of Oregon, Eugene)

J Am Acad Orthop Surg 3:309–318, 1995 4–20

Introduction.—Competitive distance runners have an injury rate of approximately 30% annually. The most common site of injury in runners is the knee. The biomechanics of running involve enormous patellar tendon force and patellofemoral joint compressive forces. The evaluation of these patients, the common knee injuries, and their management were discussed.

Evaluation.—Approximately 66% of runners' injuries are caused by training errors, including sudden changes in the duration, frequency, or intensity of training. Therefore, obtaining a history of the runner's training program is the most important aspect of the evaluation. Information on previous injuries and their treatment and the make and style of running shoes worn should also be obtained. The physical examination should involve assessment of the entire lower extremity, including evaluation of extremity length, patellar dynamics, ankle dorsiflexion, heel-leg and heel-forefoot alignment, and a thorough knee examination. The radiographic evaluation should include a weight-bearing anteroposterior view, a lateral view in 45 degrees of flexion, a tangential view of the patella, and a notch view (either weight-bearing or non–weight-bearing).

Causes of Knee Pain.—The most common causes of anterior knee pain include the excessive lateral pressure syndrome, patellar instability, quadriceps or patellar tendinopathy, and pathologic plica. Other conditions causing knee pain include meniscal lesions, bursitis, stress fractures, osteoarthritis, iliotibial band (ITB) friction syndrome, popliteal tenosynovitis, and ligamentous instability.

Management.—Most knee injuries can be managed conservatively. Evaluation and modification of the training program should be the first consideration. The anatomical and biomechanical variations of the entire lower limb should be thoroughly assessed. Shoe modifications may also be helpful: a motion-control shoe when compensatory pronation is needed, a support shoe when control is not needed, and a cushion shoe when shock absorption is needed. Careful reconditioning for restoration of muscle strength, endurance, and balance is necessary after an injury. Orthotic devices can be used to correct foot biomechanics. Nonsteroidal anti-inflammatory agents may be used to reduce pain and inflammation. Corticosteroid injection may be indicated for ITB friction syndrome, popliteal tenosynovitis, and bursitis, but is contraindicated in tendon injuries. Surgery should be reserved for patients with refractory injuries, except with conditions that can be managed well with arthroscopic surgery, such as meniscal lesion or loose body. Careful rehabilitation should be planned after surgery.

Conclusion.—Knee injuries are very common among runners. They are primarily caused by training errors. A methodologic approach to evaluation of the entire lower extremity and treatment is necessary, with carefully supervised rehabilitation.

▶ This is an excellent comprehensive review article. The original article is recommended reading for those interested in the subject matter.

J.S. Torg, M.D.

Biomechanics of Two Types of Bone-tendon-bone Graft for ACL Reconstruction

Liu SH, Kabo JM, Osti L (Univ of California, Los Angeles)

J Bone Joint Surg (Br) 77–B:232–235, 1995 4–21

Introduction.—Hamstring-tendon grafts and bone–patellar tendon–bone (BPB) grafts give similar clinical and functional results in anterior cruciate ligament (ACL) reconstruction. Each of these grafts has its disadvantages, however; these include graft site morbidity, patellar fracture, quadriceps weakness, and patellar tendon rupture with the BPB graft and inferior graft and fixation strength with the hamstring graft. A bone-hamstring-bone (BHB) graft was recently devised in an attempt to combine the advantages of the hamstring and BPB grafts while permitting interference screw fixation. Initial fixation strength was compared for the BHB and BPB grafts.

Methods.—Seventy-nine porcine stifle joints were studied: 30 with BHB grafts, 29 with BPB grafts, and 20 with intact ACLs. The BHB grafts were created by harvesting the hamstring tendons with 2 bone plugs, removing them from the upper tibia, and securing them to the tendon with sutures passed twice around each plug and longitudinally through its axis. In each group, 1 subgroup of specimens was loaded to failure and the other was subjected to cyclic loading tests to assess graft slippage.

Results.—The mean load required to cause graft failure was 1,266 N for the intact ACL, 663 N for the BPB graft, and 354 N for the BHB graft. The maximum load tolerated in all groups without failure was 235 N. After cycling to and removing this load, residual displacement averaged 0.031 for the ACL grafts, 0.078 for the BPB grafts, and 0.322 for the BHB grafts.

Conclusion.—In this porcine model, the BHB graft has a lower load to failure and greater graft slippage than the BPB graft. The findings question the clinical applicability of the BHB graft. Neither reconstruction is as strong as the intact ACL.

▶ This is a relatively straightforward study comparing 2 types of ACL reconstruction with the intact ACL. The two types of ACL reconstruction include the BHB graft and the BPB graft. The load to failure for the BPB graft was measured at about 50% of the intact ACL, whereas the BHB graft was about 30% of the intact ACL. The authors found that the BHB graft had weaker initial fixation strength than did the BPB graft, which implies that caution should be exercised during early rehabilitation when the incorporation of the hamstring graft in the bone tunnel is incomplete and the fixation site is the weak link. As a result of this study, the authors stated that they question the clinical application of the BHB graft.

Col. J.L. Anderson, PE.D.

Surgical Reconstruction of Severe Chronic Posterolateral Complex Injuries of the Knee Using Allograft Tissues

Noyes FR, Barber-Westin SD (Deaconess Hosp, Cincinnati, Ohio)
Am J Sports Med 23:2–12, 1995 4–22

Background.—There have been few publications on the treatment of knee ligament injuries of the posterolateral complex. At the authors' center, a new procedure was developed in 1986 to treat severe chronic ruptures of the posterolateral ligament complex. Allogenic tissue is used to reconstruct previously ruptured, insufficient fibular collateral ligament (FCL). The remaining posterolateral tissues are plicated or advanced. The efficacy of this reconstruction in correcting subluxations of the lateral tibiofemoral compartment was analyzed.

Methods.—Twenty patients were followed for a mean of 42 months after the procedure (Fig 4). They were 11 males and 9 females aged 14–43 years. The average time from the knee injury to the FCL reconstruction was 33 months. The patients had undergone a total of 71 surgical procedures previously. A comprehensive subjective and objective 20-factor rating system was used to assess outcomes.

Findings.—The new procedure had a success rate of 76%, as judged by knee stability assessment and stress radiographs. Three reconstructions displayed partial stretching. Two reconstructions failed completely. Functional limitations in sports activities, symptoms, and overall scores were not significantly improved compared with preoperative scores. With immediate knee motion and rehabilitation, 0 to 135 degrees of motion were restored in all knees. The rehabilitation program did not adversely affect the reconstructions.

Conclusion.—In this series, surgical reconstruction of severe chronic posterolateral complex injuries of the knee using allograft tissues was associated with a 76% success rate. Three FCL reconstructions needed additional advancement of the posterolateral complex during tibial osteotomy, and 2 reconstructions failed completely. This procedure is reserved for severe cases in which collagenous tissue is unavailable and a reconstructive procedure with an allograft or autograft is needed.

► The authors report for the first time a reconstructive procedure of the posterolateral complex using allograft tissue to restore FCL function. The procedure is designed for knees in which sufficient soft tissues are not available. It is impressive that of the 20 patients, postoperatively 11 were

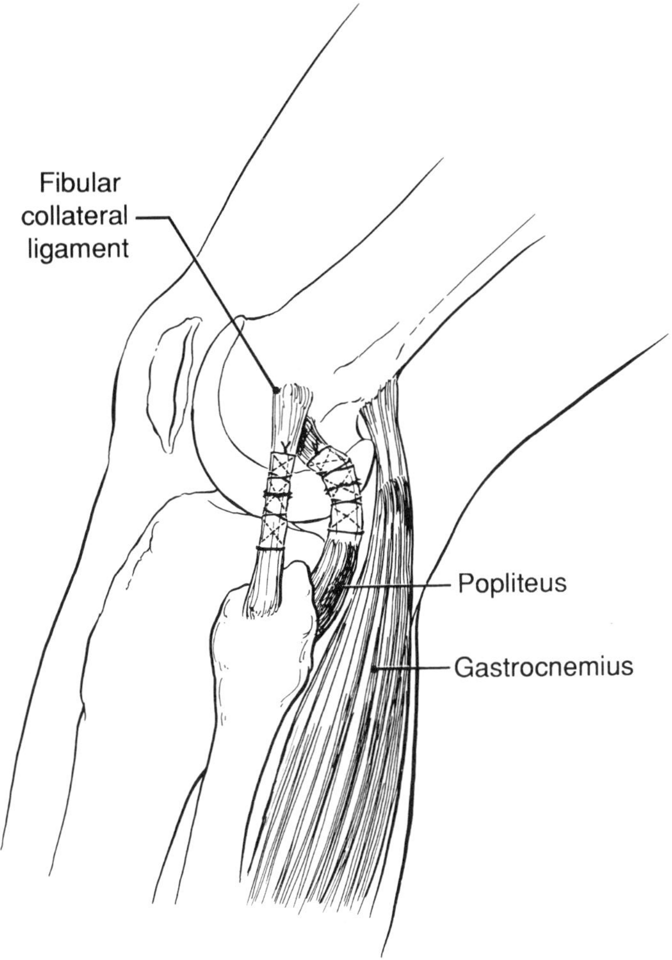

FIGURE 4.—Procedure for shortening the fibular collateral ligament and popliteus tendon after removal of a central portion for select cases in which shortening is elected in addition to the allograft reconstruction. (Courtesy of Noyes FR, Barber-Westin SD: Surgical reconstruction of severe chronic posterolateral complex injuries of the knee using allograft tissues. *Am J Sports Med* 23:2–12, 1995.)

able to increase their activity level with no symptoms, 4 were engaging in sports with some symptoms, 4 were not engaging in sports because of the condition of the knee, and 1 was not participating for non–knee-related reasons. These appear to be very impressive results.

Col. J.L. Anderson, PE.D.

Revascularization of a Human Anterior Cruciate Ligament Graft During the First Two Years of Implantation

Howell SM, Knox KE, Farley TE, Taylor MA (David Grant Med Ctr, Travis Air Force Base, Calif; Wilford Hall Med Ctr, San Antonio, Tex)

Am J Sports Med 23:42–49, 1995 4–23

Introduction.—Although the long-term survival of an anterior cruciate ligament (ACL) graft is thought to depend on its revascularization, there is controversy concerning the process of revascularization of ACL grafts. Investigators used MRI combined with the IV contrast medium gadolinium diethylenetriamine pentaacetic acid (Gd-DTPA) in an attempt to characterize the blood supply of a human ACL graft.

Methods.—The 48 patients who took part in the study had all had a double-looped, gracilis and semitendinosus ACL autograft inserted arthroscopically without roof impingement. Unimpinged grafts were defined by the low signal intensity of the graft observed on a sagittal proton density MR scan. Three patients were subsequently excluded when MRI showed impinged grafts. Five patients had their knees imaged twice, providing a total of 48 MRI studies using Gd-DTPA. Seven studies were performed at 1 month, 14 at 3 months, 11 at 6 months, 5 at 9 months, 9 at 12 months, and 7 beyond 1 year. Two radiologists evaluated each preinfusion and postinfusion scan and graded the sagittal images for degree of enhancement. Patients underwent clinical evaluation of the function and stability of the knees at an average of 21 months postoperatively.

Results.—During the 2-year period after implantation, the unimpinged ACL graft acquired no distinguishable blood supply, retaining the same hypovascular appearance as the normal posterior cruciate ligament. Although the graft itself did not acquire any significant enhancement at any of the imaging times, periligamentous soft tissues were richly vascularized and covered the graft as early as 1 month. Forty-two patients returned for clinical assessment of knee stability and function. In 90% of knees, there was less than 3 mm of anterior translation on the operated knee compared with the normal knee. Four knees were judged unstable on the pivot shift test. Overall, patients rated their knees as very functional, with a mean of 95.6% on the Lysholm scoring scale.

Conclusion.—During the first 2 years after implantation, these unimpinged, human ACL grafts remained hypovascular yet stable and functional. These findings are in agreement with those of animal studies showing that revascularization is not required for either graft viability or strength. Thus, in the unimpinged human ACL graft, viability appears to depend on synovial diffusion.

► This is an excellent study that appears to refute earlier work suggesting that the long-term survival of an ACL graft may depend on its revascularization. With continuing follow-up studies such as this, maybe we will find that these ACL grafts are really permanent.

Col. J.L. Anderson, PE.D.

Muscular and Tibiofemoral Joint Forces During Isokinetic Concentric Knee Extension

Baltzopoulos V (Univ of Liverpool, England)

Clin Biomech 10:208–214, 1995 4–24

Introduction.—With isokinetic dynamometry, muscle activation can occur during isolated joint movements at a constant joint angular velocity. Although isokinetics have been widely used to examine dynamic muscle function under normal as well as pathologic conditions, few studies have looked at the forces developed during isokinetic movements at different angular velocities. A 2-dimensional biomechanical model was used to assess the muscular and tibiofemoral forces occurring during concentric isokinetic knee extension at various angular velocities.

Methods.—The study sample comprised 5 men with no history of knee injury. All were tested on an Akron isokinetic dynamometer, which was used to measure muscular and tibiofemoral forces during isokinetic concentric knee extension at angular velocities of 30 to 210 degrees per second. The 2-dimensional biomechanical model used in this study, developed from direct video x-ray measurements of the knee, included the initial forces and resistive force developed by the dynamometer throughout the range of motion.

Results.—The mean value for maximum moment ranged from 226 Nm at an angular velocity of 30 degrees per second to 166 Nm at 210 degrees per second. Maximum muscle force ranged from 7.5 to 5.7 times body weight, respectively. Compressive tibiofemoral force ranged from 7.5 to 5.7 times body weight and shear tibiofemoral force from 0.9 to 0.8 times body weight.

Conclusion.—The forces generated during maximal isokinetic knee extension are significantly lower than those encountered in other powerful dynamic activities. However, they are still greater than the joint forces occurring during walking or cycling. The final phase of rehabilitation after joint injury should include appropriate precautions and adjustment of the isokinetic protocol.

► This author explains that the purpose of this study was to examine the muscular and tibiofemoral forces during maximum voluntary activation in individuals with no knee injury. To improve accuracy in the measurements, the author applied a manual resistive force to a distal position on the tibia during the x-ray process in order to simulate tibia translation relative to the femur during isokinetic knee extension. By using direct radiographic measurements, the author was able to obtain accurate anatomical parameters for development of the biomechanical model of the knee and measurement of the muscle and joint forces. He believes that the method used in this study is a considerable methodologic improvement in the measurement of muscle and joint forces during isokinetic concentric knee extension. He believes that the different methods used for the development of the biomechanical models, as well as the different instrumentations and procedures, are the main factors accounting for the differences in force measurements between this and previous studies.

Col. J.L. Anderson, PE.D.

Acute Exertional Anterior Compartment Syndrome in an Adolescent Female

Fehlandt A Jr, Micheli L (Children's Hosp of Boston; Harvard Med School, Cambridge, Mass)

Med Sci Sports Exerc 27:3–7, 1995 4–25

Background.—The orthopedic literature describes acute tibial compartment syndrome as a result of tibial fractures, microtrauma, minor trauma, or noncontact injury. There are also numerous reports regarding chronic exertional tibial compartment syndrome in athletic adults. There are few cases of acute tibial compartment syndrome involving women or adolescents.

Case Report.—Girl, 16 years, a soccer player, had bilateral lower leg pain during intense activity that diminished over 10–30 minutes of rest. Occasionally, the pain increased in the first few minutes of rest. She described "tingling" in her feet and "giving out and weakness" of her ankles. She had no history of an acute injury. During a game, her pain progressed and increased in spite of rest. The emergency department physician documented her symptoms of right anterior lower leg pain and dysesthesia. There was no swelling or tenderness over the lateral malleolus. The patient had decreased strength and range of motion (plantar and dorsiflexion) of her right foot. Radiograph results were normal. She received a diagnosis of ankle sprain and was given a splint, crutches, and acetaminophen with codeine.

The next day, the patient returned to the emergency department with unrelenting pain, swelling, and tenderness. A compartment syndrome was suspected. A consulting orthopedist recorded pain in the area of the tibialis anterior and extensor hallicus longus muscles. The patient was treated with narcotic analgesics, Naprosyn, rest, ice, compression, and elevation and discharged.

She returned that same day with worsening pain, swelling, and tenderness over her right anterior lower leg. A diagnosis of incipient compartment syndrome was made. The anterior compartment pressure was 54 mm Hg and the deep posterior compartment pressure was 25 mm Hg. A fasciotomy was performed after which the compartment pressures returned to normal. Within hours after the surgery, more pain developed. Pressures were again elevated. The patient was returned to the operating room, where the anterior compartment was visualized directly and the prior release extended. Primary skin closure was prevented by massive muscle swelling. Skin grafts were subsequently required and the patient had motor and sensory deficits of the superficial and deep peroneal nerves. She could barely extend her toes and could not invert or evert her foot. Three months later, she complained of pain in her left leg, similar to the initial pain in her right leg, during physical therapy. Further physical examination and compartment pressures at rest and after exercise indicated that a compartment release was necessary. She has had no pain in her left leg since the surgery. Her right leg has permanent functional deficits, but she continues to exercise.

Conclusion.—The early diagnosis of an acute exertional compartment syndrome is necessary to prevent potentially irreversible tissue damage. People who complain of "shin splints" should be evaluated for chronic exertional compartment syndrome and advised to seek immediate medical attention if the pain does not decrease after the cessation of exercise.

► Development of an acute exertional compartment syndrome in the absence of antecedent trauma is unusual in sports, as illustrated in a report of an adult male tennis player,[1] and seems to be rare in female athletes. Lower extremity compartment syndromes, however, which are also seen in athletes with sickle cell trait who collapse during "heroic" exercise bouts,[2] are getting more attention because of improved diagnostic techniques and the recognition that delayed diagnosis leads to major complications. Diagnosis of the acute compartment syndrome is mainly clinical, and this report helps the sports medicine physician to recognize the clinical clues. Compartment pressure measurement confirms the diagnosis and helps guide treatment, which includes urgent fasciotomy.

E.R. Eichner, M.D.

References

1. Shrier I: Exercise-induced acute compartment syndrome: A case report. *Clin J Sports Med* 1:202–204, 1991.
2. Eichner ER: Sickle cell trait, heroic exercise, and fatal collapse. *Physician Sportsmed* 21:51–64, 1993.

Peroneal Nerve Entrapment in Athletes

Mitra A, Stern JD, Perrotta VJ, Moyer RA (Temple Univ, Philadelphia)
Ann Plast Surg 35:366–368, 1995 4–26

Introduction.—The peroneal nerve is the nerve in the lower extremity that is most frequently injured and most vulnerable to compression. However, peroneal nerve entrapment is a relatively rare cause of exercise-induced leg pain. The preoperative histories and physical findings in 12 patients with peroneal nerve entrapment, as well as the anatomical basis for this injury, were described.

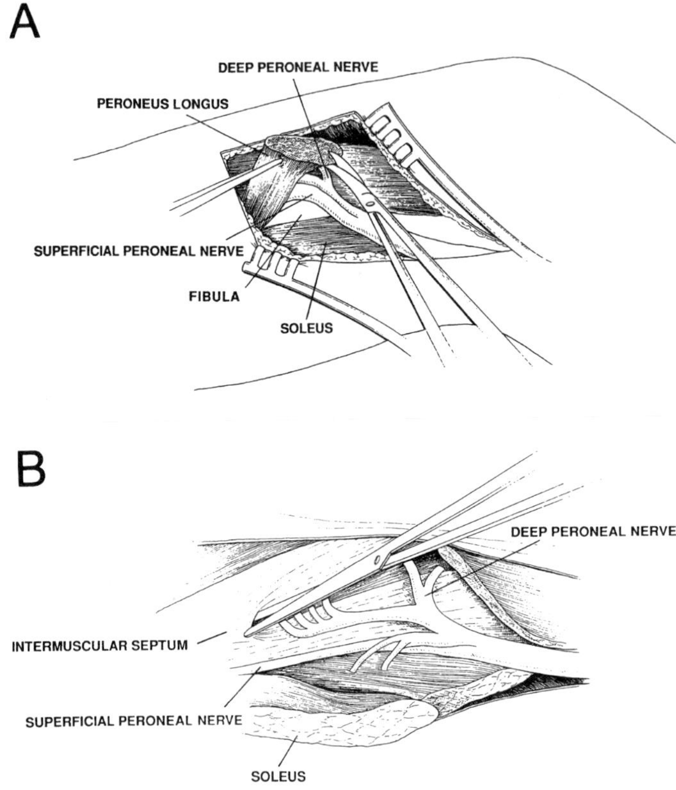

FIGURE.—**A**, division of the peroneus longus muscle origin. **B**, complete decompression requires partial division of the intermuscular septum at the entrance to the anterior compartment. (Reprinted with permission from Mitra A, Stern JD, Perrotta VJ, et al: Peroneal nerve entrapment in athletes. *Ann Plast Surg* 35:366–368, 1995.)

Methods.—The charts of 12 patients who underwent operative decompression for peroneal nerve entrapment were reviewed. To explore anatomical factors, dissections of the peroneal nerve were performed on 7 cadavers.

Results.—The patients were all competitive athletes who reported impaired performance caused by pain associated with exercise and partially relieved by rest. No nonoperative modalities, except for severe restriction of activity, brought symptomatic improvement. Physical examination revealed muscle weakness during foot dorsiflexion and eversion and a diminished muscle mass in the anterolateral leg. There was no tenderness in the anterior and lateral compartments, and there was a variable presence of Tinel's sign. There were no sensory abnormalities or abnormalities on plain radiographs. However, a focal nerve conduction velocity slowing was noted near the fibular head on electromyographic and nerve conduction studies. Intraoperative findings included constriction at the origin of the peroneus longus muscle, congestion of the vasoneurvorum, and proximal swelling pseudoneuroma formation.

Cadaveric dissection revealed a consistent path of the peroneal nerve, which passes between the biceps femoris tendon and the lateral head of the gastrocnemius muscle, pierces the deep fascia, and passes through the fibular tunnel between the fibular neck and the origin of the peroneus longus muscle. To achieve decompression of this fibular tunnel, the peroneus longus muscle and the fibrous arch within the intermuscular septum must be divided (Figure).

Conclusion.—Peroneal nerve entrapment is characterized by consistent preoperative histories, physical findings, and anatomical causes. This condition may not be as rare as is commonly assumed. Therefore, athletic trainers should be aware of the involved anatomy and the signs and symptoms of peroneal nerve entrapment to refer for prompt diagnosis and treatment, thus preventing long-term disability.

▶ Leach et al. have reported a series of 8 runners with peroneal nerve entrapment.[1] The point that they made was that electromyography and nerve conduction studies should be performed both before and after exercise as exercise apparently increases tissue pressure and compression of the nerve. They also reported the relief of symptoms in 7 of their 8 patients with surgical decompression of the nerve.

J.S. Torg, M.D.

Reference

1. Leach RE, Purnell MB, Saito A: Peroneal nerve entrapment in runners. *Am J Sports Med* 17:287–291, 1989.

Patellar Taping: A Radiographic Examination of the Medial Glide Technique

Larsen B, Andreasen E, Urfer A, Mickelson MR, Newhouse KE (Idaho State Univ, Pocatello)

Am J Sports Med 23:465–471, 1995 4–27

Background.—Patellofemoral pain, a common orthopedic complaint, is often caused by lateral tracking syndrome. Most treatment programs combine quadriceps muscle strengthening with training programs, external supports, and patient education. McConnell medial glide taping—using a small customized brace to control patellar maltracking, rotation, and tilt—has been used for nearly a decade (Fig 2). The effectiveness of this taping procedure in moving the patella medially and maintaining its alignment during exercise was studied.

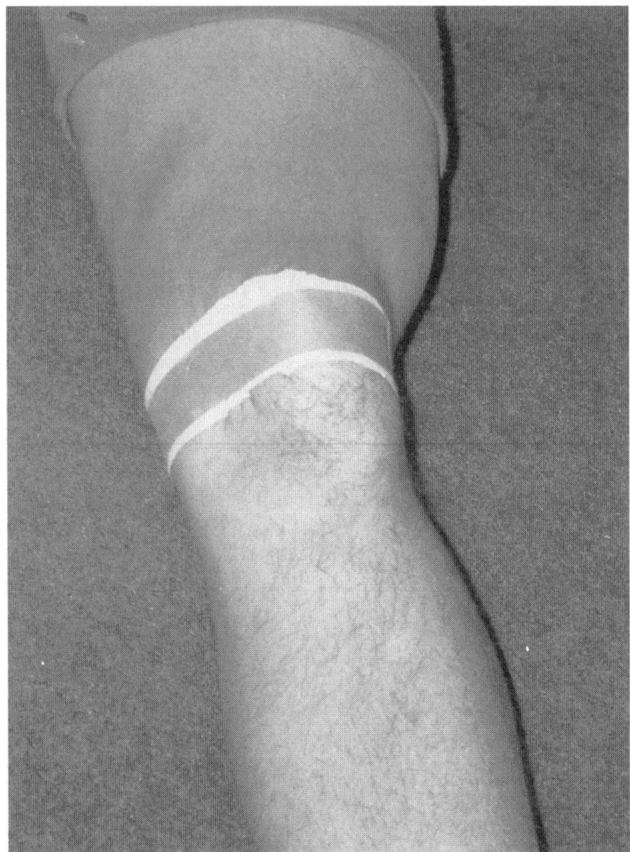

FIGURE 2.—McConnell medial glide taping technique on the left leg. (Courtesy of Larsen B, Andreasen E, Urfer A, et al: Patellar taping: A radiographic examination of the medial glide technique. *Am J Sports Med* 23:465–471, 1995.)

Methods.—Twenty male volunteers with no history of lower extremity abnormality, trauma, or surgery, underwent taping of 1 randomly selected knee, with the opposite knee serving as a control. To enable measurement of the Merchant congruent angle, radiographs were obtained before and after taping and after a standardized exercise protocol that stressed the knee and tape in several common movement planes.

Results.—Radiographic measurements revealed a significant difference in that the taped patella was moved medially an average of 9 degrees. After exercise, however, the patellae of the taped knees had returned to their pretape angles. Interestingly, exercise alone caused significant lateral displacement of control patellae by an average of 4.6 degrees. Possible causes of this effect include fatigue of the vastus medialis oblique muscle, iliotibial band tightening, and increasing elasticity of medial patellar constraints with exercise.

Conclusion.—Although the McConnell medial glide taping technique significantly displaces the patella medially, the effect does not persist during moderate exercise. Additionally, exercise tends to cause a normal patella to shift laterally.

▶ This study should be read with Abstracts 4–28 and 5–19. It appears that patellae can be realigned using the McConnell technique. Moderate exercise caused the taped patellae to return to their pretaped angles. It appears that an increase in the lateral glide of the patellae is a normal effect of exercise.

What impact will these findings and the findings from the other 2 studies have on our treatment regimens? The biomechanics of knee action must be closely scrutinized as in the following abstract. The effectiveness of taping and specific exercise in improving the vastus medialis oblique/vastus lateralis ratio must also be evaluated as they were in this study and in Abstract 5–19. An ideal situation would be to stretch the lateral retinaculum and iliotibial band, strengthen the vastus medialis oblique and develop a taping technique that would maintain correct patella alignment throughout a strenuous exercise program.

F.J. George, A.T.C., P.T.

Patellofemoral Pain in Female Ballet Dancers: Correlation With Iliotibial Band Tightness and Tibial External Rotation

Winslow J, Yoder E (Healthsouth Sports Medicine & Rehabilitation Ctr, Norfolk, Va; Old Dominion Univ, Norfolk, Va)

J Orthop Sports Phys Ther 22:18–21, 1995 4–28

Background.—Iliotibial band tightness may contribute to the development of anterior knee pain in some ballet dancers, for whom such steps as the demi-plie accentuate lateral patellar deviation and tibial external rotation (Fig 1B). The relationship between iliotibial band tightness and patellofemoral pain, with particular regard to the degree of tibial external rotation during the demi-plie, was studied in ballet dancers.

Methods.—Twelve dancers with patellofemoral pain (14 affected knees) and 12 symptom-free dancers were examined for iliotibial band tightness using the Ober test. The degree of tibial external rotation was measured in both legs of each dancer, in first position and during demi-plie.

Results.—Eleven of 14 symptomatic knees, but only 9 of 34 pain-free knees, exhibited iliotibial band tightness, a significant difference. Additionally, the mean value of tibial external rotation was significantly greater in both first position and demi-plie for dancers with iliotibial band tightness, compared with dancers with normal iliotibial band length.

Conclusion.—Iliotibial band tightness appears to predispose ballet dancers to patellofemoral pain. Affected dancers tend to compensate during the demi-plie with increased tibial external rotation, which may further accentuate the abnormal patellar deviation.

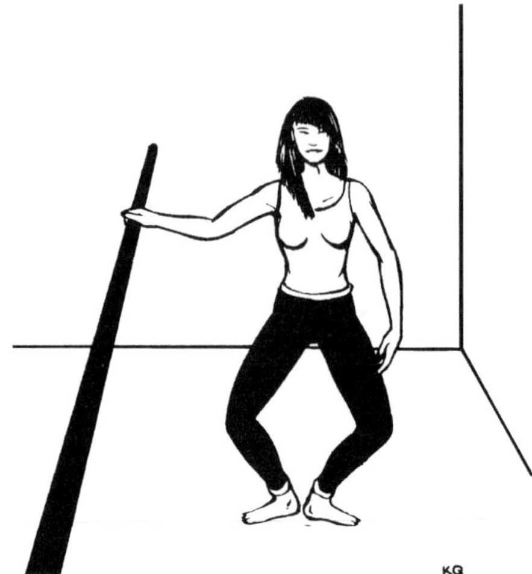

FIGURE 1B.—The demi-plie. (Courtesy of Winslow J, Yoder E: Patellofemoral pain in female ballet dancers: Correlation with iliotibial band tightness and tibial external rotation. *J Orthop Sports Phys Ther* 22:18–21, 1995.)

► Please read this study in conjunction with Abstracts 4–27 and 5–19. The authors have added another dimension to the problem of patellofemoral pain. They found a significant correlation between patellofemoral pain in ballet dancers and tightness of the iliotibial band. They explain that iliotibial band tightness plays an important role in external rotation of the tibia, which, in turn, causes an increase in the lateral tracking of the patella. Ballet dancers with patellofemoral pain should perform exercises to stretch the iliotibial band and be taught not to compensate for tight iliotibial bands by increasing external rotation of the tibia during specific dance movements. This same finding should be applied to all athletes with patellofemoral pain.

F.J. George, A.T.C., P.T.

Patellar Taping in the Treatment of Patellofemoral Pain: A Prospective Randomized Study

Kowall MG, Kolk G, Nuber GW, Cassisi JE, Stern SH (Northwestern Univ, Chicago; Northwestern Mem-Baxter Physical Therapy Ctr, Chicago; Illinois Inst of Psychology, Chicago)

Am J Sports Med 24:61–66, 1996 4–29

Background.—Both athletes and the general population must frequently contend with patellofemoral pain. Apart from acute or repetitive trauma, it may be a symptom of osteochondritis, chondromalacia, or malalignment. Initially, the pain is treated by quadriceps rehabilitation and, occasionally, by bracing. Patellar taping has been proposed as a means of passively correcting patellar subluxation, tilt, and rotation, thereby lessening pain during rehabilitation of the quadriceps. Excellent results have been reported.

Objective.—Patellofemoral taping was evaluated in a prospective series of 25 patients with pain, all of whom participated in a standardized program of physical therapy.

Patients.—The 17 women and 8 men (average age, 29 years) had had symptoms for 2 years, on average. Ten patients had symptoms in both lower extremities. None of the patients had evidence of patellofemoral dislocation or meniscal or ligament injury, and none had undergone knee surgery.

Management.—Patients received formal physical therapy twice a week for 4 weeks; the therapy featured extensive stretching and quadriceps strengthening exercises. They were also instructed in home exercises to be performed about 30 minutes a day. Twelve patients, in addition, underwent patellar taping.

Results.—Taped and control patients complied similarly with the home exercise program. Pain became less frequent in both groups of patients and less important in their daily lives. Knee strength increased to comparable degrees after treatment. In both groups, integrated electromyographic activity in the vastus medialis and lateralis muscles increased significantly.

Conclusion.—Patellar taping confers no substantial added benefit for patients with patellofemoral pain who undergo standard physical therapy that includes quadriceps strengthening exercises.

▶ On a pragmatic basis, I do not disagree with the conclusions of the authors regarding the efficacy of patella taping. However, the small size of the control and study groups, failure to categorize the clinical pathologic presentation (i.e., loose vs. tight patella), and the use of an older population with an average age of 29 years preclude clean statistical substantiation.

J.S. Torg, M.D.

Acute Dislocation of the Patella: A Correlative Pathoanatomic Study

Sallay PI, Poggi J, Speer KP, Garrett WE (Methodist Sports Medicine Ctr, Indianapolis, Ind; OFFUTT Airforce Base, Omaha, Neb; Duke Univ, Durham, NC)

Am J Sports Med 24:52–60, 1996 4–30

Introduction.—A significant number of patients who are treated nonoperatively for acute patellar dislocation have recurrences. A number of operations have failed to reliably restore a stable patella. The pathology of patellar dislocation remains incompletely understood.

Objective.—The mechanisms underlying patellar dislocation and the results of early operative repair were studied in 23 patients with clinical findings of acute dislocation who underwent MRI as well as standard radiography. The patients were 20 males and 3 females 14–46 years of age.

Nineteen patients were examined under anesthesia and underwent arthroscopic treatment of any intra-articular lesions. Sixteen patients had open exploration of the medial aspect of the knee, and 12 were followed for 2 years or longer.

Pathoanatomy.—A substantial majority of patients had a moderate-to-large effusion and significant tenderness over the posteromedial soft tissues and the adductor tubercle. Radiographs showed patellar fractures in 4 patients and a single lateral femoral condylar fracture. The MR findings included increased signal adjacent to the adductor tubercle on T2-weighted images, and a tear of the femoral insertion of the medial patellofemoral ligament (MPFL) in 20 patients, most evident on axial T2-weighted images. Ten patients had some increased signal in the parapatellar part of the medial capsule, but there was only one frank tear at this site. Osseous changes were prevalent. Exploration revealed gross lateral laxity of the patellofemoral articulation. Five patients had tears in the medial soft tissues. Osteochondral lesions were frequent. A tear of the MPFL was documented in all but 1 of the 16 patients evaluated.

Outcome.—None of the patients had recurrent dislocation after repair of the MPFL. Good-to-excellent results were achieved in 58% of patients and fair results in the remainder. Nearly 60% of patients were able to return to their previous sports activity with no major limitations. Three patients had surgical complications.

Implications.—Many operations for acute and chronic patellar instability have failed because they do not confront the major pathology: posterior rupture of the MPFL. Repairing this structure restores stability in a majority of patients. Lateral release may be indicated, in addition, if the lateral retinaculum is abnormally tight.

► This is an excellent paper that both calls attention to a generally unrecognized pathoanatomical component of acute patella dislocation and proposes the surgical remedy. The fact that 42% of the patients only had fair results is explained by the fact that a high percentage had significant chondral and osteochondral lesions involving the patella and lateral femoral condyle. In considering the results, it is important to point out that those patients who did not return to their previous level of activity for the most part elected not to do so because of fear of another knee injury rather than because of symptom-based limitations. The bottom line is that surgical repair of the MPFL predictably restored stability against further dislocation in all of the patients.

J.S. Torg, M.D.

"Aggressive" Nontreatment of Lateral Meniscal Tears Seen During Anterior Cruciate Ligament Reconstruction

Fitzgibbons RE, Shelbourne KD (Methodist Sports Medicine Ctr, Indianapolis, Ind)

Am J Sports Med 23:156–159, 1995 4–31

Background.—Complete removal of a torn lateral meniscus has a poor prognosis, but certain types of lateral meniscus tears identified at the time of anterior cruciate ligament (ACL) reconstruction appear to remain asymptomatic if excision or repair are not attempted. To determine outcome in such cases, 189 lateral meniscal tears that were left in situ at the time of ACL reconstruction were reviewed.

Methods.—At the study institution, 598 lateral meniscal tears were identified during 1,146 ACL reconstructions performed between May 1982 and July 1991. Partial excision was undertaken in 256 reconstructions, meniscal repair in 135, and 207 tears were left in situ. All but 18 of the 207 patients with lateral meniscal tears left in situ were followed for at least 1 year. Tears were classified by type, and patients completed a modified Noyes knee questionnaire.

Results.—At the time of follow-up, all patients had returned to their normal level of athletic activity and were free of symptoms related to the meniscal injury. One patient who twisted his knee 114 days after ACL reconstruction required arthroscopic surgery and medial meniscal repair, at which time the edges of the lateral meniscal tear were débrided. At an average of 3.6 years postoperatively, the average score on the Noyes questionnaire was 92.2 of 100 possible points; the knee stability score was 19.6 of 20 possible points.

Discussion.—Although lateral meniscus tears are often seen in conjunction with ACL tears, few are clinically symptomatic in the ACL-deficient knee. At present, the authors are leaving 70% of lateral meniscus tears alone when identified in conjunction with an ACL reconstruction. Vertical tears totally posterior to the popliteus tendon are asymptomatic before and after reconstruction and should be left alone or simply abraded; posterior horn avulsion tears can be left alone without becoming symptomatic; other complete and incomplete lateral meniscal tears that are stable at the time of ACL reconstruction can be safely left in situ.

▶ The observations and conclusions of the authors are in keeping with my own clinical experience.

J.S. Torg, M.D.

The Effects of Arthroscopic Partial Lateral Meniscectomy in an Otherwise Normal Knee: A Retrospective Review of Functional, Clinical, and Radiographic Results

Jaureguito JW, Elliot JS, Lietner T, Dixon LB, Reider B (Univ of Chicago)

Arthroscopy 11:29–36, 1995 4–32

Introduction.—A number of studies indicate that functional and radiographic results are poor for total lateral meniscectomy compared with total medial meniscectomy. Few data are available, however, on the results of partial lateral meniscectomy. A retrospective review of 31 patients (32 knees) who underwent arthroscopic partial lateral meniscectomy for lateral meniscus tears examined long-term outcome in the group.

Methods.—The arthroscopic procedures were performed between 1982 and June 1988. Patients eligible for the study had not undergone knee surgery before the partial lateral meniscectomy, and all had otherwise normal knees. Questionnaires were sent to obtain detailed functional information at 3 time periods: preoperatively, at the time of maximum improvement, and at the time of questionnaire completion. The mean follow-up was 8 years and the mean patient age at follow-up was 38 years.

Results.—Twenty-six patients (27 knees) returned the questionnaires and 20 (21 knees) were available for physical and radiographic follow-up. The mean preoperative Lysholm II score was 60.5. Maximum improvement occurred at an average of 5 months postoperatively; at this time, 92% of patients had good or excellent results, with a mean Lysholm II score of 92.3. At the most recent follow-up, mean Lysholm II scores showed a significant decrease (83.8), and only 62% of patients had an excellent or good result. Although 85% of patients returned to their preinjury level initially, only 48% had maintained this level at the most recent follow-up. Radiographic changes showed no correlation with subjective symptoms and functional outcome. All patients expressed satisfaction with the outcome of surgery.

Conclusion.—Total lateral meniscectomy has historically had poor results compared with total medial meniscectomy. The overall all long-term functional results are improved for arthroscopic partial lateral meniscectomy, yet functional outcome clearly degenerates with time. Patients who undergo this procedure should be advised that their activity level may be expected to decrease and their symptoms increase over the years.

► The observations and conclusions of the authors are in keeping with my own clinical experience.

J.S. Torg, M.D.

Osteoarthritis After Arthroscopic Partial Meniscectomy

Rangger C, Klestil T, Gloetzer W, Kemmler G, Benedetto KP (Univ Hosp of Innsbruck, Austria; Univ of Innsbruck, Austria)

Am J Sports Med 23:240–244, 1995 4–33

Objective.—It has been suggested that osteoarthritis may be less likely to develop after arthroscopic partial meniscectomy than after open operation. This proposal was tested by reassessing 284 patients 41–67 months after undergoing arthroscopy for meniscal injury.

Study Population.—Medial meniscal tears were treated in 247 patients (group I) and lateral meniscal tears in 37 (group II). Damage to the articular surface was observed at arthroscopy in 176 group I patients (subgroup IB) and in 25 group II patients (subgroup IIB).

Findings.—Osteoarthritic changes were evident radiographically in 35% of group I patients and 24% of those in group II at an average of 53.5 months postoperatively. Osteoarthritis was comparably frequent in the 2 subgroups of patients having medial partial meniscectomy. Arthritic changes were more prevalent after medial than after lateral meniscectomy but not significantly so. Arthritis developed or worsened in about one fourth of each subgroup. In group II, osteoarthritis worsened significantly more often when articular damage was present at the time of surgery.

Conclusion.—Osteoarthritis develops or worsens in a significant number of patients who undergo arthroscopic partial removal of either the medial or lateral meniscus.

► The literature reports osteoarthritic radiographic findings after open meniscectomy in 18% to 89% of cases. Recently, Bolano and Grana reported osteoarthritis after partial meniscectomy in 62% of their patients.[1] The lesser incidence reported in this study is attributed to the fact that non–weight-bearing radiographs were used for analysis. Most disconcerting were the findings that development of osteoarthritic changes was independent of the articular cartilage condition visualized at arthroscopy.

J.S. Torg, M.D.

Reference

1. Bolano LE, Grana WA: Isolated arthroscopic partial meniscectomy: Functional radiographic evaluation at five years. *Am J Sports Med* 21:432–437, 1993.

Osteonecrosis of the Knee Following Laser-Assisted Arthroscopic Surgery: A Report of Six Cases

Garino JP, Lotke PA, Sapega AA, Reilly PJ, Esterhai JL Jr (Univ of Pennsylvania, Philadelphia)

J Arthro Rel Surg 11:467–474, 1995 4–34

Introduction.—Five patients having significant and persistent pain in 6 knees after arthroscopic knee surgery were found to have para-articular osteonecrosis. In all cases, a laser had been used to treat diseased articular cartilage and meniscal tissue.

Case Report.—Woman, 44, reported pain in the medial side of her right knee after a fall. An MR study showed signs of degeneration in the medial meniscus. Pain persisted for 4 months after injury, at which time arthroscopic surgery was performed using a contact Nd:YAG laser in a saline medium. Exploration revealed a small radial tear of the posterior horn of the medial meniscus and an area of grade IV articular cartilage degeneration on the posterior surface of the medial femoral condyle. A minimal inner-edge partial meniscectomy was done using the laser, and the degenerated cartilage was removed mechanically. The laser probe was then used to "carmelize" the remaining abnormal femoral cartilage. A total of 54,133 J was delivered. The patient improved slowly over the next 8 months, but then marked pain and swelling developed in the medial side of the knee. X-ray studies suggested a geographic lesion of the medial femoral condyle, and a bone scan showed intense uptake. Magnetic resonance imaging demonstrated 2 geographic osseous lesions consistent with osteonecrosis (Fig 1). Arthroscopy performed 10 months after the first procedure revealed what appeared to be char marks on the femoral cortex and peeling edges of articular cartilage at the perimeter of the lesion. Core decompression and percutaneous drilling were carried out, and local autogenous cancellous bone was grafted onto the core defect in the femur. Biopsy specimens confirmed osteonecrosis. The patient remained symptomatic a year later and underwent unicompartmental knee replacement, with a good early outcome.

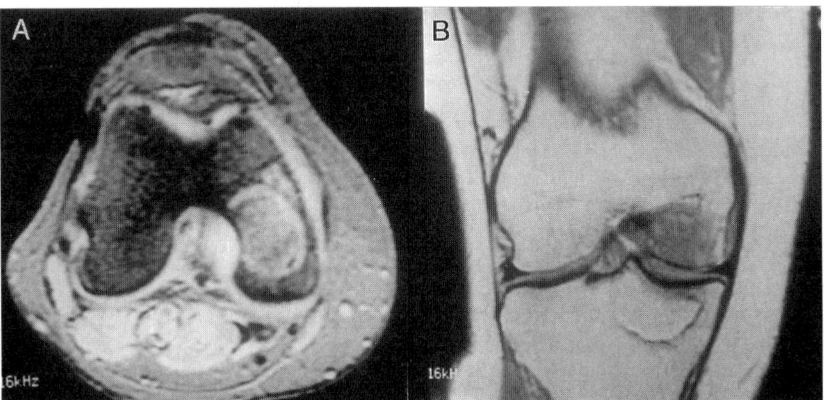

FIGURE 1.—Magnetic resonance images of the right knee 8 months after initial arthroscopic procedure. **A,** tranverse section. **B,** coronal section. (Courtesy of Garino JP, Lotke PA, Sapega AA, et al: Osteonecrosis of the knee following laser-assisted arthroscopic surgery: A report of six cases. *J Arthro Rel Surg* 11:467–474, 1995.)

Discussion.—In all 6 cases, the abnormal MR signal was found directly below or adjacent to areas of tissue that were treated with laser energy. Osteonecrosis may be a direct result of excessive temperatures or an indirect result of pressure-induced and inflammatory changes consequent to injury of the subchondral plate. Photoacoustic shock is also a possible mechanism of bone death.

► This paper brings to our attention the potentially deleterious effects of laser energy used in the knee arthroscopically. However, it is most important to point out that this article should not serve as a condemnation of this technology. What the article should have emphasized is that laser energy needs to be understood. Each wavelength has a specific tissue interaction. In 5 of the 6 cases reported, an Nd:YAG laser was reported to have been used. Apparently, this device admits light energy at a wavelength that is poorly absorbed by water and nonpigmented tissue such as meniscal tissue and hyaline cartilage. As the authors point out, "... a free beam of this type is poorly suited for most orthopaedic applications". On the other hand, the holmium:YAG laser emits energy at a wavelength that is highly absorbed by meniscal tissue and cartilage, thus delivering less energy to underlying bone.

J.S. Torg, M.D.

Nonoperative Treatment of Acute Anterior Cruciate Ligament Injuries in a Selected Group of Patients

Buss DD, Min R, Skyhar M, Galinat B, Warren RF, Wickiewicz TL (Hosp for Special Surgery, New York)

Am J Sports Med 23:160–165, 1995 4–35

Objective.—The results of conservative treatment of acute anterior cruciate ligament (ACL) injuries were examined in 61 carefully selected patients, 55 of whom were available for follow-up at an average of nearly 4 years after initial injury.

Patients.—The series included patients more than 30 years of age and those who were not interested in athletics or had sedentary jobs. The 24 males and 31 females had an average age of 31 years, compared with 26 years for a group of patients having acute ACL reconstruction at the same institution.

Management.—A knee immobilizer was used in the acute phase of injury. Weight-bearing was allowed as tolerated; patients used crutches at the outset. Rehabilitation began immediately and emphasized strengthening of the hamstring muscles. Patients used an extension-limiting brace when engaged in strenuous activities.

Outcome.—Two-thirds of patients had pain only during athletic activity. Only 4 patients had pain during daily activities. A majority of patients had symptoms of giving-way, but only 3 did so on a daily basis. Fewer than one fourth of patients noted occasional swelling. All patients but 1 were able to return to their previous work without difficulty. No patient had marked generalized ligamentous laxity. Arthrometric data did not correlate with symptoms but did correlate with the Lachman grade. Eight of the 55 patients followed (15%) had undergone surgical reconstruction and were considered to be failures.

Conclusion.—Conservative management can provide satisfactory results in older and less active patients with acute ACL injury, provided they will accept some degree of instability.

▶ The observations and conclusions of the authors regarding nonoperative treatment of ACL injuries in this selected group of patients is in keeping with my own clinical experience.

J.S. Torg, M.D.

Anterior Cruciate Ligament Injuries in Young Athletes: Recommendations for Treatment and Rehabilitation

McCarroll JR, Shelbourne KD, Patel DV (Methodist Sports Medicine Ctr, Indianapolis, Ind)

Sports Med 20:117–127, 1995 4–36

Introduction.—Three percent to 4% of skeletally immature adolescents have midsubstance tears of the anterior cruciate ligament (ACL), and the incidence may be increasing. These injuries can be serious in young athletes involved in such demanding sports as football and basketball—activities that involve twisting, cutting, and pivoting movements.

Potential Problems.—Young athletes often fail to comply with the restrictions on activity that are a critical part of conservative management. At the same time, intra-articular reconstruction through open growth plates is best avoided in order not to impede normal growth. Recurrent instability places these patients at high risk of both meniscal tears and degenerative arthritis.

Management.—It seems appropriate to attempt to salvage the menisci and to plan on a single definitive stabilizing procedure. Skeletal maturity is carefully assessed, using both clinical and radiographic criteria. Skeletally immature patients and those willing to comply with restricted activity undergo rehabilitation of the quadriceps and hamstrings as well as bracing. Surgery is indicated for patients who will not modify their activities and adolescents who are close to being skeletally mature. A positive Lachman test and a positive pivot shift test also are indications for reconstructing the ACL. Patients with chronic instability who have had repeated episodes of giving-way, pain, and swelling are considered for operative treatment.

▶ The conclusion of the authors that intra-articular ACL reconstruction in junior high school athletes, using autogenous patellar tendon grafts through femoral and tibial tunnels, provides excellent knee stability, a high rate of return to sports at the pre-injury level of competition, and a low rate of meniscal tears is in keeping with my own clinical experience. I would also agree with the authors that conservative management with bracing as well as with extra-articular ACL reconstruction is essentially ineffectual. McCarroll et al. have reported on 60 skeletally immature patients who underwent intra-articular ACL reconstruction using infrapatellar bone–tendon–bone grafts through tibial and femoral drill holes. There were no occurrences of growth disturbance, significant leg length inequality, or angular deformity in any of these patients.

J.S. Torg, M.D.

A Comparison of Outpatient and Inpatient Anterior Cruciate Ligament Reconstruction Surgery

Kao JT, Giangarra CE, Singer G, Martin S (Kaiser Permanente Hosp, San Francisco; LaCrosse, Wis; LAC/USC Med Ctr, Los Angeles; et al)

J Arthro Rel Surg 11:151–156, 1995 4–37

Background.—Various surgical procedures traditionally performed on an inpatient basis are being performed on an outpatient basis to reduce costs. Successful outpatient procedures include arthroscopic procedures, hardware removal, hand surgery, and dental surgery. There are no reports of outpatient anterior cruciate ligament (ACL) reconstruction. It may be possible to perform this procedure in an outpatient setting in selected patients because of improved surgical techniques and the availability of oral narcotics and long-acting intra-articular local anesthetics. Outpatient and inpatient ACL reconstruction were compared.

Methods.—Anterior cruciate ligament reconstruction was performed in 25 outpatients and 12 inpatients. Pain control, narcotic consumption, postoperative complications, recovery time, and costs were compared.

Results.—Of the 25 outpatients, 2 would have preferred hospitalization for pain control. There were no significant differences in severity, frequency, or relief of pain between the 2 groups; however, based on the data, the inpatients were somewhat more comfortable. Two of the outpatients were hospitalized, 1 because of nausea and vomiting and 1 because of urinary retention. There were no differences in rehabilitation or regaining full range of motion between the 2 groups. Arthrofibrosis developed in 1 inpatient; there were no other postoperative complications. Inpatient costs averaged $9,220 and outpatient costs averaged $3,905.

Discussion.—Outpatient ACL reconstruction is both feasible and safe in selected patients and is more cost-effective than inpatient procedures. Both before and after surgery, recovery time should be discussed and adequate crutch training should be provided. It is important for the patient to feel comfortable at home, have good support, and be prepared for hospitalization in case of complications.

Trends in Decreased Hospitalization for Anterior Cruciate Ligament Surgery: Double-incision Versus Single-incision Reconstruction

Nogalski MP, Bach BR Jr, Bush-Joseph CA, Luergans S (Rush-Presbyterian-St Luke's Med Ctr, Chicago)

Arthroscopy 11:134–138, 1995 4–38

Objective.—Two commonly performed methods of arthroscopy-assisted anterior cruciate ligament (ACL) reconstruction were compared for differences in total cost. As charges for such elective operations come under scrutiny, cost-effectiveness may play a role in the selection of surgical technique.

Methods.—The reconstructive methods compared were an arthroscopy-assisted double-incision technique and an endoscopic single-incision technique, both using autogenous bone tendon bone central third patellar tendon substitution. Two different surgeons operated on 151 consecutive patients between June 1989 and November 1992. Eighty-one patients underwent the double-incision procedure and 72 had the single-incision procedure. The double-incision technique was standard until mid-1991 when it was replaced with the single-incision method. Patient records were retrospectively reviewed for hospital days; total hospital charges; and charges for the operating room/hospital ward, pharmacy, and physical therapy.

Results.—The mean hospital stay was 1.47 days for the single-incision group and 2.84 days for the double-incision group. In both groups, the hospital stay tended to decrease from year to year. After adjusting for inflation, operating room/ward charges decreased significantly when the single-incision technique (average cost $9,585) replaced the double-incision technique (average cost $11,079). The 2 groups had similar charges for anesthesia and laboratory fees, but pharmacy charges were lower with the single incision. The reduction in total hospital charges achieved with the single-incision technique was strongly statistically significant.

Conclusion.—The decrease in total hospital charges associated with endoscopic single-incision ACL reconstruction can be attributed largely to a decrease in hospital days rather than to the technique itself. Patients from both single- and double-incision groups who had 2-day postoperative hospital stays had comparable hospital charges, adjusted for inflation.

► With regard to discharging patients after ACL reconstruction, I find a medium between immediate discharge as proposed by Kao et al. (Abstract 4–37) and a 2- to-3-day postoperative discharge as practiced by Nogalski et al. (Abstract 4–38) more satisfactory. Specifically, it appears reasonable to discharge the patient the morning after surgery both for patient comfort and for the surgeon's peace of mind. This is particularly true in a referral practice where many of the patients travel considerable distances to and from the hospital.

J.S. Torg, M.D.

Collagen Fibril Populations in Human Anterior Cruciate Ligament Allografts: Electron Microscopic Analysis

Shino K, Oakes BW, Horibe S, Nakata K, Nakamura N (Osaka Rosai Hosp, Japan; Monash Univ, Clayton, Australia; Osaka Univ, Japan)

Am J Sports Med 23:203–209, 1995 4–39

Background.—Anterior cruciate ligament (ACL) reconstruction with allogenic tendon grafts is popular because of the satisfactory results obtained without sacrificing normal tissue. It was previously reported that the arthroscopic macro-appearance of the ACL allografts was unchanged 11 months postoperatively and onward, and that within 18 months, the grafts reached histologic maturity. In that study, the size and density of collagen fibrils in the allogenic tendon graft were not studied. There is little information regarding the collagen remodeling process for allogenic tendons used as ACL grafts. This process was examined by quantitative electron microscopy to analyze collagen fibril populations.

Methods.—Biopsy specimens were obtained between 3 and 96 months postoperatively from 42 patients who had allograft ACL reconstruction and whose anterior stability was restored. Specimens were obtained from the superficial region of the midzone of the grafts after synovial clearance.

Results.—By 12 months postoperatively, the collagen fibril profile was almost unimodal: there were predominantly small-diameter collagen fibrils of between 30 and 80 nm within the ACL allografts. There were a small number of large-diameter fibrils of between 90 and 140 nm. Small-diameter collagen fibrils predominated in virtually all specimens older than 12 months. Several years postoperatively, the collagen fibril profiles of the ACL allografts did not resemble normal tendon grafts or normal ACLs.

Conclusion.—In these patients, predominantly small-diameter collagen fibrils were seen in allogenic tendon grafts 6 months postoperatively. A prior study also reported the loss of large-diameter collagen fibrils of the patellar tendon within 6 months after implantation.

▶ The conclusion of this study is that several years after surgery, ACL allograft collagen fibril profiles did not resemble normal tendon grafts or normal ACLs. It should be pointed out that the biopsy specimens were obtained from the superficial region of the graft and did not represent the bulk of the collagen of the graft. The clinical relevance of this observation has not been determined.

J.S. Torg, M.D.

Allograft Failure in Cruciate Ligament Reconstruction: Follow-up Evaluation of Eighteen Patients

Sterling JC, Meyers MC, Calvo RD (Texas Ctr for Sports Medicine and Orthopaedic Surgery, Sugar Land; Montana State Univ, Bozeman)

Am J Sports Med 23:173–178, 1995 4–40

Background.—Although the efficacy of cruciate ligament allograft reconstruction of the knee has been described, a high allograft failure rate also has been noted. Graft failure may be associated with graft type, size, and integrity; donor-host histocompatibility; insufficient biomechanical duplication after allograft implantation; and surgical-rehabilitative methods. The causes of overt failure of allograft material were investigated in a group of young, athletic individuals undergoing cruciate ligament allograft reconstructions.

Patients and Methods.—Eighteen patients, including 12 men and 6 women, with diagnoses of acute or chronic anterior or posterior cruciate ligament deficiency, were included in the study. All patients underwent intra-articular allograft reconstruction at a mean age of 23 years, during which deep-frozen, freeze-dried, ethylene oxide–sterilized, bone–patellar tendon–bone allografts that had been rehydrated and prestressed were implanted by open or arthroscopically assisted means. An aggressive rehabilitation program was initiated after surgery. Follow-up evaluations were completed 2–4 years postoperatively among patients with successful reconstructions and at approximately 3 months after implantation among those with failed grafts.

Results.—Graft failures occurred in 6 of the 18 patients. In the failed graft group, knee instability and roentgenographic changes were apparent. Postoperative complications also occurred more frequently among patients with failed grafts compared with those who had successful outcomes. A significant association between graft failure and time to implantation was noted. The mean time from acquisition and deep-freezing to freeze-drying and sterilization was 265.5 days for failed grafts, compared with 66.8 days for successful grafts. A significantly greater total mean time from acquisition to implantation also was noted for failed grafts, at 528.3 vs. 207.3 days for successful grafts. All grafts that had failed were obtained from the same batch number.

Conclusion.—Although cruciate ligament allograft reconstructions can be successful, the possibility of failure is high when ethylene oxide–sterilized bone–patellar tendon–bone allografts are used. A negative association between long shelf life and graft integrity also exists. The effects of long shelf life on allograft materials warrants additional investigation.

▶ Although the authors emphasize their belief that "long shelf life negatively affects graft integrity," they have failed to delineate the roles that ethylene oxide sterilization and the freeze-drying process contribute.

J.S. Torg, M.D.

Graft Failure in Intra-articular Anterior Cruciate Ligament Reconstructions: A Review of the Literature

Vergis A, Gillquist J (Univ Hosp, Linköping, Sweden)

J Arthro Rel Surg 11:312–321, 1995 4–41

Introduction.—The long-term rates of good or excellent results for patients who have undergone anterior cruciate ligament (ACL) reconstructions vary from 75% to 90%. The substantial number of patients with unsatisfactory results is of concern. Published articles for the years 1984–1994 were identified from a MEDLINE database for intraoperative and postoperative factors that probably cause graft failure.

Methods.—Search terms were used to identify articles. Additional references were collected by cross-referencing those found with search terms. Articles that only confirmed the results of earlier investigations were not included unless they added new information. Eighty-nine articles were used.

Graft Failure.—Factors contributing to graft failure include: inadequate notchplasty, improper tunnel placement, inadequate fixation, improper tensioning, improper graft selection and harvest, and overzealous rehabilitation with too-early return to activity.

Minimizing Failure Rate.—Graft failures can be minimized by following correct operative and postoperative techniques. The incidence of postoperative graft impingement—which can lead to graft abrasion and partial or complete graft rupture—can be reduced by isometric tunnel placements and the performance of an adequate notchplasty, if needed. Use of a graft with bone plugs at its ends can enhance the ability to achieve initial fixation. The use of fresh-frozen allografts harvested under sterile conditions with strict disease-screening procedures has higher success rates than those that are cleanly harvested and sterilized by exposure to ethylene oxide or gamma radiation.

Synthetic ligaments have a high incidence of failure. If an interface screw fixation is not used, adequate protection is needed for the graft during the period of graft incorporation. Autograft and allograft reconstructions undergo phases of necrosis, decrease in strength, and revascularization. Too-intense and too-early activity can contribute to graft failure.

Conclusion.—A number of factors acting either alone or in combination can increase the incidence of graft failure.

▶ This constitutes a comprehensive review of the subject matter with 89 references. The original article is recommended for the interested reader.

J.S. Torg, M.D.

Etiology of Iliotibial Band Friction Syndrome in Distance Runners

Messier SP, Edwards DG, Martin DF, Lowery RB, Cannon DW, James MK, Curl WW, Read HM Jr, Hunter DM (Wake Forest Univ, Winston-Salem, NC; Wayne Cannon Physical Therapy and Associates, Winston-Salem, NC)

Med Sci Sports Exerc 27:951–960, 1995 4–42

Introduction.—Several clinical studies have suggested numerous and varied causal factors for the iliotibial band friction syndrome (ITBFS) in runners. To investigate risk factors for ITBFS, the differences in anthropometric, biomechanical, muscular strength, and training measures between runners with ITBFS and runners without injury and the multivariate relationships among these factors were evaluated.

Methods.—Sixty-six long-distance runners with ITBFS and 70 uninjured runners underwent detailed evaluation. Training variables were investigated with a training history questionnaire. Anthropometric measurements were obtained on both legs of each runner. Knee flexor and extensor strength and endurance were evaluated with an isokinetic dynamometer. Rearfoot movement was analyzed using a high-speed video camera as the runner ran on a treadmill. Running kinetics were evaluated as the runner ran over a force platform. The findings were analyzed to identify factors that discriminated between injury and control groups.

Results.—Of the training variables, weekly mileage, training pace, number of months of using the current training protocol, percentage of time running on a track, and percentage of time swimming were significant discriminators. Of the anthropometric variables, height significantly discriminated between injured and noninjured runners. Several isokinetic strength and endurance discriminators were identified, including flexion peak torque and flexion/extension ratio at 60 degrees/sec, extension work, extension average power, flexion peak torque/BW, and flexion work at 240 degrees/sec. Calcaneal to vertical touchdown angle and maximum supination velocity were the significant discriminators among rearfoot movement variables, and maximum normalized braking force was the only significant kinetic variable. After all of these significant variables were evaluated with a combined discriminant analysis, weekly mileage and maximum normalized breaking force emerged as the significant independent discriminators.

Discussion.—Using weekly mileage and maximum normalized breaking force to predict runners with ITBFS had a specificity of 84% but a sensitivity of only 46%. However, several training, anthropometric, strength, rearfoot motion, and kinetic variables were identified in significant association with ITBFS, which could be evaluated in a prospective observational trial.

▶ Presented here is a sophisticated analysis of etiologic factors responsible for ITBFS. In addition to identifying a number of potential risk factors, the results suggests that some clinical observations concerning the cause of this problem should be viewed with caution. Specifically, the authors point out that leg length discrepancy and running on crowned roads—often cited as risk factors for ITBFS—are actually similar in healthy runners and those afflicted with the problem.

J.S. Torg, M.D.

Conservative Treatment of Isolated Injuries to the Posterior Cruciate Ligament in Athletes

Shino K, Horibe S, Nakata K, Maeda A, Hamada M, Nakamura N (Osaka Rosai Hosp, Japan; Osaka Univ, Japan)

J Bone Joint Surg (Br) 77-B:895–900, 1995 4–43

Background.—Isolated injuries of the posterior cruciate ligament (PCL) appear to do well with conservative treatment, but recent studies suggest that degenerative changes can occur later. A prospective study of young athletes treated for acute, isolated PCL injury sought to determine the effect of associated cartilage damage on subsequent outcome.

Patients and Methods.—One of the patients was 44 years of age at the time of PCL injury; the remaining 21 patients ranged in age from 16 to 26 years. Eighteen injuries occurred during sport and 4 involved motorcycle accidents. Most patients (17 of 22) were male, and all were seen within 3 months of the injury. In all cases, the affected knee had no previous injury, and in no case did radiographs reveal bony lesions or osteoarthritic changes. Arthroscopic examination was performed through the anteromedial and anterolateral portals using a 4-mm arthroscope. The severity of cartilaginous injuries was graded on a scale of 0 (normal) to IV (erosion to the subchondral bone).

Results.—In all cases, the PCL was completely torn or severely attenuated over more than 70% of the ligament. There was no damage to the anterior cruciate ligament, the medial or the lateral capsule, the popliteal tendon, or the meniscofemoral ligaments. Four patients with significant damage to the articular cartilage of the medial femorotibial compartment were advised not to return to their sport. In 3 cases, PCL reconstruction was undertaken to repair a meniscal tear or instability. The remaining 15 patients were treated conservatively and resumed athletic activities. In 1 of these patients, however, arthritic symptoms developed as the result of newly developed severe chondral damage to the medial femoral condyle. Of 14 patients who returned to their original level of sports activity, 13 were followed for a mean of 51 months. Eleven patients still participated in sports at their preinjury level and 8 of 9 who were examined radiographically had no osteoarthritic changes.

Conclusion.—Most patients with PCL injury, no severe cartilaginous lesions, and residual posterior laxity of 2+ to 3+ performed well at sports during a mean follow-up of 51 months. In 4 of 22 knees with an acute, isolated PCL injury, severe damage to the articular cartilage of the medial femorotibial compartment was present. Further athletic activity is not advisable in such cases because of the likelihood that subsequent abnormal loading will result in degenerative joint disease. Early stabilization is advised for athletically active young patients with a grade II injury to the articular surface of the medial femoral condyle or for those with a reparable longitudinal tear of the meniscus.

▶ The management of isolated injuries to the PCL remains controversial. In addition to the criteria for surgery stated by Shino et al., it appears that other considerations should be made. Specifically, we previously published a report in which the data analysis supported the thesis that individuals with unidirectional PCL instability do not require repair or reconstruction. However, there was a much less favorable prognosis for PCL-deficient knees with multidirectional instability and, in this group, consideration for surgical stabilization is in order.[1]

J.S. Torg, M.D.

Reference

1. Torg JS, Barton TM, Pavlov H, et al: Natural history of the posterior cruciate ligament-deficient knee. *Clin Orthop* 246:208–216, 1989.

Fractures of the Lateral Process of the Talus: The Value of Lateral Tomography

Whitby EH, Barrington NA (Royal Hallamshire Hosp, Sheffield, England)

Br J Radiol 68:583–586, 1995 4–44

Objective.—In the 3 case reports presented in this article, lateral tomography was required to demonstrate the fracture site and extent of bony injury in fractures of the lateral process of the talus. Routine anteroposterior and lateral radiographs may be inadequate for diagnosis of this unusual, and often overlooked, fracture.

Case Report 1.—Man, 21, was examined in the emergency department after injuring his ankle playing football. Although anteroposterior and lateral radiographs of the ankle first appeared normal, subsequent review by the radiologist indicated soft tissue swelling, a slight widening of the medial aspect of the ankle mortise, and lucency within the lateral process of the talus. Findings were similar at anteroposterior tomography. Only lateral tomography clearly revealed a fragment of bone (1 cm in diameter) displaced from the lateral process of the talus (Fig 1C). The remaining 2 cases were similar in that lateral radiographs showed no abnormality and anteroposterior radiographs revealed swelling but not the extent of the injury or the degree of bone displacement.

Discussion.—Fractures of the lateral process of the talus are rarely reported. The mechanism of injury appears to be inversion of the ankle in

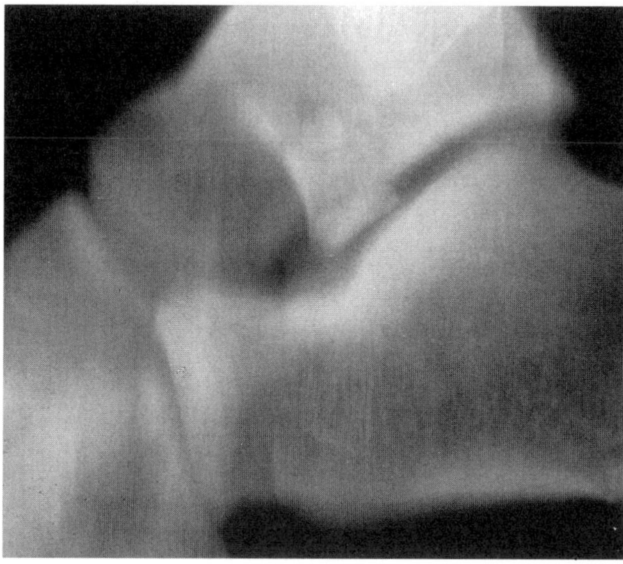

FIGURE 1C.—Lateral tomograph of the talus shows fragment of bone displaced from the lateral process. (Courtesy of Whitby EH, Barrington NA: Fractures of the lateral process of the talus: The value of lateral tomography. *Br J Radiol* 68:583–586, 1995.)

dorsiflexion or a high velocity injury. Lateral tomography is easily performed and readily available. It should be considered in patients with a significant mechanism of injury and localized acute tenderness.

▶ The relevance of this paper is seen in light of 2 large reported studies in which approximately half of the fractures were missed on initial radiographs. This apparently is caused by the fact that the fracture fragment is usually small and may be overlapped by the distal fibula and calcaneus on plain film.[1, 2]

J.S. Torg, M.D.

References

1. Heckman JD, McLean MR: Fractures of the lateral process of the talus. *Clin Orthop Rel Res* 199:108–113, 1985.
2. Mukherjee SK, Pringle RM, Baxter AD: Fracture of the lateral process of the talus: A report of thirteen cases. *J Bone Joint Surg (Br)* 56-B: 263–273, 1974.

The Tibiofibular Syndesmosis: Evaluation of the Ligamentous Structures, Methods of Fixation, and Radiographic Assessment

Xenos JS, Hopkinson WJ, Mulligan ME, Olson EJ, Popovic NA (Walter Reed Army Med Ctr, Washington, DC)

J Bone Joint Surg (Am) 77-A:847–856, 1995 4–45

Objective.—External rotation injuries disrupt the syndesmotic ligaments and result in disabling and chronic ankle instability. Evaluating ankle injuries, particularly when there is partial disruption, is difficult. Usually, the stress mortise radiograph is used to assess the degree of injury. The results of a study evaluating the role of the syndesmotic ligaments during external rotation torque, the degree of injury, the strength of fixation methods, and the value of stress mortise and stress lateral radiographs in assessing the extent of injury were presented.

Methods.—A total of 25 fresh frozen cadaver legs, amputated proximal to the knee, were dissected to expose the tibiofibular syndesmosis and mounted in neutral flexion on an external rotation instrument. In phase 1 of the study, the legs, with the ligaments intact, were tested with no load and then with 5.0 newton-meters of external rotation torque applied (Fig 3A). In phase 2, the same measurements were made after the anterior tibiofibular ligament was sectioned, again after each sectioning of the interosseous ligament in 2-cm increments to within 8 cm of the distal end, and again after the proximal sectioning of the interosseous ligament and the posterior tibiofibular ligament. In phase 3, measurements were repeated after all anterior tibiofibular ligaments were repaired with sutures and again after 12 ligaments were repaired with 1 transfixation screw and 13 were repaired with 2 transfixation screws. Mortise and lateral radiographs were done at each step under loaded and unloaded conditions.

Results.—Increase in injury was significantly related to diastasis and rotation. Under load, after all ligaments had been cut, the mean diastasis observed was 7.3 mm, and the mean increase in rotation was a significant 10.2 degrees. After suture repair, the mean torque at failure was 2.0 newton-meters with pull out of suture as the main failure mode. After repair with 1 screw, the mean torque at failure was 6.2 newton-meters, which was significantly less than the 11.0 newton-meter mean torque at failure for the 2-screw repair. Measurements of the diastasis on stress lateral radiographs were significantly correlated with measurements on the legs, and interobserver correlation was significantly higher for stress lateral radiographic measurements than for measurements on mortise radiographs.

Conclusion.—Diastasis as a result of external rotation torque is related to the degree of injury to the tibiofibular syndesmosis. Two-screw fixation for repair of the anterior tibiofibular ligament is significantly stronger than 1-screw or suture repair. The extent of diastasis in syndesmosis disruption is more highly correlated with stress lateral radiographic measurements than with stress mortise radiographic measurements.

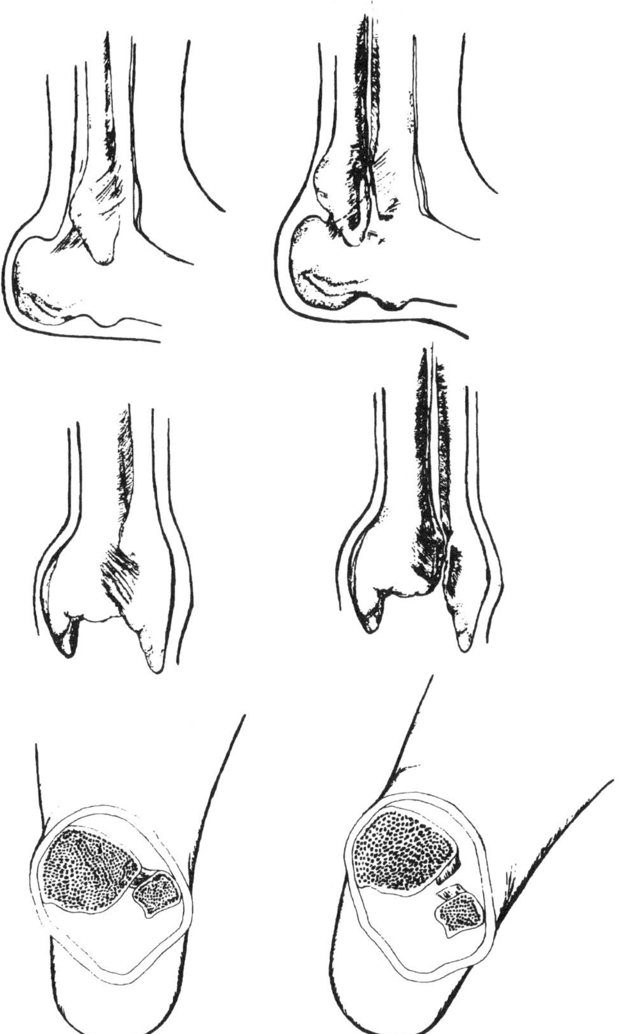

FIGURE 3A.—Schematic representation of the specimen under unloaded (**left**) and loaded (**right**) conditions. Note the posterolateral position of the fibula in relation to the tibia. (Courtesy of Xenos JS, Hopkinson WJ, Mulligan ME, et al: The tibiofibular syndesmosis: Evaluation of the ligamentous structures, methods of fixation, and radiographic assessment. *J Bone Joint Surg (Am)* 77-A:847–856, 1995.)

► As this study points out, diastasis of the distal aspect of the tibia and fibula on application of external rotation torque is related to the degree of injury to the syndesmosis. The current prevalence of syndesmotic injury associated with ankle sprains is reported in the literature to be between 1% and 11%. It is pointed out that the possible prevalence of this injury is higher because stress mortise radiographs were used in these studies, and, as the authors have pointed out, stress lateral radiographs are more reliable for assessment of the syndesmosis.

J.S. Torg, M.D.

Symptomatic Ossification of the Tibiofibular Syndesmosis in Professional Football Players: A Sequela of the Syndesmotic Ankle Sprain

Veltri DM, Pagnani MJ, O'Brien SJ, Warren RF, Ryan MD, Barnes RP (Luke AFB, Litchfield Park, Ariz; St Thomas Hosp, Nashville, Tenn; Hosp for Special Surgery, New York; et al)

Foot Ankle Intl 16:285–290, 1995 4–46

Introduction.—Studies of ankle sprain have found that injury to the syndesmotic ligaments is common among football players and that these injuries require a longer healing time than sprains involving the lateral ankle ligaments. Calcification and ossification of the syndesmosis frequently occur after syndesmotic ankle sprains. The syndesmotic ossification process in 2 professional football players was described.

Case 1.—A cornerback sustained a syndesmotic ankle sprain. Evaluation revealed no radiographic evidence of associated fractures, but there was tenderness over the anterior tibiofibular ligament. The external rotation test was performed with the patient sitting with the knee flexed 90 degrees and the ankle in a neutral position. The examiner's hands applied external rotational stress to the foot while stabilizing the proximal leg, and pain was produced, indicating positive results. After 6 weeks of aggressive physical therapy, the patient returned to competition and functioned at his pre-injury level early in the next season. However, pain in the posterolateral aspect of the ankle, induced by running and cutting, recurred approximately 1 year after the initial injury. There was radiographic evidence of ossification of the syndesmosis and cortical erosion at the posterolateral fibula (Fig 1). Uptake was significantly increased at the fibula on a bone scan. Computed tomography localized the ossification to the posterior tibiofibular syndesmosis contiguous with the tibial cortex. After surgical removal of the ossification, the player had no recurring pain at 28 months' follow-up and no recurring ossification.

Case 2.—A professional football player sustained a left syndesmotic ankle sprain with tenderness localized over the anterior tibiofibular ligament. An external rotation stress test produced positive results. Although he returned to competition 5 weeks after the injury, pain and swelling over the anterior aspect of the distal fibula recurred 8 months after the initial injury. There was radiographic evidence of an ossified mass in the anterior region of the distal syndesmosis with corresponding cortical hypertrophy of the

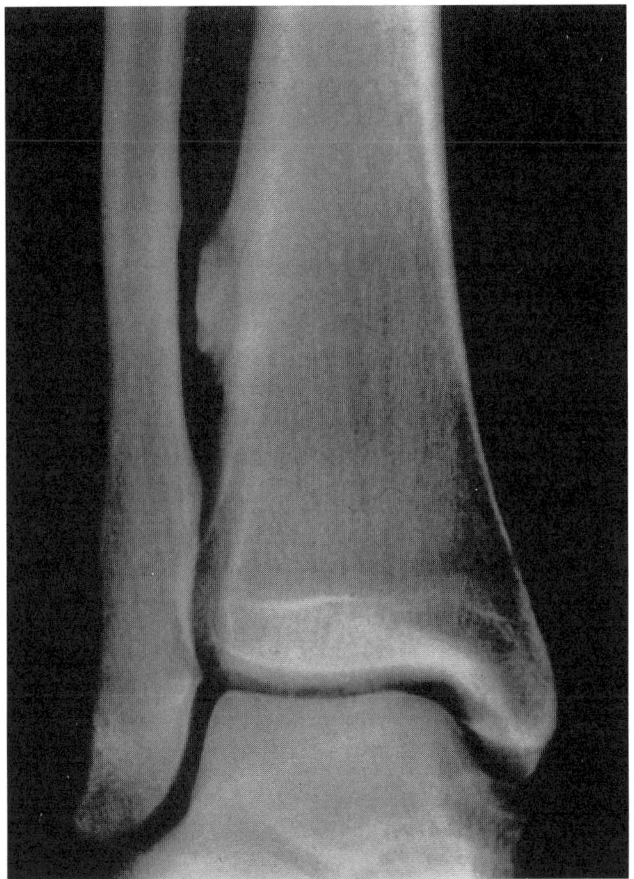

FIGURE 1.—Anteroposterior radiograph of the right ankle demonstrates ossification of the tibiofibular syndesmosis. (Courtesy of Veltri DM, Pagnani MJ, O'Brien SJ, et al: Symptomatic ossification of the tibiofibular syndesmosis in professional football players: A sequela of the syndesmotic ankle sprain. *Foot Ankle Intl* 16:285–290, 1995.)

tibia. Computed tomography scanning showed the presence of a frank synostosis (Fig 5). The ossification was removed, followed by immobilization in a posterior splint for 3 days. After 2 months of progressive physical therapy, the patient returned to competition and remained free of pain and ossification at the 1-year follow-up.

Discussion.—Repeat radiographs are recommended for patients with syndesmotic ankle sprains to monitor the development of syndesmotic calcification or ossification in the absence of frank synostosis. Bone scans can reveal increased osseous metabolic activity, and excision of symptomatic ossified masses should be delayed until bone scan activity is normalized.

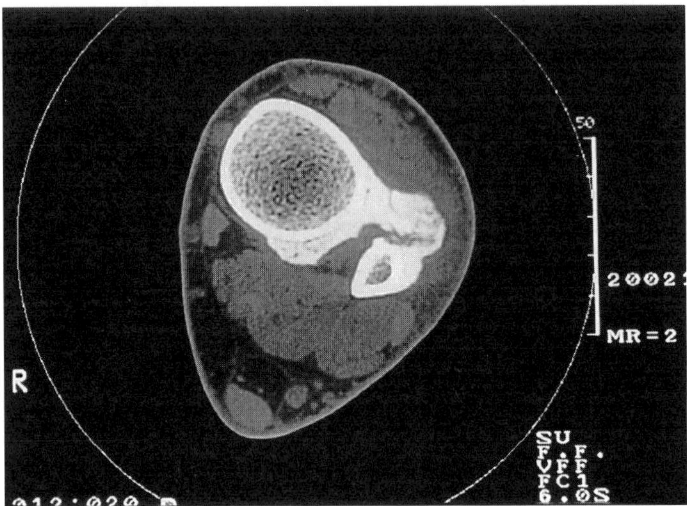

FIGURE 5.—Computed tomography scan shows ossification of the syndesmosis of the left ankle, resulting in a frank tibiofibular synostosis. (Courtesy of Veltri DM, Pagnani MJ, O'Brien SJ, et al: Symptomatic ossification of the tibiofibular syndesmosis in professional football players: A sequela of the syndesmotic ankle sprain. *Foot Ankle Intl* 16:285–290, 1995.)

▶ The observations and conclusions of the authors are in keeping with my own clinical experience in dealing with ossification of the tibiofibular syndesmosis.

J.S. Torg, M.D.

Effect of Maintained Stretch on the Range of Motion of the Human Ankle Joint

Kirsch RF, Weiss PL, Dannenbaum RM, Kearney RE (McGill Univ, Montréal)
Clin Biomech 10:166–168, 1995 4–47

Introduction.—A slow, maintained stretch to the end of the pain-free range is accepted as the best means of permanently augmenting range of motion. Its efficacy has not, however, been demonstrated under controlled experimental conditions.

Objective.—The ability of maintained stretch to increase the passive range of motion of the ankle joint was studied in 12 healthy adults 20–60 years of age.

Methods.—A rotary actuator configured as a position servo imposed controlled angular displacements on the ankle joint of the supine subject. A rigid glass fiber boot clamped the foot to the actuator. The voluntary pain-free range of motion was determined by peak dorsiflexion movements. Triangular movements then were applied, during each of which the joint was stretched to the dorsiflexion range of motion and held there for

1 minute. The electromyogram of the triceps surae and tibialis anterior was monitored to ensure that only passive movement generated ankle torque.

Results.—Seven of the 12 subjects had enough muscle activity to distort the subjective assessment of change in range of motion. In the other 5 subjects, the maintained stretch led to a small decrease in the torque subsequently generated by imposed dorsiflexion motion. The effect was largely absent after 5 minutes of rest at the neutral position.

Implication.—The viscoelastic properties of collagenous tissue that is stretched will produce a transient decrease in the joint resistance to motion, and this may influence judgments of altered joint mobility.

▶ The results of the authors' study do not support the hypothesis that maintained stretch affects a permanent change in ankle range of motion. This agrees with my observations during the past 25 years when I have attempted to increase my own range of motion or flexibility to little or no avail. About the only thing I can report is that I am also apparently not losing any range of motion.

Col. J.L. Anderson, PE.D.

Taping and Semirigid Bracing May Not Affect Ankle Functional Range of Motion

Lindley TR, Kernozek TW (Hamline Univ, St Paul, Minn; Univ of Minnesota)
J Athletic Train 30:109–112, 1995 4–48

Introduction.—After a sports injury, selected supportive devices can allow the athlete to return to training while preventing reinjury. The traditional taping methods have recently been replaced by commercial ankle stabilizers, resulting in some debate over the relative effectiveness of the 2 methods. Taping has its limitations, such as hindering running and agility in uninjured athletes as well as being unable to provide consistent support during extended exercise. Most of the current data use open kinetic chain testing, which does not mimic functional activities. How the functional range of motion of the ankle is affected by taping and semirigid orthoses was investigated.

Methods.—Eleven male football players with no history of ankle injury (confirmed by physical examination by the team orthopedist) volunteered to be subjects. Four variables were measured: functional range of motion, maximum ankle dorsiflexion and plantar flexion, and time in stance phase. There were 5 treatments: control (no support), Active Ankle Trainer, Airstirrup Ankle "Training" Orthosis, Ankle Ligament Protector (ALP), and the closed basketweave with moleskin stirrup technique. The order of treatments was counterbalanced through a Latin square design. The same brand of socks and shoes (Nike BBX Low-top) were used by all subjects. The subjects were videotaped while they ran a series of 40-yard sprints at

85% of maximum speed. Ankle ranges of motion, from markers placed on the lower leg and foot, and stance time were determined using the Peak 2D Manual Acquisition System.

Results.—The maximum plantar flexion occurred at the end of the stance phase. Maximum dorsiflexion occurred at various times in the various individuals. Plantar flexion was significantly lower when the subjects wore the ALP. There was no difference in dorsiflexion among the supportive methods. The functional range of motion was significantly lower for the ALP. Because the speed of running was controlled, there was no difference in stance time.

Conclusion.—The running required in this study did not test the range-restrictive characteristics of the devices tested. The use of open chain kinetic testing may not be appropriate for determining how the devices will respond to functional athletic activities. Of the devices tested, only the ALP restricted functional range of motion. The other 3 methods offer support to the ankle without compromising plantar flexion or dorsiflexion during running.

▶ The authors have stated, "Because range of motion demands are not as great during the running stance phase, the range restrictive characteristics of these supportive devices are not reached during running". The best way to test the effectiveness of these braces is to have the athletes wear them in controlled sport-specific activities. The athlete and athletic trainer can then determine which brace provides adequate support and is comfortable enough to be worn for an entire game or practice. Fitting of these ankle braces is also very important. Because of foot width, an athlete may be more comfortable in a larger or smaller brace than is indicated by sizing charts. Athletic trainers have reported on the successful use of a combination of tape and brace worn at the same time for acute ankle sprains. Please read Abstract 4–49.

F.J. George, A.T.C., P.T.

Ankle Ranges of Motion During Extended Activity Periods While Taped and Braced

Paris DL, Vardaxis V, Kokkaliaris J (Concordia Univ, Montreal; McGill Univ, Montreal)

J Athletic Train 30:223–228, 1995 4–49

Introduction.— The ankle sprain, particularly the inversion type, is the most common injury seen in sports. Supportive devices have been affixed to this area to reduce the incidence of ankle trauma, including cloth ankle wrap, elastic and nonelastic tape combinations, and nonelastic adhesive tape. There is still inconclusive information regarding the effects of taped ankle support compared to braced ankle support. The effects of nonelastic adhesive ankle tape and commercial ankle braces were examined on the range of motion after various periods of activity.

Methods.—Thirty males volunteered to have their plantar flexion–dorsiflexion and inversion-eversion range of motion compared with unsupported, nonelastic adhesive taped, Swede-O–braced, and SubTalar Support–braced ankles. Before activity, measurements were taken and were then repeated after 15, 30, 45, and 60 minutes of activity on a motorized treadmill.

Results.—Compared with unsupported ankles, all supports significantly reduced preactivity range of motion in all directions. Fifteen minutes after the initiation of activity with tape or the SubTalar Support brace, the ankle significantly increased its plantar flexion range of motion. After 30 minutes, the ankle increased its plantar flexion range of motion with the Swede-O brace. More increases in plantar flexion range of motion were seen with tape with continued activity. By 15 minutes of activity, all 3 supports had caused significant increases in inversion range of motion.

Conclusion.—Before activity, all 3 methods offer support in all directions. Both braces offer longer support than tape after activity is begun. The Swede-O brace resulted in longer support than the SubTalar Support brace during inversion range of motion and plantar flexion range of motion, actions that are prevalent in ankle sprains.

► This study should be read in conjunction with the study outlined in Abstract 4–48. The conclusions of the previous study and my comments should be considered when reading this study. There has been a great deal of controversy among athletic trainers regarding the effectiveness of ankle taping and bracing. Many factors should be considered, such as expense (both for tape and manpower for application of the tape), comfort, effect on function, the psychological effect, and the amount of time that the tape or brace will provide support during activity. Future studies should address the common practice of using a combination of tape and brace to provide a more effective support system that may last for longer periods of time.

F.J. George, A.T.C., P.T.

A Modified Low-dye Taping Technique to Support the Medial Longitudinal Arch and Reduce Excessive Pronation

Schulthies SS, Draper DO (Brigham Young Univ, Provo, Utah)

J Athletic Train 30:266–268, 1995 4–50

Background.—The low-dye arch support taping technique is commonly used in athletic training. A modified low-dye taping technique designed to support the medial longitudinal arch was described.

Technique.—With the athlete sitting or supine with the lower leg supported by a table and the foot extending past it, an anchor is applied around the metatarsal heads. Figure-eight strips are placed on the sole of the foot in a manner similar to a longitudinal arch support taping technique. The clinician attaches the tape to the

> dorsomedial aspect of the first metatarsal head, encircles the posterior aspect of the calcaneus, pulls the tape obliquely along the plantar aspect of the foot, then attaches the tape again to the dorsomedial aspect of the first metatarsal head. When applying the tape to the first metatarsal head, the clinician passively everts the forefoot and plantarflexes the first metatarsal (Fig 3) by simply twisting the forefoot so that the sole is turned out.

The clinician is careful not to passively pronate the subtalar joint during this procedure by keeping tension on the tape while applying the figure-eight strip around the posterolateral aspect of the calcaneus. Three to 5 figure eights are then applied to the first metatarsal head while the forefoot is twisted each time to evert, plantar flex, and adduct the forefoot on the rearfoot. The clinician may also apply alternating figure eights to the fifth metatarsal head but should not attempt to evert the forefoot during their application. Lateral to medial strips are then applied to the plantar aspect of the foot, beginning on the calcaneus and moving toward the forefoot until the first cuneiform is reached. The direction of the tape is then reversed and pulled from medial to lateral to further evert the forefoot and plantar flex the first metatarsal (Fig 4). The taping method is completed by the application of strips around the transverse plane of the foot. Strips of tape are applied over the dorsum of the forefoot to secure the tape on the plantar surface of the foot.

Conclusion.—As with many taping methods, the long-term use of this technique is precluded by cost, skin breakdown, and the possible creation

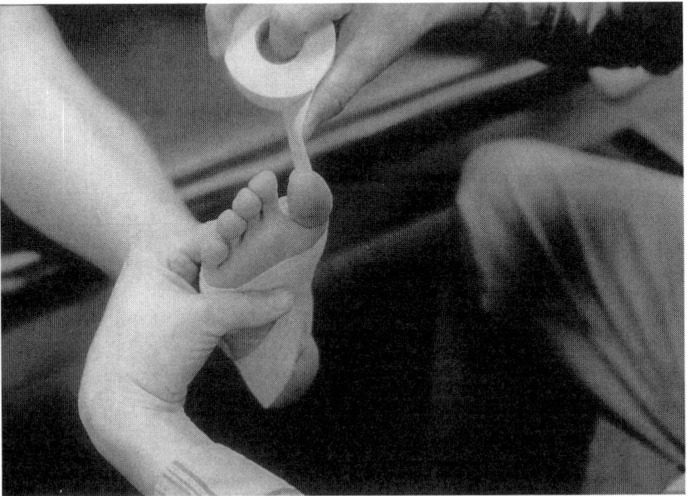

FIGURE 3.—Application of the figure-eight strips. The forefoot is passively everted and the first metatarsal is plantar flexed by the athletic trainer's left hand. The pull of the tape on the lateral calcaneus provides a counterforce to allow the subtalar joint to remain in the neutral position. (Courtesy of Schulthies SS, Draper DO: A modified low-dye taping technique to support the medial longitudinal arch and reduce excessive pronation. *J Athletic Train* 30:266–268, 1995.)

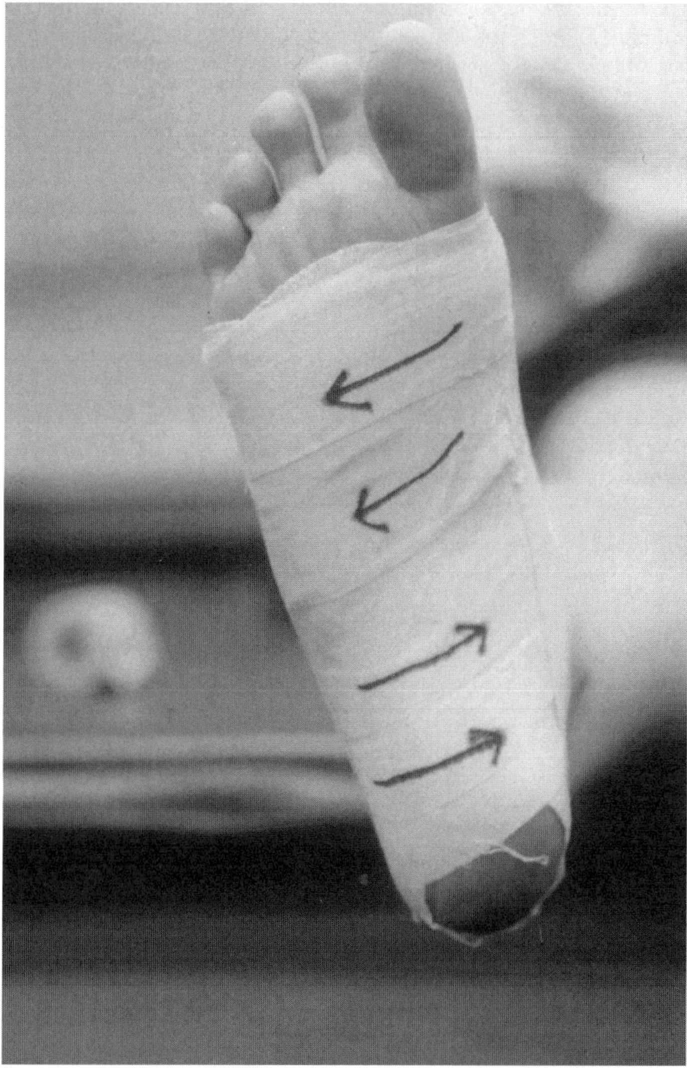

FIGURE 4.—A view of the plantar aspect of the foot showing the direction of pull of the tape. Note the lateral to medial pull on the calcaneus and the medial to lateral pull on the forefoot, thus stabilizing the midtarsal joint in eversion and the first metatarsal in plantar flexion. (Courtesy of Schulthies SS, Draper DO: A modified low-dye taping technique to support the medial longitudinal arch and reduce excessive pronation. *J Athletic Train* 30:266–268, 1995.)

of new overuse injuries. Foot orthotic intervention is indicated for long-term reduction of subtalar joint pronation or long-term arch support.

▶ Some very important points are emphasized in describing this taping procedure to reduce subtalar joint pronation. The authors caution, "Take care not to excessively evert the forefoot and plantar flex the first metatarsal.

This may cause the first metatarsal head to strike the ground first during early midstance which may cause abnormally high pressures under the first metatarsal head. This may also cause the subtalar joint to supinate excessively during weight bearing."

As in other taping techniques, a good deal of practice is required to perfect this procedure. Always evaluate the athlete in the standing position after taping is completed to determine the effectiveness of the procedure. A slight splaying of the toes may occur. If the desired results are not achieved, the tension of the tape may be increased or decreased.

F.J. George, A.T.C., P.T.

Late Versus Early Repair of Achilles Tendon Rupture: Clinical and Biomechanical Evaluation

Boyden EM, Kitaoka HB, Cahalan TD, An K-N (Mayo Clinic and Found, Rochester, Minn)

Clin Orthop 317:150–158, 1995 4–51

Background.—Authorities disagree on how best to treat acute Achilles tendon ruptures. Few reports have critically analyzed patient function after late Achilles tendon reconstruction is performed. One experience with late reconstruction of Achilles tendon rupture was reviewed, and the findings were compared with those of patients who had early repair.

Methods.—Eleven patients undergoing late reconstruction and 10 who had immediate repair were included in the study. Both groups were followed for 8 years.

Findings.—Based on a clinical score, all patients but 1 had excellent or good outcomes. Manual testing showed normal plantar flexion strength in all but 1 patient. However, significant differences were observed in isometric and isokinetic plantar flexion strength of the involved sides, compared with the uninvolved sides. In the patient with an unsuccessful outcome, abnormalities in vertical, foreaft, and medial-lateral force components of the ground reaction force were observed. Three-dimensional motion analysis in this patient showed reduced total motion in the sagittal plane on the operated side, compared with the unoperated side.

Conclusion.—The clinical outcomes of patients undergoing late reconstruction of Achilles tendon rupture are comparable with those of patients undergoing immediate repair. Outcomes in both groups are successful. The indications for immediate repair of the Achilles tendon rupture have yet to be determined.

▶ It has been my experience that late repair of Achilles tendon rupture has successful clinical results, comparable with those of earlier repair. That is to say, it is not necessary to augment the repair with adjacent soft tissue such as the plantaris tendon or an Achilles tendon turned down. The important point in late repair is that the procedure be performed with the patient supine so that maximal knee flexion and ankle dorsiflexion can be achieved to approximate the disruption.

J.S. Torg, M.D.

Achilles Tendon Ruptures: A New Method of Repair, Early Range of Motion, and Functional Rehabilitation

Mandelbaum BR, Myerson MS, Forster R (Santa Monica Orthopaedic and Sports Medicine Group, Calif; Union Mem Hosp, Baltimore, Md)

Am J Sports Med 23:392–395, 1995 4–52

Background.—The authors' approach to Achilles tendon ruptures includes a technique previously used for patellar tendon repair, using early, aggressive postoperative motion and weight-bearing to enhance tendon healing and strength. The results of this treatment protocol were evaluated prospectively.

Methods.—Twenty-nine athletes with Achilles tendon ruptures were treated. The patients were 25 men and 4 women aged 19 to 56 years. Repairs were done with a Krackow suture of no. 2 nonabsorbable polyfilament (Fig 1), and range-of-motion exercises were begun 72 hours later. The patients used a posterior splint for 2 weeks and began ambulating in a hinged orthosis. Orthosis use was discontinued 5 weeks after surgery,

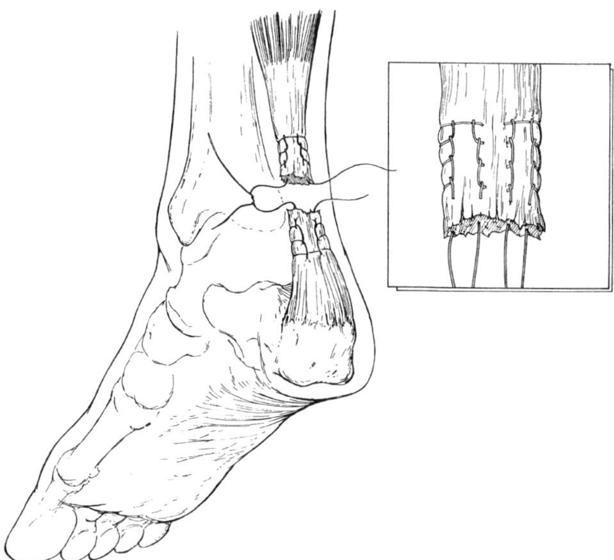

FIGURE 1.—The suture repair technique is shown. A second suture may be inserted in the center of the tendon to strengthen the repair (**inset**). (Courtesy of Mandelbaum BR, Myerson MS, Forster R: Achilles tendon ruptures: A new method of repair, early range of motion, and functional rehabilitation. *Am J Sports Med* 23:392–395, 1995.)

and full weight-bearing was allowed. Progressive resistance exercises were begun. Three, 6, and 12 months after surgery, isokinetic strength and endurance testing were done.

Outcomes.—No ruptures recurred. In 2 patients, superficial wound infections developed and were successfully treated with débridement or local wound care. A pulmonary embolism occurred in another patient. At the 3-month assessment, isokinetic assessment demonstrated mean functional deficits of 2.9% at 60 degrees/sec and 2.3% at 120 degrees/sec. At a mean of 4 months after surgery, all patients returned to their pre-injury activity levels. No significant differences in ankle motion, isokinetic strength, or endurance compared with the uninvolved side were found 12 months after surgery.

Conclusion.—Achilles tendon repair using this suture technique is effective. No postoperative ruptures occurred in this series, and patients had regained 94% of their pre-injury functional level by 6 months after surgery. This treatment approach is also cost-effective and has an acceptable complication rate.

▶ The results reported by the authors using early range-of-motion and functional rehabilitation in Achilles tendon rupture repairs is in keeping with my own clinical experience.

J.S. Torg, M.D.

5 Fitness, Muscle Training, and Exercise Prescription

Physical Activity and Public Health: A Recommendation From the Centers for Disease Control and Prevention and the American College of Sports Medicine

Pate RR, Pratt M, Blair SN, Haskell WL, Macera CA, Bouchard C, Buchner D, Ettinger W, Heath GW, King AC, Kriska A, Leon AS, Marcus BH, Morris J, Paffenbarger RS Jr, Patrick K, Pollock ML, Rippe JM, Sallis J, Wilmore JH (Univ of South Carolina, Columbia; Ctrs for Disease Control and Prevention, Atlanta, Ga; Cooper Inst, Dallas; et al)

JAMA 273:402–407, 1995 5–1

Introduction.—A healthy lifestyle includes regular physical activity. There is increasing evidence that exercise is related to numerous physical and mental health benefits. Although the public is increasingly aware of such benefits, millions of North Americans remain essentially sedentary. Public education is needed to encourage such individuals to participate in regular physical exercise.

Physical Activity and Health.—Epidemiologic research has demonstrated that chronic exercise is beneficial in patients with coronary heart disease, hypertension, non–insulin-dependent diabetes, osteoporosis, colon cancer, anxiety, and depression. Low levels of physical activity are associated with high all-cause mortality rates, which are reduced when middle-aged people take up exercise. Twelve percent of the annual deaths in the United States can be attributed to a lack of physical activity. These conclusions meet the epidemiologic criteria of causality: consistency, strength, temporal sequencing, dose response, plausibility, and coherence.

Demographics of Exercise.—The goal of Healthy People 2000 was to get 30% of the U.S. population exercising. Currently, only 22% of the population meet these goals and 24% remain totally sedentary. Men are more likely to exercise, than women, but the percentage of active individuals decreases with age in both sexes. Ethnic minorities are less active than white Americans, this difference being greater for women than for men. Regular exercisers are likely to be well educated.

Determinants of Participation.—"No time" is the primary excuse for not exercising, and an injury is the most frequently cited reason for stopping exercise. Smokers are more likely to drop out of an exercise program. There is less compliance with high- than with low-intensity programs. Positive influences are family and friend role models, whereas a lack of community facilities (e.g., paths, bicycle trails) works against continued exercise participation.

Activity Recommendations.—Every adult should accumulate 30 minutes or more of moderate intensity (the equivalent of a 3- to 4-mph walk) on most, if not all, days. This averages out to about 200 calories of energy expenditure per day. The activity can be continuous or accumulated through short bursts of exercise be it formal, structured exercise or work around the home (e.g., housework, gardening, playing with the children). This differs from an earlier recommendation that suggested the exercise be continuous and at a higher intensity. Health benefits increase according to the total amount of activity performed (Fig 2). The higher the level of fitness or activity, the lower the relative risk of cardiovascular mortality. Four features need to be emphasized. First, the total time spent on exercise is negatively associated with cardiovascular mortality. Second, the

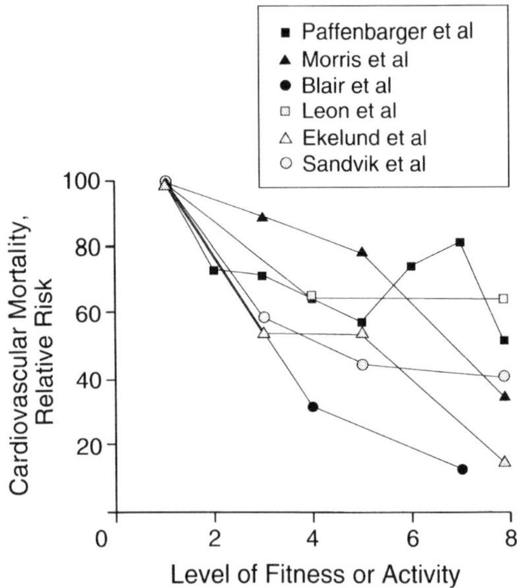

FIGURE 2.—The relationship between level of physical activity (Paffenbarger et al., Morris et al., and Leon et al.) or exercise capacity (Blair et al., Ekelund et al., and Sandvik et al.) and coronary heart disease mortality. Values for more active or fit persons are expressed as the ratio of the event rate for more active or fit divided by the event rate for least active or fit. (Courtesy of Pate RR, Pratt M, Blair SN, et al: Physical activity and public health: A recommendation from the Centers for Disease Control and Prevention and the American College of Sports Medicine. *JAMA* 273:402–407, Copyright 1995, American Medical Association.)

association is dose-dependent. Third, moderate exercise will bring about these effects. Fourth, intermittent activity (bouts, as short as 8–10 minutes that total 30 minutes a day) is effective in achieving the health benefits. An emphasis on flexibility and strength seems to improve balance, coordination, and agility and is of particular importance in programs for the elderly.

Call to Action.—A coordinated effort from public health agencies, health professionals, special populations, communities, educators, individuals, and families is necessary to increase the proportion of North Americans who engage in regular physical activity as a part of a healthy lifestyle.

► There have been a large number of consensus meetings concerned with physical activity and health over the past 4 years. Many have involved the same group of investigators, and most have reached essentially similar conclusions regarding the benefits to be derived from a physically active lifestyle. There has been less agreement on the minimum dose of activity needed to achieve such benefits, and the primary concern of the present panel was to examine this specific question. The available evidence is still somewhat sketchy, but it points to the conclusion that the greatest public health benefit would occur if those who are currently totally sedentary were to initiate a modest activity program. Some additional benefit would be derived from more vigorous effort, but as the intensity of physical activity increased, returns would diminish, and at the highest intensities adverse effects might be observed.

When the Healthy People 2000 program was begun, more ambitious goals were set, and indeed were believed to be important. Cynics may argue that the targets are merely being reduced downward to something that health educators can achieve. However, given the potential of vigorous programs to cause musculoskeletal injuries and a high drop-out rate, modest targets may actually have a greater impact upon public health than overambitious goals. Cost-effectiveness is also likely to be enhanced by the new approach, because much of the required exercise can be incorporated into ordinary daily activities without a need for expensive structured and supervised programs.

R.J. Shepard, M.D., Ph.D., D.P.E.

Health Promotion by Encouraged Use of Stairs

Blamey A, Mutrie N, Aitchison T (Greater Glasgow Health Board, Scotland; Univ of Glasgow, Scotland)

BMJ 311:289–290, 1995 5–2

Background.—The American College of Sports Medicine recommends that sedentary adults participate in 30 minutes or more of accumulated moderate physical activity on most days of the week. The use of stairs may make an important contribution toward achieving this target. Whether

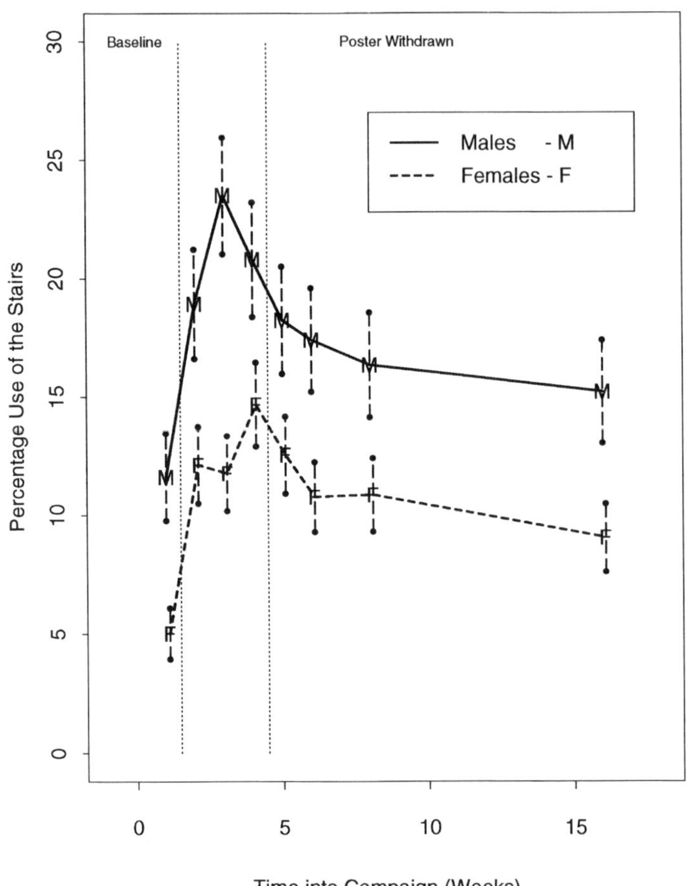

FIGURE.—Pattern of stair use among men and women during study. Values are weekly sample percentages with 95% confidence intervals. (Courtesy of Blamey A, Mutrie N, Aitchison T: Health promotion by encouraged use of stairs. *BMJ* 311:289–290, 1995. Reprinted with permission from the American College of Cardiology.)

members of a Scottish community would respond to signs prompting them to use the stairs rather than an escalator was examined.

Methods.—Signs reading "Stay Healthy, Save Time, Use the Stairs" were posted in a city center underground station featuring 2 flights of 15 steps that were adjacent to an escalator. The number of individuals using the stairs and escalator were recorded 3 times a week during a 16-week period. Observations were made during the week preceding the posting of signs, for 3 weeks after signs were placed, for 2 weeks immediately after signs were removed, and again during the fourth and twelfth week after sign removal. Stair use at baseline was compared with that noted during each of the subsequent observation periods.

Results.—The number of observations totaled 22,275. Stair use at baseline was approximately 8%, which increased to 15% to 17% during the 3 interventional weeks. Stair use by both men and women remained significantly higher than baseline levels during the 3 weeks that signs were posted, but a decrease was observed during the 2 weeks after signs were removed. Although stair use remained significantly higher than baseline 12 weeks after posters were removed, a downward trend suggesting a possible eventual return to baseline values was noted (Figure). Overall, women were more likely to use the escalator than men at all points during the study.

Conclusions.—The posting of motivational signs led to an improvement in stair use. Additional studies are needed to determine whether sedentary individuals or those who are currently active take note of these cues.

► The humble staircase has for too long been hidden behind marble paneling in our modern office towers. There is little doubt that if people were encouraged to use the stairs, not only by signs, but also by tricks of architectural design (making the stairs an attractive short-cut), a substantial amount of physical activity could be added to the day of many office workers. It is worth emphasizing that younger workers who can run up stairs two at a time can beat an elevator over several stories—I used to amuse some of my more sedentary colleagues by doing so over a distance as much as 13 floors!

R.J. Shepard, M.D., Ph.D., D.P.E.

Randomised Controlled Trials of Physical Activity Promotion in Free Living Populations: A Review

Hillsdon M, Thorogood M, Anstiss T, Morris J (West London Healthcare NHS Trust, Middlesex, England; London School of Hygiene and Tropical Medicine)

J Epidemiol Community Health 49:448–453, 1995 5–3

Background.—In a recent meta-analysis of physical activity as a risk factor for coronary heart disease, the relative risk in the least active subjects compared with the most active was 1.9. Randomized controlled trials of the promotion of physical activity in apparently healthy adults were reviewed systematically.

Methods.—Computerized databases and references were searched, and experts were contacted for information about existing research. The studies included were required to be randomized controlled trials of healthy, free-living adults in which exercise behavior was the dependent variable.

Findings.—Only 10 trials were found for the analysis, limiting the strength of conclusions and underscoring the need for more studies. In addition, the methodology of the trials varied greatly, as did the definitions of compliance. The data suggest that increasing activity levels and maintaining these levels at a frequency and intensity sufficient for long-term health benefits is possible. The best way to achieve this is through home-based exercise of moderate intensity that can be done alone or with others, is enjoyable, convenient, and can be completed in 3 sessions per week. Walking meets all these criteria. Early compliance may be improved

TABLE 2.—Summary of Results

Study	*Quality score (0–3)*	*No in study*	*Subjects*	*Post intervention follow up*	*Actual frequency intensity and duration of exercise intervention group*	*Main outcomes p <0.05*
1	2	50	Wives of graduate students	Nil	Mean frequency = 1.7 wk.	Subjects in *relevant* balance sheet group attended approximately twice as frequently as the *irrelevant* balance sheet and control group.
2	1	124	Male firefighters aged 24–56 y	3&6 mth	Not stated.	No significant difference between groups at 2 mth follow up.
3	1	58	18–20 y old, previously sedentary, female psychology students	2 mth	Mean frequency JAR and G = 2.4/wk; GR = 1.4/wk.	83% of jogging alone + relapse subjects still exercising at follow up compared with 36% of control subjects. No significant difference between groups on post study fitness levels.
4	1	315	Males aged 53–72 y with one or no risk factors for CHD	12 y	Mean hours jogging/wk at year 13 = 0.3 h.	No difference between exercise and control conditions at follow up on jogging hours per week.
5	2	229	Post menopausal women aged 50–65 y	Annually	Mean miles walking/wk = 8.4. Mean energy expenditure = 1514 kcal/wk.	Self reported walking level significantly higher at year 1 & 2 compared with controls.
6	1	103	52 male and 51 female, middle aged subjects	Nil	Adoption arm = mean of 3 sessions/wk for 32 min. Maintenance arm = mean of 2.9 sessions/wk for 37 min.	Adoption arm = subjects receiving telephone support showed significant increase in VO_{2max}. Maintenance arm = daily self monitoring resulted greater exercise frequency than weekly self monitoring.
7	1	77	28 men (mean age 40) and 49 women (mean age 36)	Nil	Self monitoring group = mean of 2.4/wk for 26 mins. Reinforcement group = mean of 2.5/wk for 29 mins.	Increase in VO_{2max} in all three conditions. Behavioural interventions increased frequency of exercise compared to controls.
8	2	357	160 women and 197 men aged 50–65 y Predominantly white and well educated	On-going	Mean frequency = HIG ~ 1.2/wk HIH ~ 2/wk LIH ~ 3/wk	Increase in VO_{2max} in all exercise groups. Higher adherence in both home based conditions. No changes in other CHD risk factors.
9	1	61	Middle or upper class, middle aged, apparently healthy, male bank workers	4 mth	Mean of 12.9 km/wk.	Only changes in vigour on psychometric test significantly correlated with 8 mth activity levels. No significant differences in lipids, blood pressure, body composition or endurance capacity.
10	1	120	Previously sedentary, female university employees with a mean age of 35 y and mean body mass index of 25	2 mth	Percentage of classes attended during the 18 wk RP = 51%, R = 49%.	No significant difference in attendance at 18 wk or 2 mth follow up.

Abbreviations: JAR, jogging alone plus relapse prevention; *G*, group jogging; *GR*, group jogging plus relapse prevention; *HIG*, high-intensity group; *HIH*, high-intensity home; *LIH*, low-intensity home; *RP*, relapse prevention; *R*, reinforcement.

(Courtesy of Hillsdon M, Thorogood M, Anstiss T, et al: Randomised controlled trials of physical activity promotion in free living populations: A review. *J Epidemiol Community Health* 49:448–453, 1995.)

through self-monitoring and relapse prevention training. Continuing support and reinforcement may improve long-term compliance. The most effective compliance strategy may be an initial brief instructional session followed by short, frequent telephone support. Such interventions are not as costly as facility-based group exercise interventions. The barriers and costs associated with attendance at facility-based programs may result in high drop-out rates. Increasingly popular prescription-for-exercise schemes are unlikely to increase population activity levels effectively (Table 2).

Conclusions.—Previously sedentary adults are able to increase and sustain increased activity levels. Personal instruction, continued support, and exercise of moderate intensity that does not rely on attending facility-based programs are needed to promote these changes. Such exercise should be enjoyable and easily included into existing lifestyles. Walking is most likely to meet these criteria.

► There is now little discussion that North Americans need to take more exercise. The problem is, how can this be accomplished? The "medicalization" of moderate activity is increasingly considered as a possible factor contributing to the current prevalence of sedentary lifestyles. People do not need extensive medical examination and attendance at a costly, distant, and specialized facility to get moderate amounts of exercise. One would even question the assumption in this paper that a brief instructional session is needed so that people find out how to walk, although it may be useful to talk about ideas like walking a couple of bus stops or one subway station on the way to work.

A number of studies have shown that "lack of time" is the most common reason for not exercising, and an important component of this "lack of time" is the perception that precious hours must be spent in traveling to and from fitness centers to exercise. One important issue is whether the usual home-based exercise of walking provides sufficient physical activity for health. The answer depends on the individual's age and initial fitness—fast walking can be quite a challenge for an elderly unfit adult, but it will amount to only 35% to 40% of maximal oxygen intake in a fit young adult. The metabolic demands of walking can be augmented by increasing the speed from perhaps 4–5 km/hr to 6–7 km/hr, including a route with hills, and carrying a substantial load, such as a briefcase with several books.

R.J. Shepard, M.D., Ph.D., D.P.E.

Cardiorespiratory Fitness and Coronary Heart Disease Risk Factor Association in Women

Kokkinos PF, Holland JC, Pittaras AE, Narayan P, Dotson CO, Papademetriou V (Veterans Affairs Med Ctr, Washington, DC; Georgetown Univ, Washington, DC; Natl Defense Univ, Washington, DC; et al)

J Am Coll Cardiol 26:358–364, 1995 5–4

Background.—A sedentary lifestyle is associated with increased risk for myocardial infarction and coronary heart disease. Coronary heart disease is the leading cause of death in women. There is little reliable information on the effects of increased physical activity on coronary risk factors in women. The correlation between physical fitness and coronary risk factors in healthy women was assessed.

Methods.—The subjects were 478 nonsmoking, healthy women between 22 and 79 years of age. A medical history was obtained, and examination included a rest ECG, blood pressure, fasting blood chemistry, and lipoprotein analyses. Fitness was determined by the Bruce graded exercise test. Three fitness categories were established based on treadmill exercise time to exhaustion and were adjusted for age. Among these categories, body weight, body mass index, and sum of skinfolds differed significantly.

Results.—Triglyceride and low-density lipoprotein cholesterol levels, ratio of total cholesterol to high-density lipoprotein cholesterol, glucose levels, and rest systolic and diastolic blood pressures were directly correlated with age, body mass index, and body weight; these measurements were inversely correlated with exercise time. High-density lipoprotein cholesterol levels were inversely correlated with body mass index, body weight, and glucose levels and directly correlated with treadmill time and alcohol consumption. Treadmill time was directly correlated with weekly

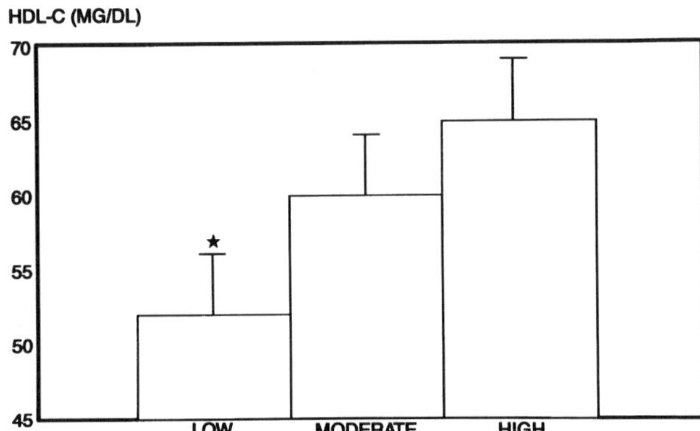

FIGURE 2.—High-density lipoprotein cholesterol *(HDL-C)* levels for women in the low, moderate, and high fitness categories. *Different from one another ($P < 0.001$). (Courtesy of Kokkinos PF, Holland JC, Pittaras AE, et al: Cardiorespiratory fitness and coronary heart disease risk factor association in women. *J Am Coll Cardiol* 26:358–364, 1995. Reprinted with permission from the American College of Cardiology.)

mileage and length of training. Weekly mileage, body mass index, and length of training were the strongest independent determinants of treadmill time. The lipoprotein-lipid profiles of the 3 fitness categories differed significantly. There was a correlation between more favorable profiles and higher fitness (Fig 2).

Discussion.—Cardiorespiratory fitness is independently and strongly correlated with all the coronary risk factors that were examined. Even moderate fitness levels can improve coronary risk factor profiles in women. The fitness level that was correlated with significant improvement in coronary risk factors can easily be met by women engaging in activity of moderate intensity, such as a brisk, daily walk of 30–60 minutes. Such physical activity is feasible for and within the ability of most women and has a low risk/benefit ratio.

► Many women are unaware that heart disease is the leading cause of mortality among women. This is probably not surprising in view of the fact that until recently women were usually excluded from studies relating risk factors to cardiovascular disease. The Multirisk Factor Intervention Trial, aptly called MR FIT, enrolled 15,000 men but no women. Now that attention is being directed to the prevention of cardiovascular disease in women, it is encouraging to see that physical activity has the same positive effect on risk factors for women that it does for men. Although these authors did not obtain information on diet, oral contraceptive use, or hormone replacement therapy, their data from a different population of women confirms the results reported by Blair and colleagues for women tested at the Cooper Institute for Aerobics Research.

B.L. Drinkwater, Ph.D.

Long Term Effects of Smoking on Physical Fitness and Lung Function: A Longitudinal Study of 1393 Middle Aged Norwegian Men for Seven Years

Sandvik L, Erikssen G, Thaulow E (Central Hosp of Akershus, Nordbyhagen, Norway)

BMJ 311:715–718, 1995 5–5

Purpose.—Physical fitness, an important predictor of mortality, is mainly a function of the status of the cardiovascular and respiratory systems. Although smoking is known to hasten the decline of lung function, there are few data concerning its effects on physical performance. The link between smoking and long-term declines in physical fitness and lung function was studied in healthy middle-aged men.

Methods.—The study included 1,393 apparently healthy Norwegian men aged 40–59 years at baseline. All underwent a detailed evaluation, including cardiovascular examination, first in 1972–1975 and again in 1980–1982. Seven hundred ninety-one men were nonsmokers and 347 were smokers at both examinations; the remainder either quit or started

TABLE 4.—Physical Fitness (J/kg) of Healthy Middle-Aged Men by Smoking Habit

	Unchanged smoking habits		Changed smoking habits	
	Non-smokers	Smokers	Stopped smoking	Started smoking
All subjects:				
No of men	791	347	199	56
Baseline fitness	1618 (630)	1349 (413)*	1477 (520)	1565 (457)
Follow up fitness	1532 (639)	1132 (439)*	1307 (593)	1362 (471)
Difference	86 (384)	217 (307)*	170 (338)	203 (338)
95% Confidence interval of difference	59 to 113	185 to 149	123 to 217	114 to 292
Men aged 40–49 at baseline:				
No of men	437	182	95	32
Baseline fitness	1808 (653)	1488 (392)*	1645 (567)	1613 (391)
Follow up fitness	1761 (659)	1280 (430)*	1546 (654)	1473 (487)
Difference	47 (411)	208 (332)*	99 (355)	139 (351)
95% Confidence interval of difference	8 to 86	160 to 256	28 to 170	17 to 261
Men aged 50–59 at baseline:				
No of men	354	165	104	24
Baseline fitness	1384 (513)	1195 (380)*	1324 (423)	1501 (535)
Follow up fitness	1250 (483)	968 (389)*	1088 (430)	1214 (412)
Difference	134 (341)	227 (277)*	236 (308)	287 (307)
95% Confidence interval of difference	98 to 170	185 to 269	177 to 195	164 to 410

Note: Values are mean (± 1 SD) unless stated otherwise.
* $P < 0.001$ compared with persistent nonsmokers.
(Courtesy of Sandvik L, Erikssen G, Thaulow E: Long term effects of smoking on physical fitness and lung function: A longitudinal study of 1393 middle aged Norwegian men for seven years. *BMJ* 311:715–718, 1995.)

smoking during the interval. The long-term effects of smoking on physical fitness, as reflected by total work performed during a symptom-limited cycle ergometer test, divided by body mass, and on lung function—as measured by forced expiratory volume in 1 second—were assessed.

Results.—Initial work performed to exhaustion was 1,349 J/kg in the persistent smokers compared to 1,618 J/kg in the persistent nonsmokers. Initial forced expiratory volume was 3,341 vs. 3,638 mL. Over the 7-year period between evaluations, work performance declined by a mean of 217 J/kg in smokers vs. 86 J/kg in nonsmokers (Table 4). The decrease in forced expiratory volume was 271 vs. 116 mL. Adjustment for age and physical activity had little influence upon the smoking-related differences. Men who quit smoking had fitness and pulmonary function changes similar to those of the persistent nonsmokers, whereas men who started smoking had changes similar to those of the persistent smokers.

Conclusions.—Middle-aged men who smoke have lower levels of physical fitness than men who do not smoke, and smokers show significantly greater declines in fitness over time. Comparable differences are noted in pulmonary function, but the difference in forced expiratory volumes does not fully account for smoking's effects on fitness. The major factors limiting maximal exercise performance in healthy subjects appear to be cardiovascular in nature.

► It has been known for a number of years that the aging of lung volumes proceeds more rapidly in the smoker than in the nonsmoker. But there is less information concerning the impact of smoking on a person's tolerance of exhausting work. It will be important to check that the differences observed in this paper do not reflect some extraneous factor, such as socioeconomic status, diet, or exposure to air pollutants. However, there are a number of possible explanations of the observed effects that are related more directly to smoking history. Carbon monoxide may block oxygen transport, not only by a high-affinity binding with hemoglobin and a resultant leftward shifting of the oxygen dissociation curve, but also by combining with cytochrome. The effects of such binding would be particularly evident in an all-out, exhausting exercise test, of the type used in the present study. Moreover, smoking has many effects upon the lungs. Not only are spirometric volumes reduced, but the distribution of inspired gas is impaired and pulmonary diffusing capacity decreases, so that the uptake of oxygen in the pulmonary capillaries may be limited in smokers. Finally, there could be a downregulation of inotropic mechanisms in the myocardium response to repeated catecholamine release during smoking.[1]

R.J. Shephard, M.D., Ph.D., D.P.E.

Reference

1. Laustiola KE, Lassila R, Kaprio J, et al: Decreased beta-adrenergic receptor density and catecholamine response in male cigarette smokers. A study of monozygotic twin pairs discordant for smoking. *Circulation* 78:1234–1240, 1988.

The Mechanics of Torso Flexion: Situps and Standing Dynamic Flexion Manoeuvres

McGill SM (Univ of Waterloo, Ont, Canada)

Clin Biomech 10:184–192, 1995 5–6

Background.—Because of the lack of knowledge of tissue force-time histories during torso flexion exercise performance, the mechanics of torso flexion has not been studied thoroughly. The loads on low back tissues were documented in addition to the kinematics of the torso during the performance of various flexion maneuvers.

Methods and Findings.—Twelve young healthy men volunteered for the study. None had had low back pain for at least the 1 preceding year nor any disabling back injury. Tissue load distribution was determined using an anatomically detailed, three-dimensional model sensitive to lumbar curvature and muscle activation patterns. Assessments were made during the performance of isometric and dynamic situps as well as standing flexion maneuvers. The sit-ups were done beginning with the torso flexed, which was lowered to horizontal, then raised again. Instrumentation limitations did not permit the volunteers to rest their torsos in the lowered position. Air flow during inhalation-exhalation; intra-abdominal pressure; myoelectric activity of the torso muscles, intercostals, and rectus femoris;

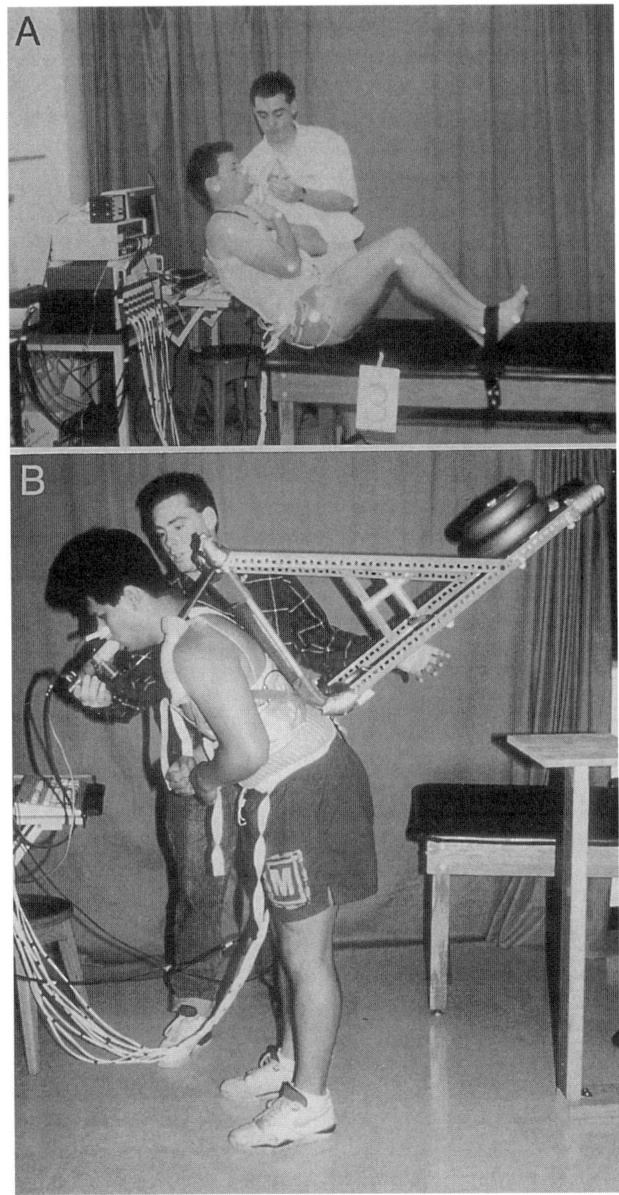

FIGURE 1.—**A**, with the subject in a sit-up posture, lung air was measured with a pneumotach in series with the mouth, intra-abdominal pressure was measured with a catheter through the nose and anchored in the stomach, myoelectric electrodes over the torso and rectus femoris monitored muscle activity, and lordosis was measured with a 3-SPACE ISOTRAK secured over the sacrum and T12–L1. **B**, isometric and dynamic flexion efforts were conducted with the subject in a standing posture with a pack frame loaded with weight to produce a flexion challenge. (Reprinted from *Clinical Biomechanics*, Vol. 10, McGill SM: The mechanics of torso flexion: Situps and standing dynamic flexion manoeuvres. pp 184–192, Copyright 1995, with kind permission from Elsevier Science Ltd, The Boulevard, Langford Lane, Kidlington 0X5 1GB UK.)

three-dimensional dynamic curvature of the lumbar spine; and body segment displacements were determined (Fig 1). The predicted lumbar compressive loads predicted for straight-leg and bent-knee sit-ups exceeded 3,000 N. Bent-knee and straight-leg sit-up techniques were not significantly biologically different.

Conclusions.—Performing dynamic and quasistatic sit-ups seems to impose high levels of compressive loading on the low back. The question of whether to recommend the straight-leg or bent-knee technique is probably not as important as that of whether sit-ups should be prescribed at all.

▶ The author questions whether the sit-up exercise should ever be used for training or for physical fitness testing. This comment gets my attention immediately because in the U.S. Army the sit-up exercise is 1 of the 3 test events in the Army Physical Fitness Test that all soldiers must take twice each year. He bases his finding on the compressive loading on the low back. However, he does not explain how he arrived at the conclusion that 3,000 N must be considered to constitute a significant risk for some people. What about healthy, physically fit people? It has been my experience that most people suffering from low back pain are not people who are involved in a balanced exercise program, but rather are people who have no exercise program or one that is seriously out of balance. We have noticed that most individuals with low back pain will get significant relief when they include proper back extension exercises to help strengthen the erector spinae muscles. I must admit that although this research appears to be well done, I am constitutionally opposed to placing limits on functional physical activities that the body is capable of performing. It certainly should take a number of replications of studies such as this before we arrive at a definitive decision.

Col. J.L. Anderson, PE.D.

Benefits and Practical Use of Cross-Training in Sports

Loy SF, Hoffmann JJ, Holland GJ (California State Univ, Northridge; Univ of California, Davis)

Sports Med 19:1–8, 1995 5–7

Introduction.—The popularity of triathlons is partly responsible for new research into the benefits of cross-training. In this article, cross-training means training in an activity or mode that is not task- or sport-specific. The purpose of cross-training or combining cross-training with task-specific training is to attain a level of performance as good as or better than the performance level achieved by sport-specific training alone.

Dissimilar Modes.—Various studies have examined specific cardiovascular and peripheral changes associated with cross-training using dissimilar activities or modes, and how training in one activity affects performance in others. Other studies have examined transfer effects of arm or leg exercise to the untrained muscle. These studies and their findings are discussed in detail.

Similar Modes.—To apply cross-training successfully, the physiologic needs of the single-event athlete must be understood so that the results of cross-training can be compared with those of sport-specific training. One study reported that the physiologic demands of running and stair-climbing are similar for the specific muscles involved. In treadmill and track running performance, subjects who trained in stair-climbing increased the maximum oxygen consumption ($\dot{V}O_{2max}$) by 2% and decreased their initial run time by 8%. Likewise, subjects who trained in running increased the $\dot{V}O_{2max}$ by 16% and decreased their initial run time by 11%. The group that trained in stair-climbing lost fewer days to injuries related to exercise. The study concluded that stair-climbing was a practical alternative to running. Additional studies of cross-training in activities that use similar muscle groups were also reviewed.

Conclusions.—Research suggests that cross-training benefits most athletes, especially cross-training in similar activities. It may be beneficial to use an alternative mode alone or combined with the primary training mode. Athletes must evaluate their own strengths and weaknesses as well as the demands of specific athletic events to determine how best to apply the various methods of cross-training.

▶ Cross-training can be a very beneficial tool in an athletic trainer's injury prevention and alternate workout program. Cross-training can be used to reduce the number of stress-related injuries and to help prevent "staleness" in athletes with extended seasons. It is very difficult for an injured athlete to understand that rest is an important component of healing. Cross-training will help athletes accept the prescription if they still believe they are getting a good workout.

F.J. George, A.T.C., P.T.

Influence of Breathing Technique on Arterial Blood Pressure During Heavy Weight Lifting

Narloch JA, Brandstater ME (Loma Linda Univ Med Center, Calif; Jerry L Pettis Mem VA Hosp, Loma Linda, Calif; SPORT Clinic, Riverside, Calif)

Arch Phys Med Rehabil 76:457–462, 1995 5–8

Purpose.—Intracerebral hemorrhage and other health risks associated with blood pressure (BP) elevation during heavy weight lifting have been reported. The risk of stroke would likely be reduced by any training intervention that would lessen the pressor effect of exercise. Two cases of intracerebral hemorrhage were recently seen in previously healthy recreational weight lifters. This experience prompted a study of the effects of breathing technique on arterial BP during heavy weight lifting.

TABLE.—Subject Data of Maximal Blood Pressure

Subject	Resting BP	Resting BP VALSALVA	85% Exercise Breathing	85% Exercise VALSALVA	100% Exercise Breathing	100% Exercise VALSALVA
1	100/60	130/100	130/100	210/180	140/110	240/200
2	130/90	200/150	170/150	300/250	200/180	350/320
3	130/70	200/180	190/170	270/250	250/230	360/340
4	130/70	170/150	190/170	290/280	180/160	310/280
5	140/30	200/180	210/180	300/270	240/210	330/300
6	140/110	180/160	170/150	270/250	200/170	300/280
7	100/70	140/120	110/90	200/170	140/120	200/170
8	140/70	210/170	190/170	260/220	200/180	300/270
9	120/90	180/170	200/170	280/250	230/200	350/320
10	140/110	190/170	220/200	290/270	200/190	370/360
Average	127/82	180/155	178/156	267/239	198/175	311/284

Note: Blood pressure readings at rest and peak values during exercise using Valsalva's maneuver and open glottis technique.

Abbreviation: BP, blood pressure.

(Courtesy of Narloch JA, Brandstater ME: Influence of breathing technique on arterial blood pressure during heavy weight lifting. *Arch Phys Med Rehabil* 76:457–462, 1995.)

Methods.—Radial artery catheterization for BP recording was performed in 10 male athletes who regularly used free weights. All the athletes performed double-leg press sets at 85% and 100% of maximum. These exercises were performed once with a closed-glottis Valsalva maneuver and again with slow exhalation during concentric contraction. Mean and maximal blood pressures were compared for these 2 breathing techniques.

Results.—At 100% maximum, the mean BP with Valsalva was 311/284, rising to 370/360 for 1 individual. In contrast, at the same level of lifting, mean BP with slow exhalation was 198/175. Breathing out also lowered the pressor response at 85% maximal lifting (Table).

Conclusions.—Heavy weight lifting with a closed-glottis Valsalva maneuver causes extreme arterial hypertension. This change can be dramatically reduced by slow exhalation during lifting, without a Valsalva maneuver. Breathing with an open glottis during heavy resistance exercise may reduce the risk of stroke.

► It is widely recognized that performance of the Valsalva maneuver can cause a substantial elevation of blood pressure during weight lifting, but it is useful to have careful documentation of both the extreme pressures that can develop and a direct comparison showing the extent to which such dangers can be avoided by the simple expedient of slow expiration during the lift. Other factors influencing the extent of the rise in blood pressures are the mass of muscle that is exerted[1] and weight-lifting experience.[2] MacDougall et al.[3] found even higher pressures (up to 480/350 mm Hg) when subjects exhaled against a mouthpiece.

There seems to be a need to examine more carefully the risk of adverse response to such high pressures. The literature contains scattered case reports of cerebrovascular accidents, but nothing from which one could form a clear estimate of risk.

R.J. Shephard, M.D., Ph.D., D.P.E.

References

1. Lewis SF, Snell PG, Taylor WF, et al: Role of muscle contraction mass and mode of contraction in circulatory response to exercise. *J Appl Physiol* 58:146–151, 1985.
2. Fleck SJ, Dean LS: Resistance training experience and the pressor response to heavy resistance exercise. *J Appl Physiol* 63:116–120, 1987.
3. MacDougall JD, Tuxen D, Sale D, et al: Arterial blood pressure response to heavy resistance exercise. *J Appl Physiol* 58:785–790, 1985.

Spontaneous Pneumothorax in Weightlifters

Marnejon T, Sarac S, Cropp AJ (St Elizabeth Hosp, Youngstown, Ohio; North-Eastern Ohio Univ, Rootstown)

J Sports Med Phys Fitness 35:124–126, 1995 5–9

Introduction.—Infrequently, pneumothorax can be caused by exertion. Weight lifting appears to be an extremely rare cause of spontaneous pneumothorax, with only 1 previously published case. Three patients with spontaneous pneumothorax associated with weight lifting were seen.

Case 1.—Man, 64, with a history of mild chronic obstructive pulmonary disease, was hospitalized with dyspnea and chest pain radiating to the left shoulder. The pain started the day before his admission while he was lifting weights. The only remarkable finding of the physical examination was diminished breath sounds on the left side. Left-sided pneumothorax was seen on the chest radiograph. He was treated successfully with tube thoracostomy. However, the left-sided pneumothorax recurred 4 weeks later while he was lifting a garage door and he required open thoracotomy.

Case 2.—Boy, 14 years, complained of pleuritic chest pain and dyspnea. He had no history of respiratory illness, but reported starting weight lifting 1 week before his admission. He had subcutaneous emphysema from the right sternal border into the neck. A small right apical pneumothorax, pneumomediastinum, and subcutaneous air extending into the neck were seen on the chest radiograph. He was successfully treated with oxygen and acetaminophen.

Case 3.—Man, 18, complained of right-sided neck pain radiating to the right chest wall and exacerbated by deep inspiration. He had lifted weights the day before his admission. He had subcutaneous emphysema along the border of the right sternocleidomastoid muscle. Chest radiography demonstrated a small apical right-sided pneumothorax and pneumomediastinum, which resolved with supplemental oxygen.

Discussion.—Spontaneous pneumothorax can result from either a visceral tear caused by the rupture of a subpleural bleb or from a partial bronchial obstruction leading to progressive distal hyperinflation and dissection of air into the lung hilum and mediastinum and possibly into fascial planes. The pneumothoraces in these 3 patients may have been caused by improper breathing techniques during weight lifting. Performing a concentric contraction against a closed glottis causes an additive increase in intrathoracic pressure, which, if continuous, can lead to progressive airway hyperinflation.

► To be noted, the authors "postulate that spontaneous pneumothorax in these patients may be secondary to improper breathing techniques." They further point out that the proper breathing technique is to inspire at the beginning of an eccentric contraction and exhale during the last two thirds of a concentric contraction. During a bench press, one would inhale while lowering the weight to the chest and exhale while pushing it back to the starting position. They further point out that physicians and weight trainers should be aware of the association between weight lifting and spontaneous pneumothorax and provide proper instruction to athletes who are involved in weight lifting.

J.S. Torg, M.D.

Effects of Electromyostimulation and Strength Training on Muscle Soreness, Muscle Damage and Sympathetic Activation

Moreau D, Dubots P, Boggio V, Guilland JC, Cometti G (Université de Bourgogne, France)

J Sports Sci 13:95–100, 1995 5–10

Background.—Muscular strength and hypertrophy can be developed through electromyostimulation (EMS). The effects of an EMS session were compared with those of a concentric exercise bout in terms of plasma creatine kinase activity (CK), lactate dehydrogenase (LDH) activity, subjective ratings of muscle soreness, and urinary catecholamine excretion.

Methods.—By random assignment, 12 male athletes performed 5 sets of 6 voluntary contractions or 30 contractions of 6 seconds each with 20 seconds of rest between contractions, both at 80% of maximal isometric force. The athletes were assessed 1 day before and for 3 days after exercise.

Findings.—Athletes in the EMS group had significantly elevated catecholamine urinary excretion. Adrenaline, plasma CK activity, and plasma LDH activity were particularly increased (Table 4). Those performing concentric exercise had less pronounced changes with nonsignificant differences. Athletes in the EMS group also reported greater muscle soreness.

TABLE 4.—Mean (± SEM) Plasma Creatine Kinase Activity and Plasma Lactate Dehydrogenase Activity (IU^{-1}) From 1 Day Before to 3 Days After Exercise

Group	D_{-1}	D_0	D_{+1}	D_{+2}	D_{+3}
CK activity					
CONC (n=6)	93 ± 24	88 ± 24	126 ± 39	120 ± 22	110 ± 13
EMS (n=6)	108 ± 17	119 ± 11	156 ± 27	185 ± 30*	154 ± 27
LDH activity					
CONC (n=6)	337 ± 23	298 ± 6	311 ± 8	313 ± 13	294 ± 11
EMS (n=6)	315 ± 10	304 ± 7	358 ± 22*	356 ± 13*	315 ± 11

* $P < 0.05$ vs. D_{-1}.

Abbreviations: CK, creatine kinase; *LDH*, plasma lactate dehydrogenase; D_{-1}, 1 day before exercise; D_{+3}, 3 days after exercise; *CONC*, concentric; *EMS*, electromyostimulation.

(Courtesy of Moreau D, Dubots P, Boggio V, et al: Effects of electromyostimulation and strength training on muscle soreness, muscle damage and sympathetic activation. *J Sports Sci* 13:95–100, 1995.)

Conclusions.—Muscle contractions during EMS sessions may injure skeletal fibers, as evidenced in the current study by enzyme release. Elevated adrenaline excretion may contribute to the changes in plasma enzyme concentrations, possibly through modifications to muscle membrane permeability.

▶ Electromyostimulation has some popularity among trainers, as it is reputed to induce greater gains of muscle strength than can be realized by voluntary concentric exercise. However, this study by Moreau and associates confirms an earlier report[1] that EMS also causes greater muscle soreness than voluntary contractions, with substantial increases in various markers of muscle damage.

R.J. Shephard, M.D., Ph.D., D.P.E.

Reference

1. Enoka RM: Muscle strength and its development: New perspectives. *Sports Med* 6:146–168, 1988.

Improving Rehabilitation Effectiveness by Enhancing the Creative Process

Pitney WA, Bunton EE (Northern Illinois Univ, DeKalb; American Rehabilitation Network, Southgate, Mich)

J Athletic Train 30:261–264, 1995 5–11

Background.—Although creativity is a key aspect of many different tasks, it has been rarely mentioned in the literature on athletic rehabilitation. Nevertheless, creativity is an implicit part of rehabilitation; it is essential for disseminating technology, management resources, and solving problems. The value of creativity in athletic rehabilitation was discussed, including a new technique to facilitate creative thinking.

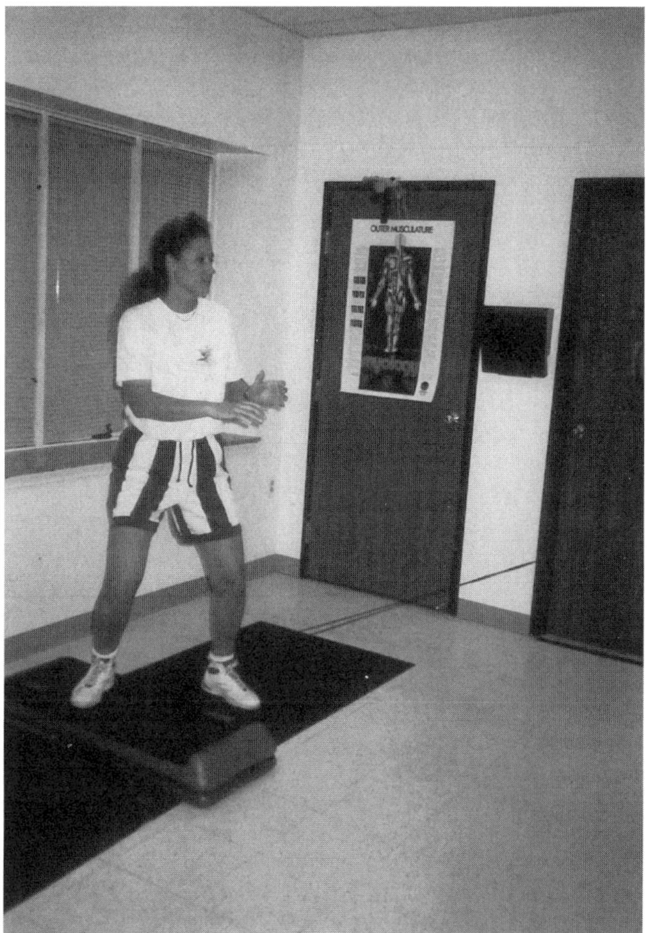

FIGURE 3.—Step and resistive tubing can be creatively combined to promote control of function of the right knee in the transverse/frontal plane. (Courtesy of Pitney WA, Bunton EE: Improving rehabilitation effectiveness by enhancing the creative process. *J Athletic Train* 30:261–264, 1995.)

Enhancing Creativity.—The functional rehabilitation program includes not only the patient and injury but also the innovation of the clinician. However, it takes effort and persistence to enhance individual creativity. The authors have developed a new technique, called the CLEAR method, to help enhance the creative process. The CLEAR strategy, based on various strategies and concepts from the literature, is a 5-step process. The first step is challenging old routines, that is, overcoming obstacles that limit professional creativity. The second step, learning new attitudes or characteristics, is essential to the creative process. The third step is enlisting specific cognitive exercises, such as brainstorming, to help generate

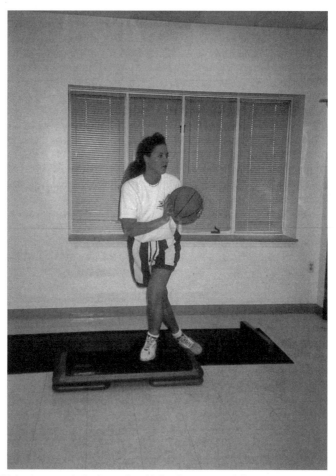

FIGURE 4.—An external stimulus can be added to the exercise to help remove conscious effort during movement and also to make the exercise more fun and creative. (Courtesy of Pitney WA, Bunton EE: Improving rehabilitation effectiveness by enhancing the creative process. *J Athletic Train* 30:261–264, 1995.)

new ideas. The fourth step is to assess the new idea for clinical relevance and, most importantly, safety. The final step is revision, especially if the idea is not biomechanically safe.

Implementing Creativity.—In the rehabilitation process, simply having the athlete perform the same exercises again and again may result in noncompliance. In contrast, developing alternative, creative exercises through the CLEAR method provides a new and innovative avenue for achieving results. The authors consider the common example of knee instability. Rather than general lower extremity strengthening and proprioceptive exercises, creative exercises would focus on challenging movement into the transverse/frontal plane, with an emphasis on eccentric control. Thus the slide board could be used to facilitate safe movement into the transverse/frontal plane. Control and function in this plane could be enhanced by the use of a step and resistive tubing (Fig 3). An external stimulus could be used to make the movement less conscious and to make the exercise more enjoyable (Fig 4).

Conclusions.—Clinicians must use their creativity to prevent functional rehabilitation from becoming a stagnant process. Potential benefits include a more dynamic work place, better compliance by the athlete, improved problem-solving ability, and better therapeutic results. The CLEAR method provides an easy to follow process for enhancing clinical safety and for assessing the clinical relevance and safety of innovations.

▶ Why do we as clinicians need to use the creative process in developing rehabilitation programs? There are numerous reasons, the most important being optimum therapeutic results for the patient. Patients will certainly benefit from an individualized program that is both dynamic and varied. They will be more compliant with a program that is designed to meet the demands of their specific injury, the sport in which they participate, and the changes made as they progress. Utilizing the creative process also prevents the clinician from becoming bored with "cookbook-type" rehabilitation programs. Available resources are better utilized, and the need for expensive rehabilitation equipment can be minimized.

F.J. George, A.T.C., P.T.

Relationship of Knee Extensor Strength and Hopping Test Performance in the Assessment of Lower Extremity Function

Greenberger HB, Paterno MV (Ithaca College, New York; Cincinnati Sports Medicine and Orthopaedic Ctr, Ohio)

J Orthop Sports Phys Ther 22:202–206, 1995 5–12

Introduction.—Until recently, isokinetic strength testing was used to determine a patient's ability to return to a maximum level of function; however, little is known about the correlation between isokinetic strength testing and functional performance. The relationship between knee extensor strength of the quadriceps, or isokinetic strength testing, and performance on a one-legged hop for distance test was determined on individuals with no history of knee injury.

Methods.—Twenty volunteers, 7 males and 13 females, participated in two 20-minute sessions, separated by at least 72 hours. The functional test consisted of a one-legged hop for distance. The isokinetic test consisted of maximal concentric extensions of the quadriceps at 240 degrees/sec.

Results.—No significant difference was found when the mean distance hopped in centimeters was compared with the isokinetic test at 240 degrees/sec in the dominant or nondominant legs.

Conclusion.—Isokinetic strength does not correlate strongly with functional tasks. More functional performance tests, such as the one-legged hop for distance, should be developed to help better assess a patient's dynamic functional level and readiness to return to activity.

▶ This is another study that indicates the importance of functional testing to evaluate an injured athlete's ability to return to activity. Isokinetic testing may be done to determine isolated muscle weakness but should never be the sole criterion for return to activity.

It is uncertain whether a deficit in isokinetic strength can be related to a deficit in functional performance. A recent study by Greenberger and Paterno indicates that, "Isokinetic strength does not correlate strongly with functional tests."[1] T.A. Blackburn, Jr, M.Ed., A.T.C., P.T., made some very interesting comments on this study.[2]

F.J. George, A.T.C., P.T.

References

1. Greenberger HB, Paterno MV: Relationship of the knee extensor strength and hopping test performance in the assessment of lower extremity function. *J Sports Med Phys Fitness* 22:202–206, 1995.
2. Blackburn TA: *Athletic Training Sports Health Care Perspectives* Vol. 2, p 166, 1996.

Relationship Between Strength Qualities and Sprinting Performance

Young W, McLean B, Ardagna J (Australian Inst of Sport, Belconnen, ACT, Australia)

J Sports Med Phys Fitness 35:13–19, 1995 5–13

Background.—The importance of strength qualities for sprinting performance is not clear. Disparity in the results of studies on this topic may be attributable to the multiple variables involved in sprinting, the type of strength performance analyzed, and in the sex, age, weight, and other characteristics of the study participants. Sprinting involves 3 phases—the start, acceleration, and attainment of maximum speed. Strength performance may be assessed by tests of concentric, isometric, or stretch-shortening cycle (SSC) muscular activity. The correlations between these sprint and strength variables were investigated.

Methods.—The subjects were 11 male and 9 female trained track-and-field athletes with ages between 16 and 18 years. Sprint performance was evaluated by detailed analyses of two 50-m sprints. Sprint times were recorded at various distances and measurements of force exerted by the hands and feet at the sprint start were obtained. Strength was assessed by having the participants perform 3 tests: (1) maximum height jumping from a vertical position and measurement of displacement of a 9-kg shoulder bar; (2) measurement of displacement of a 19-kg shoulder bar after a vertical jump from a 120-degree knee angle position; and (3) drop jumps from various heights (30, 45, 60, and 75 cm) with correlation of height with contact time. Appropriate measuring techniques were used to quan-

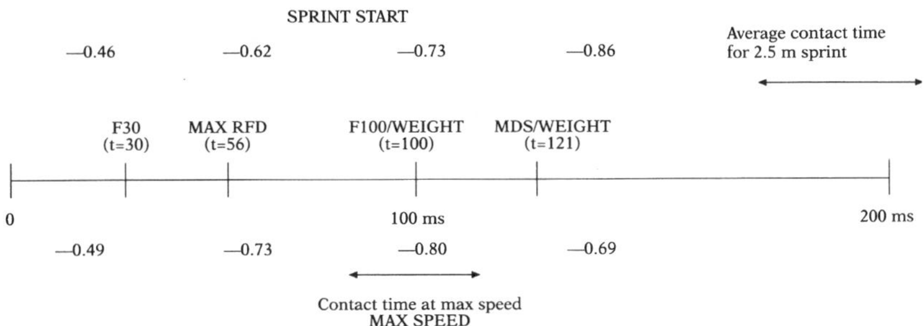

FIGURE 1.—Relationships between selected variables and sprint performance in relation to contact/movement times. The negative numbers represent the correlation coefficients describing the relationships between each strength measure and start (t 2.5) and maximum speed (tmax 10) performance. (Courtesy of Young W, McLean B, Ardagna J: Relationship between strength qualities and sprinting performance. *J Sports Med Phys Fitness* 35:13–19, 1995.)

titate strength from the results of these tests. The presence or absence of correlations between sprint performance and strength was then determined.

Results.—Sixteen of the 27 strength measurements correlated significantly with sprint starting ability. The best predictor of starting ability was the peak force (related to body weight) generated during a jump from a 120-degree knee angle, and represented concentric muscular contraction. Twenty strength parameters correlated significantly with maximum sprinting speed attained. The single best correlate with maximum speed was the force applied at 100 msec (related to body weight) from the start of a loaded vertical jumping action, and represented concentric muscular contraction. None of the drop jump variables were significantly correlated to either starting ability or maximum sprinting speed. Stretch shortening cycle measurements and maximum absolute strength were better related to maximum sprinting speed than to starting ability. Figure 1 presents the relationships between selected variables and sprint performance in relation to contact/movement times.

Conclusions.—Strength qualities measured under varying muscular contraction conditions (concentric, stretch-shortening cycle, and isometric) are significantly correlated with sprinting performance. Maximum attainable sprinting speed is better correlated with strength variables that are different from those correlated with starting ability.

▶ We continue to search for measurable qualities that may affect functional performance. How much weight can an athlete lift? How much height can an athlete attain in a vertical jump test? How much distance can an athlete attain in a horizontal one-legged hop test? Can performance be predicted by any test or measurement? The authors have concluded that strength qualities are related to sprinting performance in trained sprinters. These qualities are more related to maximum speed than they are to starting times. This study should be read in conjunction with the following study. (See Abstract 5–14.)

F.J. George, A.T.C., P.T.

Influence of High-resistance and High-velocity Training on Sprint Performance

Delecluse C, Van Coppenolle H, Willems E, Van Leemputte M, Diels R, Goris M (Katholieke Universiteit Leuven, Belgium)

Med Sci Sports Exerc 27:1203–1209, 1995 5–14

Background.—There is general agreement that strength exercises are important in sprint training, but the appropriate program to accomplish this is still under discussion. The effects of high resistance (HR) and high velocity (HV) exercise training on the different phases of 100-m sprint performance were studied.

Methods.—Forty-three male physical education students were divided into 2 groups. The first, numbering 22, underwent a 9-week program involving HR exercises 2 days a week and sprinting for 1 day a week. The second group, numbering 21, underwent a similar program except that HV exercises were employed. The HR group worked with free weight lifting and exercise machines with variable resistance. The HV group participated in a program of exercises that involved speed of motion, primarily jumping exercises. Each program was defined, standardized, and closely supervised. Additionally, 2 groups of 12 and 11 physical education students, respectively, comprised groups who participated only in the weekly running (RUN group), whereas the other (PAS group) did not participate in any component of the training program. The participants in each of the 4 groups were matched for height, weight, and physical ability including sprint performance. Comparisons between groups were made at the end of the 9-week program.

Results.—Both the HR and the HV groups manifested significant improvement in the performance of their specific exercises. In the case of the HR group, however, this did not significantly affect sprint performance. High velocity training resulted in a highly significant improvement in sprint starting and acceleration, as a result of which it was the only group to manifest improved 100-m sprint time. Surprisingly, however, the HV group experienced a greater decrease in speed endurance than the RUN and PAS groups. It was theorized that the marked increase in initial sprint speed and acceleration experienced by the HV group might have jeopardized its speed endurance.

Conclusions.—A 9-week special training program evaluating the effects of high resistance and high velocity exercises resulted in improvement in sprint performance in 2 comparable groups of physical education students. Both groups manifested signficant improvement in the performance of the specific exercises used by these groups. However, in the case of the HR program, there was no significant effect on sprint performance. Although HV exercises significantly improved initial speed, acceleration, and total sprint speed, this group experienced a decrease in speed endurance. A more prolonged or alternative training program may be indicated.

► This study should be read in conjunction with Abstract 5–13. The previous study has important findings regarding initial speed and maximum speed and relationships of these to strength. To improve sprint performance, the sprint should be divided into different segments—the start, acceleration, attainment of maximum speed, and speed endurance. Each segment should be worked on with specific exercises designed to improve that segment and thereby the whole.

F.J. George, A.T.C., P.T.

Examining Warm-up Decrement as a Function of Interpolated Open and Closed Motor Tasks: Implications for Practice Strategies

Anshel MH (Univ of Wollongong, NSW, Australia)

J Sports Sci 13:247–256, 1995 5–15

Introduction.—The term warm-up decrement (WUD) refers to the phenomenon in which level of physical performance declines after resting and before subsequent trials. One proposed explanation for WUD is the activity-set hypothesis, which links the length of the post-rest decline in performance to the athlete's ability to adjust the underlying systems to the level they were at in the immediate pre-rest period. This hypothesis suggests that the amount of WUD depends on the type of activities performed at the end of the rest period, just before performance starts again.

Objectives.—The efficacy of the activity-set hypothesis was examined, along with the ability of performing closed or open interpolated tasks to reduce WUD.

Methods.—Twenty elite-level tennis players were studied. The criterion task was hitting ground strokes to a specified area in the opponent's court in response to a ball-tossing machine. The same task was used as an open interpolated task between trials. The closed interpolated task was hitting a stationary tennis ball that was suspended from the ceiling with a rope. The athletes performed the criterion task, then practiced 1 of these 2 tasks or rested, then performed the criterion task again. The athletes performed each of the 3 interpolated tasks in separate sessions 1 week apart in a repeated-measures design.

Results.—The athletes showed a marked reduction in WUD when performing the closed interpolated task. However, their performance after the rest period was significantly better when they performed the open, criterion task. They showed a clear WUD under the rest condition. At least for the first 2 trials after resting, post-rest scores were significantly better for the open skill condition than for the closed, interpolated task condition.

Conclusions.—The findings partially support the activity-set hypothesis in that both open and closed interpolated tasks decrease WUD. Thus certain relevant features of both open and closed interpolated tasks appear to be important parts of the open criterion tasks. Future studies should seek to identify these features and to determine how they influence WUD.

The inherent characteristics of open interpolated tasks may promote general somatic arousal, thus producing a warm-up effect, thus reducing WUD.

▶ The more sport-specific the warm-up after a rest, the less effect warm-up decrement will have on performance. Baseball batters might have an advantage if they could swing a few times at a pitched ball before they stepped into the batter's box. The same is true of most athletes who have a rest period between warm-up and activity.

F.J. George, A.T.C., P.T.

Comparative Effectiveness of Accommodating and Weight Resistance Training Modes

O'Hagan FT, Sale DG, MacDougall JD, Garner SH (McMaster Univ, Hamilton, Ont, Canada)

Med Sci Sports Exerc 27:1210–1219, 1995 5–16

Background.—Accommodating resistance devices (ARD) are becoming increasingly popular in strength training. However, one drawback is that they require only concentric actions, unlike weight resistance devices (WRD), which require both concentric and eccentric actions in the exercise cycle. The effectiveness of ARD, compared to WRD, was studied over a 20-week training program.

Methods.—Six male and 6 female volunteers trained the elbow flexors of 1 arm on an ARD and the other arm on a WRD. Training was similar, but not identical, in terms of exertion and duration of exercise. Six trained the dominant arm on ARD, the others the dominant arm on WRD. Strength and muscle cross-sectional area were measured regularly. Needle biopsy of the biceps brachii was obtained before and after the program to evaluate the ratio of type I and type II muscle fibers.

Results.—Significant strength improvement was noted for both ARD and WRD, beginning at the fifth week, with no difference in the percentage improvement between the groups. By week 5, WRD produced a significantly greater one-repetition maximum weight lifting performance than ARD. Improvement in isokinetic concentric peak torque was similar for both methods. Cross-sectional area of biceps, brachialis, and total elbow flexors increased in both groups, with a significantly greater increase in brachialis size in the WRD-trained arms. Muscle fiber area increased more for type II than for type I fibers in both methods, and to a similar degree.

Conclusion.—Use of ARD for weight training is an acceptable alternative to the use of WRD, although WRD may produce greater muscle hypertrophy, possibly because of the combined concentric and eccentric forces used in WRD.

▶ This is another study that indicates a combination of concentric and eccentric exercises against resistance may have advantages over concentric training alone. The authors' explanation is that "the eccentric action of each repetition would be borne preferentially by the type II fibers, but the type I fibers would be abruptly thrown into greater action in the transition from eccentric to concentric phases. Perhaps the abrupt coupling between eccentric and concentric phases provided a special training stimulus". The authors comment on a study that does not support this theory and another that studied "isolated" eccentric actions.

F.J. George, A.T.C., P.T.

Randomised Controlled Trial for Evaluation of Fitness Programme for Patients With Chronic Low Back Pain

Frost H, Moffett JAK, Moser JS, Fairbank JCT (Nuffield Orthopaedic Centre, Oxford, England)

BMJ 310:151–154, 1995 5–17

Introduction.—Exercise programs have been found to reduce disability in patients with low back pain. A randomized trial was designed to test the hypothesis that a supervised, progressive fitness program would be more effective than home exercise alone in improving function, reducing pain, and enhancing the confidence of patients with chronic low back pain.

Patients and Methods.—Participants were recruited from patients referred to a physiotherapy department between 1991 and 1993. Criteria for inclusion were age between 18 and 55 years, somatic low back pain for at least 6 months, no serious medical illness, and a plain radiograph of the lumbar spine obtained within the past year. All patients were taught specific exercises to carry out at home; in addition, those randomized to the supervised group attended 8 exercise classes over 4 weeks. A blinded observer assessed patients before and after the treatment period using a battery of validated measures. Patients kept pain diaries and completed a questionnaire 6 months after treatment.

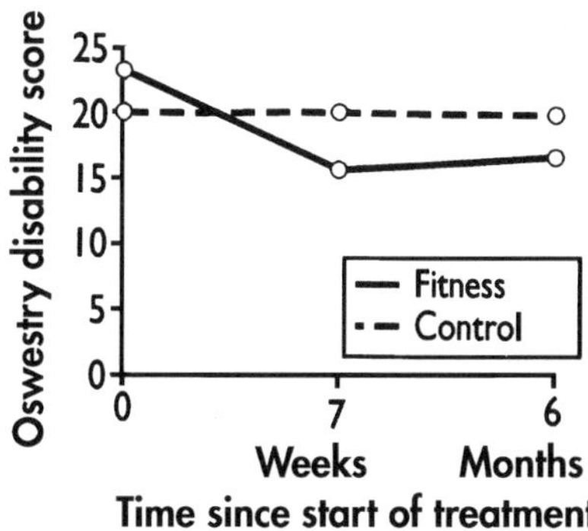

FIGURE 1.—Scores on low back pain disability index for all patients included in intention to treat analysis. Higher scores on index correspond to greater disability. (Courtesy of Frost H, Moffett JAK, Moser JS, et al: Randomised controlled trial for evaluation of fitness programme for patients with chronic low back pain. *BMJ* 310:151–154, 1995.)

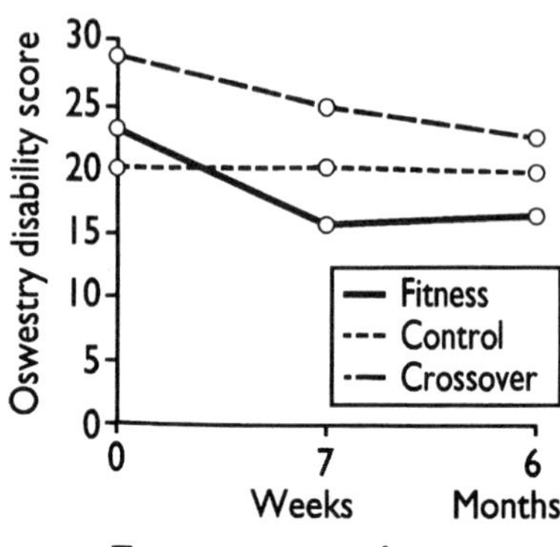

FIGURE 2.—Scores on Oswestry low back pain disability index, including crossover data. Higher scores correspond to greater disability. (Courtesy of Frost H, Moffett JAK, Moser JS, et al: Randomised controlled trial for evaluation of fitness programme for patients with chronic low back pain. *BMJ* 310:151–154, 1995.)

Results.—Seventy-one patients were available for analysis, 36 in the supervised program group and 35 in the control group. The 2 groups were similar in baseline measures and both reported considerable improvements in general health after the treatment period. Immediately after the program, patients in the supervised group scored significantly higher than controls on a subjective scale of benefit (mean 65.6 vs. 45.0, on a scale of 0–100). At 6 months' follow-up, 86% of patients completed the questionnaire. Scores on the Oswestry low back pain disability index showed that the supervised group maintained a benefit of about 6 percentage points over the control group (Figs 1 and 2). Patients who crossed over from the control group to the supervised fitness group reported reduced disability at 6 months, although the difference was not significant.

Conclusion.—Moderately disabled patients with chronic low back pain achieved greater benefits when they attended a supervised fitness program than similar patients who were advised to exercise at home. The additional support of a supervised program is necessary to improve pain, reduce disability, and restore patient confidence.

▶ Many fitness organizations offer low back exercise programs. It seems logical to assume (as do the authors of this paper) that if the spinal muscles are strengthened by a course of vigorous exercises, the demands that are made upon a weakened vertebral column will be reduced and low back pain will be corrected. However, results of formal trials of the value of exercise programs in the prevention and treatment of lower back pain have been somewhat equivocal.[1, 2] Part of the problem is that the condition is very chronic, with no good method of objective diagnosis. Often compensation is involved (for example, as a result of an automobile accident), or an employee may be receiving insurance payments for work that is not very attractive. Both of these circumstances encourage continued symptom reporting.

The present study showed a decrease in the Oswestry pain score with both supervised and home treatment, in contrast to controls, whose scores were unchanged. It is also suggested that the supervised program was more effective than the home program. Certainly, the reduction in pain score was greater in supervised classes, but this conclusion is weakened somewhat by an initial difference in pain ratings that favored the supervised treatment group.

R.J. Shephard, M.D., Ph.D., D.P.E.

References

1. Biering-Sorensen F, Bendix T, Jorgensen K, et al: Physical activity, fitness, and back pain, in Bouchard C, et al. (eds): *Physical Activity, Fitness and Health,* Champaign, Ill, Human Kinetics Publishers, 1994, pp 737–748.
2. Nachemson AL Exercise, fitness, and back pain, in Bouchard C, et al (eds): *Exercise, Fitness and Health,* Champaign, Ill, Human Kinetics Publishers, 1990, pp. 533–540.

Static Back Endurance and the Risk of Low-back Pain

Luoto S, Heliövaara M, Hurri H, Alaranta H (Invalid Found (ORTON), Helsinki; Social Insurance Inst, Helsinki)

Clin Biomech 10:323–324, 1995 5–18

Background.—The spinal muscles are intended to maintain a fixed truncal posture while allowing controlled spinal motions. The static back endurance test measures isometric fatigue of the back muscles as the point where contraction cannot be maintained at a given level. A short endurance time reportedly predicts first-time low back pain (LBP).

Objective.—The predictive value of the static back endurance test was studied in 508 adults 35–54 years of age who were having a comprehensive physical examination that included detailed tests of physical capacity. Of 167 individuals who denied having LBP in the past year, 75% were followed prospectively for 1 year.

TABLE 1.—Odds Ratios and 95% Confidence Intervals of Low Back Pain for Tertiles of Static Back Endurance, Adjusted for Age, Sex, and Occupation

Tertile of back endurance	*No. of subjects examined*	*Incident cases of low-back pain*	*Odds ratio*	*95% CI*
I (good performance)	43	7	1.0	
II (medium performance)	40	9	1.4	0.4–4.2
III (poor performance)	43	17	3.4	1.2–10.0
P for trend		0.04		
P for heterogeneity		0.04		

Abbreviation: CI, confidence interval.

(Reprinted from *Clinical Biomechanics*, Vol. 10, Luoto S, Heliövaara M, Hurri H, et al: Static back endurance and the risk of low-back pain, pp 323–324, Copyright 1995, with kind permission from Elsevier Science Ltd, The Boulevard, Langford Lane, Kidlington 0X5 1GB UK.)

The Test.—The subject lay prone with the arms along the sides, with the upper trunk unsupported horizontally and the inguinal region at the edge of the test table. The time for which the horizontal position could be maintained was recorded up to a maximum of 4 minutes.

Results.—New LBP developed in 33 of the 126 assessable individuals. The only physical measure that correlated significantly with new LBP was the static back endurance test. The adjusted relative risk of new LBP in poorly performing subjects was more than 3 times greater than in those performing at a medium or good level (Table 1).

Conclusion.—A simple test of static back endurance may prove useful in predicting the subsequent development of low back pain.

▶ Many fitness facilities include low back programs among their offerings, but the objective evidence supporting the value of such programs as a means of preventing low back pain is sparse. This paper by Luoto and colleagues suggests a substantial association between a poor initial endurance of the trunk muscles and the risk of subsequent back pain. The test of muscle endurance is simple to perform and might be considered in screening workers in jobs where there is a high risk of back injury. The success of the test in predicting risk also supports the continued use of specific exercise programs to strengthen the lower back as part of campaigns of primary and secondary prevention.

R.J. Shephard, M.D., Ph.D., D.P.E.

Vastus Medialis Oblique/Vastus Lateralis Muscle Activity Ratios for Selected Exercises in Persons With and Without Patellofemoral Pain Syndrome

Cerny K (California State Univ, Long Beach)

Phys Ther 75:672–683, 1995 5–19

Objective.—Patellofemoral pain (PFP) is a common problem that may be caused by lateral malalignment of the patella. Studies of exercise programs for the treatment of PFP syndrome differ as to which exercises will preferentially activate the vastus medialis oblique (VMO) muscle, with its medial pull on the patella. One author has suggested that medial taping of the patella or tensor fascia lata muscle will increase the activity of the VMO over the vastus lateralis (VL) muscle, i.e., the VMO/VL activity ratio. Various exercises were studied to determine whether they increased the VMO/VL activity ratio in subjects with and without PFP syndrome.

Methods.—The study included 10 patients with a physician's diagnosis of PFP syndrome and 21 subjects with no known musculoskeletal problems of the lower limb. The mean age was 26 years; in the PFP group, women outnumbered men 9 to 1. Subjects in both groups were studied while performing various closed and open chain exercises. The normalized, integrated electromyographic (IEMG) activity of the VMO and VL muscles, and the VMO/VL ratio, were determined using wire electrodes.

Results.—Activation of VMO over VL activity was not enhanced by any of the commonly used exercsies or by patellar or fascia lata medial glide taping. Just one exercise demonstrated a higher VMO/VL ratio compared to similar exercises in subjects without PFP syndrome. Terminal knee extension with the hip in medial rotation was associated with a VMO/VL activity ratio of 1.2, compared to a ratio of 1.0 for knee extension with the hip in lateral rotation. The patients with PFP reported an average 94% decrease in pain with patellar taping during step-down exercise, but there was no change in the VMO/VL ratio.

Conclusions.—The exercises commonly prescribed for patients with PFP syndrome do not preferentially activate the VMO over the VL. Also, medial-glide taping of the patella or tensor fascia lata does not appear to affect the VMO/VL ratio. The findings raise questions as to whether it is possible to train the VMO to increase its activity selectively. There are also questions about the magnitude of change in the VMO/VL ratio that would be necessary to achieve a therapeutic effect. Patellar taping does appear to decrease pain; this should be studied further to examine the possibility of a placebo effect.

▶ This study may have a significant impact on how patients with patellofemoral pain are treated. Current treatment protocols for these patients have included a regimen of taping and exercise, which we assumed was increasing the ratio of VMO/VL activity. This study did not have a large number of patients with patellofemoral pain. However, it did indicate that a number of exercises being used and the McConnell taping technique may not be as effective as we thought. The study did not address the use of biofeedback to increase the VMO/VL activity ratio. It did state that 94% of subjects with PFP who were taped with the McConnell technique had a decrease in pain with step-down exercises. This significant finding should be considered when developing a rehabilitation program for these patients.

F.J. George, A.T.C., P.T.

Energy Expenditure in Adolescents During Low Intensity, Leisure Activities

Horswill CA, Kien CL, Zipf WB (Ohio State Univ, Columbus; Children's Hosp Research Found, Columbus, Ohio)

Med Sci Sports Exerc 27:1311–1314, 1995 5–20

Objective.—There is an association between time spent viewing television and the amount of body fat in children and adolescents. Because some children do not like vigorous exercise, a study was designed to determine whether low levels of activity such as playing a musical instrument could elevate the metabolic rate in a manner comparable to walking at modest pace.

Methods.—Energy expenditure (EE) was measured on 3 separate days in each of 8 adolescents (1 male), average age 14 years, while they were watching television for 1 hour, playing a stringed instrument for 1 hour, and walking on a treadmill at 40% of the peak oxygen uptake for 43 minutes. Each individual maintained a similar diet for 24 hours before testing and recorded that diet. Calorimetry was done before and at 15- to 20-minute intervals during the test sessions to measure EE. Heart rates, fractional concentrations of oxygen and carbon dioxide, and minute volume of expired air (VE) were measured. Energy expenditure was calculated from Weir's equation.

Results.—Oxygen consumption, heart rate, and EE increased significantly from television viewing to playing an instrument to walking. Respiratory quotient was significantly greater for walking than for either instrument playing or watching television. Mean EE for television viewing was as predicted from body surface area calculations. Metabolic rate increased significantly by 41% for instrument playing and by 235% for walking.

Conclusion.—Although playing a stringed instrument significantly increased metabolic rate over the level measured while watching television, it is not a substitute for more vigorous physical exercise in adolescents attempting to lose or control their weight.

► As we have reviewed before, prior studies suggest that too much television viewing promotes obesity and hypercholesterolemia in children, and that parents can boost physical activity in their kids by playing with them and taking them to games.[1] A remarkable 55-year follow-up of some 500 Bostonians shows that being chubby in adolescence predicts a broad range of adverse health effects in adulthood (including early death in men) that are largely independent of adult weight.[2] Yet, American adolescents, like American adults, grow ever fatter. This novel study shows that playing the violin makes you a better person in more ways than one. As expected, walking at 40% of peak oxygen uptake increased the metabolic rate by 235% compared with television viewing. But a beneficial 41% increase in metabolic rate (compared with television viewing) also occurred when these adolescents played the violin or cello. The violin is good for body, brain, and soul.

E.R. Eichner, M.D.

References

1. 1994 Year Book of Sports Medicine, pp 288–289.
2. Must A, Jacques PF, Dallal GE, et al: Long-term morbidity and mortality of overweight adolescents: A follow-up of the Harvard Growth Study of 1922 to 1935. *N Engl J Med* 327:1379–1380, 1992.

6 Cardiovascular and Respiratory Systems

The Chronotropic Response of the Sinus Node to Exercise: A New Method of Analysis and a Study of Pacemaker Patients

Crook B, Nijhof P, van Der Kemp P, Jennison C (Univ of Bath, England)

Eur Heart J 16:993–998, 1995 6–1

Purpose.—Chronotropic incompetence of the sinus node is one of the main indications for the use of a rate responsive pacemaker. Estimates of the incidence of chronotropic incompetence and the need for rate responsive pacemaking vary. The intercepts and slopes of the regression lines of sinus heart rate response to cycle ergometer exercise were examined as a possible means of investigating normal and abnormal chronotropic responses.

Methods.—Regressions of sinus heart rate were plotted for 223 normal and 93 subjects with pacemakers during progressive cycle exercise to exhaustion. The pacemaker group consisted of 46 patients with symptomatic sick sinus syndrome and 47 with second or third degree atrioventricular (AV) block.

Results.—The regression lines were sufficiently linear to permit calculation of the intercept and slope value for both normal and pacemaker groups. Multiple regression analysis of these values indicated that the AV block group was not significantly different from the normal group; however, the intercepts were significantly lower than normal in the sick sinus group (Fig 1). The patients with sick sinus syndrome appeared to have an abnormality of sinus node function such that the base rate setting was too low for all levels of exercise, although the acceleration was normal with exercise. Among the sick sinus syndrome group, only 4 had intercept values more than 2 standard deviations below that of the normal control group and were considered to be chronotropically incompetent.

Conclusions.—The results of this study suggest that patients with sick sinus syndrome have an abnormally low base rate setting at all exercise levels but accelerate normally with exercise. Very few of these patients appear to be chronotropically incompetent. There was no evidence of a need for rate responsive pacing in patients with AV block. Therefore, chronotropic incompetence of the sinus node during exercise appears to be

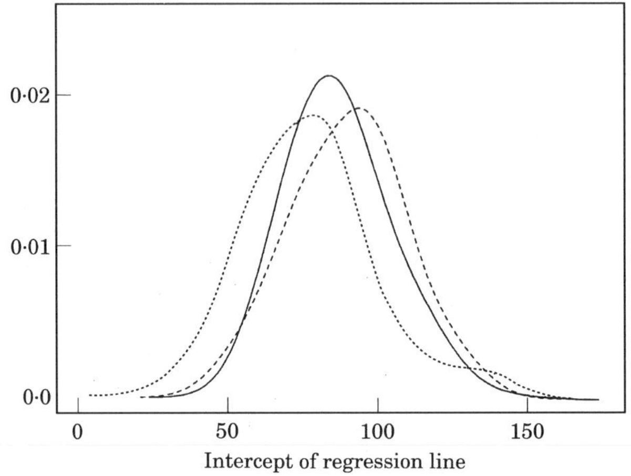

FIGURE 1.—The curves are density estimates of the distribution of intercept values (beats/min^{-1}) in the normal subjects (*solid line*) and the 2 pacemaker groups: sick sinus subjects (*dotted line*); heart block subjects (*dashed line*). Note the slightly lower intercept values in the patients with sick sinus. (Courtesy of Crook B, Nijhof P, van Der Kemp P, et al: The chronotropic response of the sinus node to exercise: A new method of analysis and a study of pacemaker patients. *Eur Heart J* 16:993–998, 1995.)

uncommon. The question of how to identify those few patients with chronotropic incompetence and how to program the rate response of their pacemakers remains unanswered.

▶ The concept of the sick sinus syndrome is that the rate of the cardiac pacemaker is low and/or fails to increase normally with exercise because blood flow to the sinus is inadequate. Diagnosis is commonly based on a maximal heart rate that falls substantially below some arbitrary (and dubious!) figure for a "normal" person of similar age. One would anticipate that any problem of sinus oxygenation would be exacerbated by exercise, and it is puzzling to find that in the present series of patients there was a normal acceleration despite a low resting rate (as gauged from the linear plot of heart rate against work rate). There has been much discussion about the prevalence of sick sinus syndrome, and the present paper adds to skepticism regarding those who maintain that it is a common condition. In the sample of 46 patients who supposedly had the sick sinus syndrome, only 4 individuals had a resting heart rate intercept that was more than 2 standard deviations below that for the normal control group. This is not much more than the expectation from a chance distribution of resting heart rates. Certainly, some endurance athletes have rates slower than the suggested cutoff value (a resting heart rate less than 45 beats/min), and many clinics are making excessive use of pacemakers.

R.J. Shephard, M.D., Ph.D., D.P.E.

The Prevalence and Significance of Post-exercise (Postural) Hypotension in Ultramarathon Runners

Holtzhausen L-M, Noakes TD (Univ of Cape Town, South Africa)

Med Sci Sports Exerc 27:1595–1601, 1995 6–2

Objective.—Prolonged exercise can result in a striking postexercise postural hypotension associated with tachycardia usually lasting only a few seconds. Such findings are common in ultramarathon runners with exercise-associated collapse (EAC). Because the prevalence and incidence of these blood pressure changes have not been well studied, the prevalence and magnitude of these changes in blood pressure among ultramarathon runners were measured and the relationship to fluid status and symptoms was determined.

Methods.—Before and after an 80-km footrace, systolic and diastolic blood pressure, weight, and plasma volume were determined and compared with symptoms of postexercise hypotension in 31 runners (average age, 39 years). Asymptomatic postural hypotension was defined as a decrease in systolic blood pressure of > 20 mm Hg between the supine and erect position.

Results.—Mean weight was 73.9 kg and race time averaged 498 minutes. Average weight loss during the race was 3.5 kg, representing a mean dehydration of 4.6%. Blood glucose, potassium, total protein, creatinine, urea, serum osmolality, hemoglobin, hematocrit, and white blood cell values increased significantly. All blood pressure levels, except diastolic blood pressure measured in the supine position, were significantly lower after the race. After the race, there was an erect systolic blood pressure drop exceeding 20 mm Hg in 68% of runners and 23% had systolic blood pressure below 90 mm Hg. No runners had syncope, but all runners with systolic blood pressure below 90 mm Hg experienced nausea and dizziness. The variation in systolic blood pressure resulting from posture changes was not associated with changes in a decrease in weight or plasma volume.

Conclusion.—The runners had dehydration, and the majority experienced asymptomatic postexercise hypotension that was not entirely attributable to dehydration and plasma volume reduction but rather to a blood volume shift to the periphery.

► Last year we reviewed an earlier report from this group[1] showing that, in a very long race on a cool day, most runners who collapse do so after finishing. Many have a normal cardiovascular status while supine and are not notably dehydrated or hyperthermic. They seem "benign" medically and respond to leg elevation and oral fluids. The thesis is that this form of exercise-associated collapse is syncope from venous pooling after the cessation of running. This report extends that thesis by studying a race in which all runners had dehydration, usually marked, with two thirds of them having postexercise (postural) hypotension. Because the fall in postural blood pressure correlated poorly with the degree of dehydration or plasma volume change, the authors conclude that the postural hypotension was likely multifactorial—also influenced by venous pooling and by a training-induced impairment in the sympathetic nervous system response to any acute hypotensive challenge. They argue that even in such a race, with major dehydration resulting, the medical tent physician can begin treating the collapsed athlete with pelvic and lower limb elevation and oral fluids, monitoring for recovery of a stable cardiovascular status before resorting to IV fluids. Given the vagaries of field measurements, however, just because a significant correlation between dehydration and postural hypotension was not found, does not mean that it did not exist. In general, the advice to begin with leg elevation and oral fluids seems suited more to long, slow races on cool days than to short, fast races on hot days. In my opinion, if a runner collapses during a fast, hot 10-km race, the physician should act fast, get a rectal temperature immediately, cool the runner quickly, and judiciously use IV fluids.

E.R. Eichner, M.D.

Reference

1. 1995 Year Book of Sports Medicine, pp 284–285.

The Diagnostic and Prognostic Importance of Ambulatory ST Recording Compared to a Predischarge Exercise Test After an Episode of Unstable Angina or Non-Q Wave Myocardial Infarction

Larsson H, Areskog M, Areskog N-H, Jonasson T, Rinqvist I, Fellenius C, Wallentin L (Univ Hosp Linköping, Sweden)

Eur Heart J 16:888–893, 1995 6–3

Objective.—It is known that ST-segment depression on Holter monitoring has prognostic importance in patients with stable or unstable angina. This measure was compared with a symptom-limited predischarge exercise test in 170 men with either unstable angina or non–Q-wave myocardial infarction who were participating in a trial of aspirin vs. low-dose heparin. Men less than 70 years of age were entered into the study within 72 hours of admission to coronary care.

Methods.—Patients without contraindications received metaprolol as well as nitrates, and those whose chest pain continued also received calcium inhibitors. The patients were randomly assigned to placebo-controlled treatment with 75 mg of acetylsalicylic acid daily and/or 7,500–10,000 IU of IV heparin every 6 hours. ST-segment monitoring was performed for 24 hours during the coronary care unit stay and before discharge. The symptom-limited cycle ergometer test usually preceded the predischarge ST recording.

Results.—No tests were associated with side effects or complications. The predischarge exercise test identified two thirds of patients who had 1–10 minutes of ST depression in the coronary care unit, and all of those with longer-lasting ST depression. Patients with ST depression in the

TABLE 4.—Occurrence of Myocardial Infarction or Death Over 1 Year in Relation to Findings at ST Recordings and at an Exercise Test Before Discharge After an Episode of Unstable Coronary Artery Disease in Men

	Time of Follow-up		
	30 Days	90 Days	365 Days
ST recording			
No ST depression (n=140)	2.9%	7.1%	15.9%
ST depression (n=30)	16.7%	23.3%	23.3%
P	0.009	0.019	0.46
Predischarge exercise test*			
No ST depression (n=82)	2.4%	6.1%%	13.4%%
ST depression (n=88)	8.0%	13.6%	20.5%
P	0.21	0.17	0.06
Predischarge exercise test†			
No ST depression (n=356)	3.7%	5.1%	9.0%
ST depression (n=374)	8.3%	13.1%	18.2%
P	0.013	0.0003	0.0005

* Results of predischarge exercise test in patients with an ST recording before discharge.
† Result of predischarge exercise test in all patients.
(Courtesy of Larsson H, Areskog M, Areskog N-H, et al: The diagnostic and prognostic importance of ambulatory ST recording compared to a predischarge exercise test after an episode of unstable angina or non-Q wave myocardial infarction. *Eur Heart J* 16:888–893, 1995.)

predischarge test had a threefold to fivefold increase in the risk of myocardial infarction or death in the next 3 months, but subsequently the prognostic value of the ST recording declined (Table 4). ST-segment depression on the predischarge exercise test correlated with both continued severe angina and the need for coronary angiography.

Recommendations.—ST-segment recording is appropriate before patients with unstable coronary disease are discharged to identify those who might benefit the most from early revascularization. Patients whose symptoms stabilize and who have no ST-segment depression on Holter monitoring should have a symptom-limited exercise test before being discharged.

► It is generally accepted that exercise-induced ST-segment depression is associated with an adverse prognosis, both in clinically healthy patients (those with "silent" myocardial ischemia) and those who have already sustained myocardial infarction.[1] The increase of risk, although statistically significant, is generally only about twofold, which makes it somewhat difficult to advise the individual on prognosis. The risk demonstrated here (a threefold to fivefold increase) is more important, probably because the patients were more severely affected; 40% had noted angina in the last month, and in about 30% the angina had been increasing in severity. The predischarge exercise test seems a safe way of distinguishing those patients who will benefit from early surgical treatment.

R.J. Shephard, M.D., Ph.D., D.P.E.

Reference

1. Shephard RJ: *Ischemic Heart Disease and Exercise.* London, Croom-Helm Publications, 1981.

Exercise Echocardiography Is an Accurate and Cost-efficient Technique for Detection of Coronary Artery Disease in Women

Marwick TH, Anderson T, Williams MJ, Haluska B, Melin JA, Pashkow F, Thomas JD (Cleveland Clinic Found, Ohio)

J Am Coll Cardiol 26:335–341, 1995 6–4

Background.—Cardiovascular disease is the leading cause of death among American women. Recent studies have suggested that women receive too few coronary interventions, which may be attributable, in part, to the lower specificity of the standard exercise stress test, exercise ECG, in women than in men. Exercise echocardiography accurately identifies coronary artery disease in women but is a more expensive procedure than ECG. The accuracy and cost implications of using exercise echocardiography or exercise ECG for the detection of coronary artery disease was examined in women.

Methods.—The study group included 161 women from The Cleveland Clinic Foundation; St. Luc Hospital, Brussels; and St. Mary's Hospital, London. Symptom-limited exercise testing was performed by patients on either a treadmill or a cycle ergometer. An ECG was recorded at rest and at the end of each stage of exercise. The ECG findings were considered positive in the presence of horizontal or downsloping ST-segment depression of at least 0.1 mV at 0.08 seconds after the J point in any lead. Echocardiographic images were recorded before and immediately after treadmill stress testing or before, during, at peak, and immediately after cycle stress

TABLE 3.—Accuracy, Rate of Angiography, and Cost of 7 Diagnostic Strategies for Diagnosis of Coronary Disease

Strategy	Cost/Pt ($)	Angiography (%)	Inappropriate Angiography (%)	False Negative Results (%)
I/Angiography	1,434	100	63	0
II/Exercise ECG	1,023 ± 43	69 ± 3	56 ± 4	11 ± 3
III/Exercise echo	828 ± 44	41 ± 3	29 ± 5	13 ± 4
IV/Selective ECG/echo	836 ± 45	51 ± 3	44 ± 5	14 ± 4
V/Stepwise ECG/echo	663 ± 36	31 ± 2	26 ± 4	22 ± 6
VI/Bayesian ECG	740 ± 29	50 ± 2	32 ± 2	29 ± 1
VII/Bayesian echo	641 ± 24	37 ± 2	25 ± 1	25 ± 1

Note: Data presented are mean value ± 1 SD.
Abbreviations: echo, echocardiography; *Pt*, patient.

testing. Echocardiography findings were considered positive in the presence of new or worsening wall motion abnormality. Patients also underwent coronary angiography.

Results.—Coronary artery stenosis of greater than 50% was present in 59 patients. The sensitivity of exercise echocardiography was 80%. In 48 patients with an interpretable ECG, the sensitivity of exercise echocardiography was 81%, whereas that of exercise ECG was 77%. In 102 patients without coronary artery disease, the specificity of exercise echocardiography was 81%. In 70 patients with an interpretable ECG, the specificity and accuracy of exercise echocardiography significantly exceeded that of exercise ECG. Exercise echocardiography had the best balance between accuracy and cost for the diagnosis of coronary artery disease in women (Table 3).

Conclusions.—Exercise echocardiography was superior to exercise ECG in specificity and accuracy of diagnosis of coronary artery disease in women. The use of exercise echocardiography is justified on a cost basis as it avoids unnecessary coronary angiography.

▶ This paper provides a useful reminder of the fiscal cost that is generated by the need to undertake further laboratory exploration of patients with false positive ECG test results. To this fiscal cost must be added a great deal of anxiety and iatrogenic disease from the unnecessary restriction of physical activity. Such problems can be minimized by using only screening procedures with a high specificity and restricting testing to high-risk individuals for whom there is a substantial pretest probability that disease is present.

R.J. Shephard, M.D., Ph.D., D.P.E.

Incremental Value of Exercise Electrocardiography and Thallium-201 Testing in Men and Women for the Presence and Extent of Coronary Artery Disease

Morise AP, Diamond GA, Detrano R, Bobbio M (West Virginia Univ, Morgantown; Cedars-Sinai Med Ctr, Los Angeles; Univ of California, Los Angeles; et al)

Am Heart J 130:267–276, 1995 6–5

Background.—A growing number of studies have assessed the incremental diagnostic value of a given test over data acquired before or at the same time as the test in question. This approach is warranted, because clinicians make decisions based on the integration of all available data. Previous research has demonstrated a significant incremental value to the use of exercise ECG both for diagnosing coronary disease (when considered in its appropriate clinical context) and for prognosis. The incremental value of exercise ECG and thallium-201 testing for diagnosing and determining the extent of coronary artery disease was studied in both male and female patients.

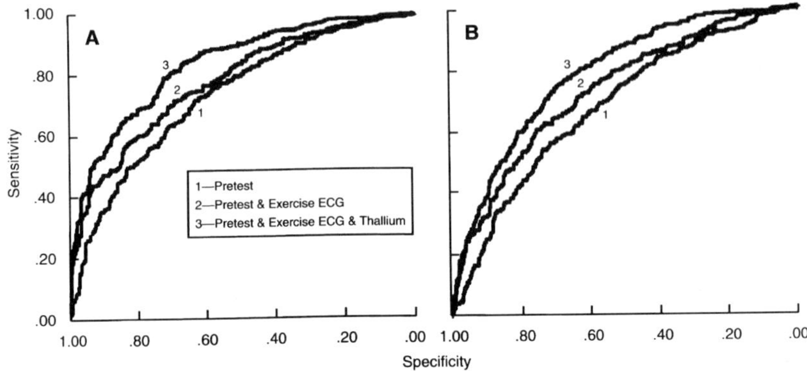

FIGURE 1.—Receiver operating characteristic curves of 3 incremental models for coronary disease presence (**A**) and extent (**B**) derived from validation population. Performance of pretest model (*1*) was significantly improved by addition of exercise ECG variables. Likewise, performance of combined pretest and exercise ECG model (2) was improved by addition of thallium-201 scintigraphy variables (*3*). (Courtesy of Morise AP, Diamond GA, Detrano R, et al: Incremental value of exercise electrocardiography and thallium-201 testing in men and women for the presence and extent of coronary artery disease. *Am Heart J* 130:267–276, 1995.)

Methods.—Data from 1 center were used to develop incremental logistic algorithms. These were then assessed in another group of 865 patients, seen at 4 centers. Pretest variables included were age, sex, symptoms, diabetes, smoking, and cholesterol concentrations. Exercise ECG and thallium-201 scintigram features were also included.

Findings.—Incremental receiver operating characteristic curve areas for disease presence were 0.75 for pretest variables, 0.82 for postexercise ECG, and 0.85 for post-thallium scintigram. For disease extent, the incremental ROC curve areas were pretest, 0.71; postexercise ECG, 0.76; and post-thallium scintigram, 0.78 (Fig 1). Women and men had similar incremental increases in accuracy.

Conclusions.—A significant incremental increase in accuracy was associated with exercise testing for the presence and extent of coronary artery disease when multivariable algorithms derived from 1 center were applied to a different group of patients. This increased accuracy was comparable for men and women.

▶ The important feature of this paper seems not that additional information about myocardial ischemia was obtained by an exercise ECG and thallium-201 scintigram, but rather that the increase in diagnostic information was so limited. It is also interesting that the amount of new knowledge added by exercise ECG was similar in men and in women. Several previous authors have suggested that ST-segmental depression is a less valid indicator of coronary vascular disease in women. The explanation of this paradox seems that the present analysis was based on a detailed analysis of the ECG, rather than a simple consideration of ST-segmental voltages.

R.J. Shephard, M.D., Ph.D., D.P.E.

Electrocardiographic Monitoring During Cardiac Rehabilitation
Keteyian SJ, Mellett PA, Fedel FJ, McGowan CM, Stein PD (Henry Ford Heart and Vascular Inst, Detroit)
Chest 107:1242–1246, 1995 6–6

Objective.—There is a lack of prospective controlled trials to determine the value of continuous ECG monitoring during cardiac rehabilitation. For this reason, the frequency of cardiovascular events was reviewed in 289 patients with heart disease who participated in an ECG-monitored phase 2 cardiac rehabilitation program during a 10-month period in 1992–1993. Patients exercised aerobically for approximately 30 minutes per session, using a variety of modalities. The number of sessions averaged 14.

Findings.—No major cardiovascular events were recorded during exercise training. Minor events occurred in 27% of patients and were more frequent in those who met the American College of Cardiology criteria for ECG monitoring. Asymptomatic new-onset events were not, however, more frequent in these patients. In all, 11 of the 289 patients (3.8%) had at least one new-onset asymptomatic event (Table 4). In only 4 instances was management known to have been altered because of an ECG-identified event. Two patients had medical treatment changed, and 2 had their exercise heart rate range reduced.

Conclusion.—The rarity with which management is altered because of ECG monitoring should be considered when deciding whether patients should be monitored continuously during participation in a phase 2 cardiac rehabilitation program.

▶ Treatment should be kept as simple as possible during cardiac rehabilitation to minimize costs and make the programs applicable to a wide segment of the public with coronary vascular disease. Continuous ECG monitoring of the "postcoronary" patient is one luxury that has been promoted vigorously by some segments of the medical technology industry. Although not presented in such terms, the study by Keteyian et al. is useful in showing that such monitoring has a very limited cost-effectiveness. More than 2,000 hours of exercise monitoring led to only 2 changes of drug treatment and 2 changes in exercise prescription. It still remains unclear whether even these changes altered prognosis, or whether the need for them could have been determined by the much simpler approach of talking to the patient!

R.J. Shephard, M.D., Ph.D., D.P.E.

TABLE 4.—Characteristics and Clinical Findings of Patients Who Experienced a New-onset, Asymptomatic* Event

Subject No./ Age, yr/Sex	MET Level at Entry Into Phase 2	Met ACC Criteria	Session No. When Event Occurred/ Total Sessions	Event	Comment/Action
156/71/M	4.4	Yes	3/12	ST segment depression	Lowered THRR
248/58/M	4.4	Yes	11/12	Ventricular bigeminy	THRR violator
260/67/M	3.0	Yes	1/12	RBBB	Physician-no change in therapy
5/64/F	2.8	No	1/12	ST segment depression	THRR violator
25/60/M	3.3	No	1/9	Nonsustained VT	Physician-no change in therapy
59/59/M	2.2	No	2/12	Inverted T waves	None taken
100/63/M	3.8	No	7/12	ST segment depression	None taken
118/57/M	8.2	No	18/18	Nonsustained VT	Physician-no change in therapy; THRR violator
148/48/F	3.6	No	7/20	Wandering pacemaker	None taken
162/68/F	3.9	No	4/18	SVT	Physician-β-adrenergic blocking agent added
270/45/M	5.8	No	10/12	Pacemaker related 3 to 1 AV block	Physician-THRR violator

* An asymptomatic event is defined as one likely not detectable without ECG monitoring.

Abbreviations: AV, atrioventricular; *MET*, metabolic equivalent; *RBBB*, right bundle branch block; *THRR*, target heart rate range; *VT*, ventricular tachycardia; *SVT*, supraventricular tachycardia.

(Courtesy of Keteyian SJ, Mellett PA, Fedel FJ, et al: Electrocardiographic monitoring during cardiac rehabilitation. *Chest* 107:1242–1246, 1995.)

Training Room Evaluation of Chest Pain in the Adolescent Athlete
Billups D, Martin D, Swain RA (West Virginia Univ, Charleston; Marshall Univ, Huntington, WVa)
South Med J 88:667–672, 1995 6–7

Introduction.—Chest pain in young athletes is only rarely caused by cardiac problems. It is a common complaint that cannot be specifically diagnosed in 21% to 45% of the patients. The most common diagnoses are musculoskeletal or respiratory difficulties, but chest pain may also be caused by gastrointestinal problems and psychological factors. Although the majority of the etiologic factors will be benign, syncopal episodes or severe dizziness during exercise may be signs of a more serious disorder. Specific etiologic factors and pointers for athletic trainers in the management of chest pain in young athletes were reviewed.

Cardiac Causes.—Sudden death, which occurs rarely, is most often caused by congenital heart disease. Diagnosis is based on a complete medical history. Pain described as heavy tightness or squeezing in the chest or a history of diabetes, cigarette smoking, hypertension, or high cholesterol may raise suspicion of coronary artery disease, especially in athletes with Kawasaki disease or an anomalous coronary arterial system. Patients with hypertrophic cardiomyopathy may have vague chest pain, dizziness, or syncope, or may have a systolic murmur at the left apex. Cardiac tamponade can occur with a wound to the chest or upper abdomen; patients may have low blood pressure, distant heart sounds, and distended neck veins. Pain in athletes with mitral valve prolapse is usually sharp, nonradiating, and accompanied by palpitations. Aortic stenosis (revealed by a loud, harsh systolic crescendo murmur), pericarditis (examination may reveal a sandpaper-like friction rub), or myocarditis (possibly with symptoms of congestive heart failure) are other rare causes of chest pain in young athletes. A drug use history should be obtained. Cocaine, anabolic steroids, and amphetamine can all affect the cardiovascular system.

Other Causes.—Musculoskeletal injuries include muscle strains, costochondritis (characterized by pain on palpation of the juncture of the rib and sternum), or a fractured rib or sternum. The mechanism of injury is most helpful in determining the cause in these cases. Gastrointestinal causes of chest pain include esophageal reflux, dysmotility, a hiatal hernia, peptic ulcer disease, or esophageal spasm. Many patients can be managed with antacids, but when this is insufficient, the patient should be referred to a physician. Pulmonary causes include asthma or exercise-induced asthma (suggested by wheezing, "burning" chest, or breathing difficulty), pneumonia (indicated by fever and persistent cough), bronchitis (in patients with a productive cough without fever), spontaneous or traumatic pneumothorax (which causes chest discomfort and shortness of breath), pleurisy (often viral), pulmonary embolus (characterized by severe pleuritic chest pain, shortness of breath, and tachycardia), or spontaneous pneumomediastinum (particularly during weight lifting). Psychogenic causes, most often panic disorder, are usually diagnosed by exclusion.

Conclusion.—Chest pain in young athletes can have many causes. The athletic trainer should rule out or identify the most serious causes first and/or refer the athlete to a physician. Prompt evaluation and treatment can enable an efficient and safe return to competition.

▶ This practical review is useful to team physicians and athletic trainers because it presents in a clear and thoughtful fashion the telltale clinical features of the most common causes of chest pain in adolescents. It emphasizes that in adolescents, unlike in adults, exertional chest pain is rarely cardiac, but is often from musculoskeletal or pulmonary causes, and is sometimes from gastrointestinal or psychogenic causes. It does highlight, however, when to suspect cardiac pain in adolescents. Other recent articles also emphasize that activity-related chest pain in youngsters can be from asthma,[1] hyperventilation,[2] or psychogenic causes.[3]

E.R. Eichner, M.D.

References

1. Wiens L, Sabath R, Ewing L, et al: Chest pain in otherwise healthy children and adolescents is frequently caused by exercise-induced asthma. *Pediatrics* 90:350–353, 1992.
2. Bernhardt DT, Landry GL: Chest pain in active young people: Is it cardiac? *Physician Sportsmed* 22:70, 1994.
3. 1993 Year Book of Sports Medicine, pp 273–274.

Nontraumatic Sports Death in High School and College Athletes

Van Camp SP, Bloor CM, Mueller FO, Cantu RC, Olson HG (Univ of California, San Diego; Natl Ctr for Catastrophic Sports Injury Research, Univ of North Carolina, Chapel Hill)

Med Sci Sports Exerc 27:641–647, 1995 6–8

Introduction.—Since 1982, the National Center for Catastrophic Sports Injury Research has compiled data on catastrophic injuries that resulted in death or serious disability in men and women in high school and college athletics in the United States. Using these data, the largest study to evaluate comprehensively the frequency and causes of nontraumatic sports deaths in high school and college athletes during a 10-year period was undertaken.

Findings.—From July 1983 through June 1993, nontraumatic sports deaths were reported in 126 high school athletes and 34 college athletes, for an annual fatality rate of 16 per year. The estimated death rates in male athletes were more than fivefold higher than in female athletes (7.47 vs. 1.33 per million athletes per year) and more than twofold higher in male college athletes than in male high school athletes (14.50 vs. 66.60 per million athletes per year). The latter trend was also noted in female athletes, but the sample of women was too small to carry out a valid test of significance. Deaths were most frequently attributable to cardiovascular conditions, particularly hypertrophic cardiomyopathy and coronary artery

TABLE 3.—Causes of Nontraumatic Sports Deaths in High School and College Athletes

Nontraumatic Sports Deaths	Total (*N* = 136)	Male (*N* = 124)	Female (*N* = 12)
Athletes with cardiovascular conditions	100*,†	92*,†	8
Hypertrophic cardiomyopathy	51‡,§	50‡,§	1
Probable hypertrophic cardiomyopathy	5	5	0
Coronary artery anomaly	16*,‡	14*,‡	2
Myocarditis	7‖	7‖	0
Aortic stenosis	6	6	0
Dilated cardiomyopathy	5	5	0
Atherosclerotic coronary artery disease	3	2	1
Aortic rupture	2	2	0
Cardiomyopathy-nonspecific	2‖	2‖	0
Tunnel subaortic stenosis	2¶	2¶	0
Coronary artery aneurysm	1	0	1
Mitral valve prolapse	1	1	0
Right ventricular cardiomyopathy	1	0	1
Ruptured cerebellar arteriovenous malformation	1	0	1
Subarachnoid hemorrhage	1	0	1
Wolff-Parkinson-White syndrome	1§	1§	0
Athletes with noncardiovascular conditions	30*	27*	3
Hyperthermia	13	12	1
Rhabdomyolysis and sickle cell trait	7*	6*	1
Status asthmaticus	4	3	1
Electrocution due to lightning	3	3	0
Arnold-Chiari II malformation	1	1	0
Aspiration-blood-GI bleed	1	1	0
Exercise-induced anaphylaxis	1	1	0
Athletes with cause of death undetermined	7	6	1

* One male athlete had a cardiovascular condition (coronary artery anomaly) and a noncardiovascular condition (rhabdomyolysis and sickle cell trait).
† Five male athletes had multiple cardiovascular conditions.
‡ Three male athletes had hypertrophic cardiomyopathy and a coronary artery anomaly.
§ One male athlete had hypertrophic cardiomyopathy and Wolff-Parkinson-White syndrome.
‖ One male athlete had myocarditis and a nonspecific cardiomyopathy.
¶ One male athlete had hypoplasia of the aortic arch associated with tunnel subaortic stenosis.
(Courtesy of Van Camp SP, Bloor CM, Mueller FO, et al: Nontraumatic sports death in high school and college athletes. *Med Sci Sports Exerc* 27:641–647, 1995.)

anomalies (Table 3). Noncardiovascular conditions accounted for 22% of deaths, almost half of which were the result of exertional hyperthermia. Death in 7 black athletes with sickle cell trait resulted from exertional rhabdomyolysis.

Summary.—Nontraumatic sports deaths in high school and college athletes are, fortunately, quite infrequent. Male athletes are at increased risk for nontraumatic sports deaths compared to females, even after adjustment for participation frequency. College male athletes are at greater risk than their high school counterparts. Nontraumatic sports deaths are primarily caused by cardiovascular conditions.

► The sudden death of any athlete is a tragedy and an irony. Invariably, the public impact is stark and profound. We say to others, surely this can and must be prevented. And we think to ourselves, if the best among us—the fittest of all—collapse and die, what does this imply about the rest of us? This is the most recent national study of nontraumatic sports deaths in high school and college athletes. As in prior studies of young athletes,[1] hypertrophic cardiomyopathy (HCM) was the most common cause of sudden exertional death. Cardiac conditions comprised about 70% of the deaths; after HCM in frequency came anomalous coronary arteries, myocarditis, and aortic stenosis. Noncardiac causes of death included rupture of the aorta (Marfan's syndrome) or of a cerebral vessel, heat stroke, asthma, and rhabdomyolysis with sickle cell trait.[2] An intriguing mystery is the "gender gap" in sports deaths: men are more apt to die than women. In this study, 50 of the 51 HCM deaths were in males and, in general, after adjusting for gender trends in sports play, the estimated death rates in males were fivefold higher than in females. Do women know when to quit, or does testosterone accelerate the consequences of HCM in men? See also Abstract 6–9.

E.R. Eichner, M.D.

References

1. Maron BJ: Sudden death in young athletes: Lessons from the Hank Gathers affair. *N Engl J Med* 329:55–57, 1993.
2. Eichner ER: Sickle cell trait, heroic exercise, and fatal collapse. *Phys Fit Sports Med* 21:51–64, 1993.

Blunt Impact to the Chest Leading to Sudden Death From Cardiac Arrest During Sports Activities

Maron BJ, Poliac LC, Kaplan JA, Mueller FO (Minneapolis Heart Inst Found; Dartmouth Med School, Lebanon, NH; Natl Ctr for Catastrophic Sports Injury Research, Chapel Hill, NC; et al)

N Engl J Med 333:337–342, 1995 6–9

Background.—Although most cases of sudden death in young athletes result from unsuspected cardiovascular diseases, this is not always the case. Athletes with no structural cardiovascular disease or traumatic injury may die suddenly of cardiac arrest after a blow to the chest. This condition is known as cardiac concussion or commotio cordis. Twenty-five cases of sudden death resulting from a blunt impact to the chest in young sports participants were reported.

Findings.—The patients were identified by review of registry data and other sources, including news media reports. All but 1 of the patients were male; the age range was 3–19 years. All experienced cardiac arrest and collapse immediately after an unexpected blow to the chest.

Most of the injuries were inflicted by a projectile, such as a baseball or hockey puck. Sixteen occurred during organized competitive sports (Fig 1). In no case did the chest impact seem excessive for the sport involved, nor did the impact have sufficient force to be fatal. Twelve of the victims collapsed immediately, and 13 were conscious and physically active for a

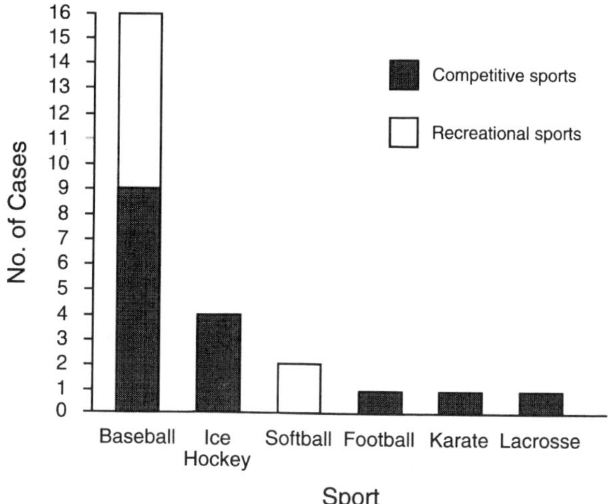

FIGURE 1.—Participation in competitive and recreational sports at the time of sudden cardiac death induced by blunt impact to the chest. (Reprinted by permission of The *New England Journal of Medicine,* Maron BJ, Poliac LC, Kaplan JA, et al: Blunt impact to the chest leading to sudden death from cardiac arrest during sports activities. *N Engl J Med* 333:337–342, Copyright 1995, Massachusetts Medical Society.)

while. Nineteen of the victims received CPR within about 3 minutes; however, only 2 regained normal cardiac rhythm, and both of these patients died of irreversible brain damage. Twenty-eight percent of the victims were wearing protective chest padding when injured (Fig 2). Twelve patients had small contusions that were judged to result from blunt impact (Fig 3).

Discussion.—Blunt impact to the chest can cause sudden death of cardiac arrest in young athletes. Most of these deaths probably result from a ventricular dysrhythmia induced by a sudden, blunt precordial blow. The impact most likely occurs at an electrically vulnerable phase of ventricular excitability. It is hoped that these findings will stimulate a better clinical understanding of commotio cordis, as well as efforts to define its mechanism and to prevent it.

▶ This article, the most comprehensive description of "cardiac concussion" or commotio cordis, will likely become a classic. Each of 25 young victims collapsed in cardiac arrest just after a blow to the chest, usually from a baseball or puck. This tragedy seems to result from ventricular fibrillation triggered by impact over the heart at an electrically vulnerable phase of ventricular excitability. As reviewed in 1994,[1] even beginning CPR within 1 minute tends to be of no avail here, and deaths like this have wrongly been regarded as criminal acts (as when a stick-slash to the chest killed an Italian

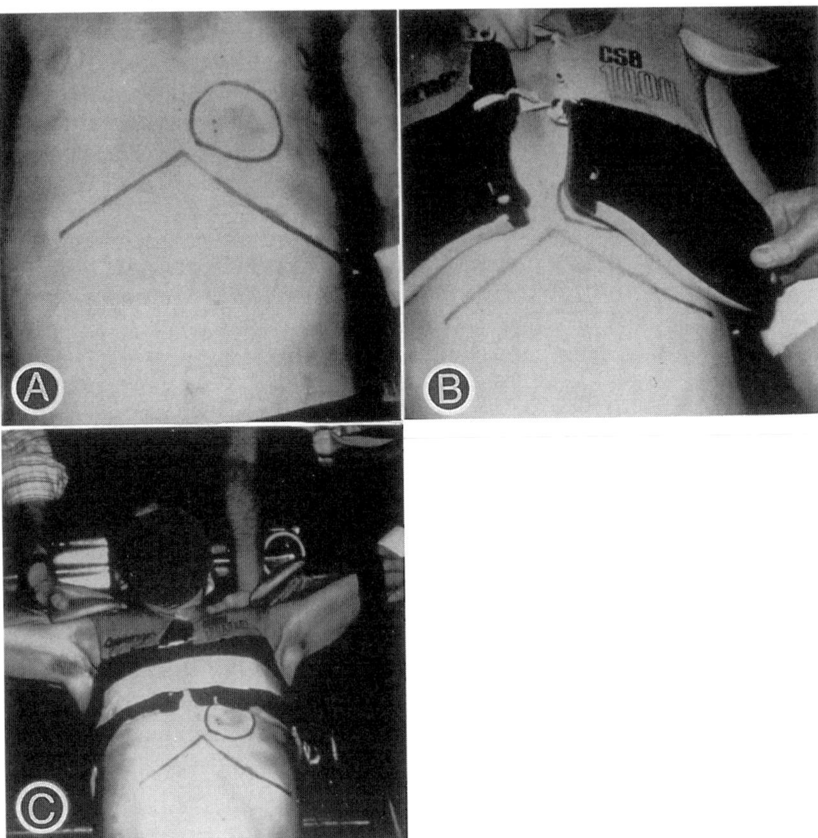

FIGURE 2.—A 15-year-old patient with blunt nonpenetrating impact to the chest delivered by a hockey puck during a competitive interscholastic hockey game in which the boy rose from a prone position after a melee in front of the goal, raised his arms above his head, and was struck in the chest at close range by a puck from a forehand shot toward the goal. **A,** the patient with his protective chest gear removed. A relatively small midprecordial contusion (3 cm in diameter) produced by the impact of the puck is present just to the left of the sternum, demarcated by the *circle*; the *line* delineates the inferior margins of the rib cage. **B,** the plastic-and-foam chest and shoulder protector in its proper position as worn by the patient (with arms at his sides); here, the contusion appears to be covered by the chest protector. **C,** the patient's arms are raised (to simulate their position at the moment of the accident, when the patient was attempting to break the flight of the puck), elevating the chest and shoulder padding and leaving the area of impact unprotected. (Reprinted by permission of The *New England Journal of Medicine,* Maron BJ, Poliac LC, Kaplan JA, et al: Blunt impact to the chest leading to sudden death from cardiac arrest during sports activities. *N Engl J Med* 333:337–342, Copyright 1995, Massachusetts Medical Society.)

hockey player and led to a manslaughter charge). We need better chest protectors. See also Abstract 6–8.

E.R. Eichner, M.D.

Reference

1. 1994 Year Book of Sports Medicine, pp 421–422.

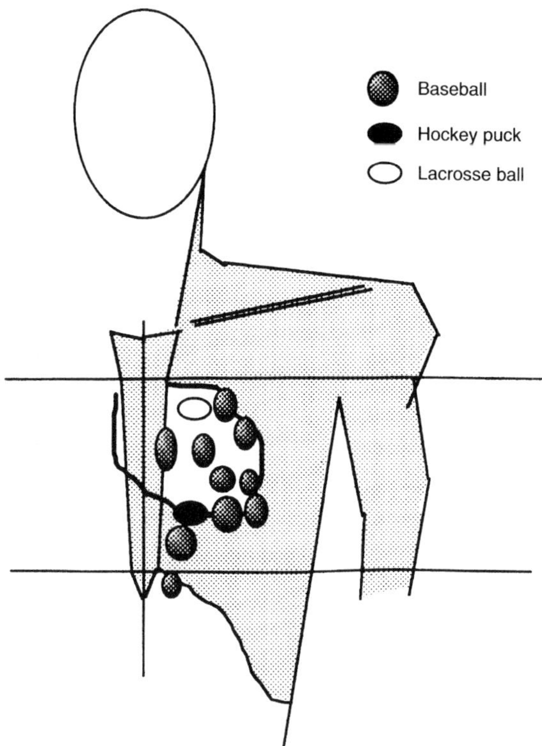

FIGURE 3.—Schematic representation of the locations of impact points (contusions) judged to have been produced by baseballs (n =10), a hockey puck, and a lacrosse ball on the anterior chest walls of 12 victims of commotio cordis. The estimated contour of the heart is indicated by the heavy line. (Reprinted by permission of The *New England Journal of Medicine,* Maron BJ, Poliac LC, Kaplan JA, et al: Blunt impact to the chest leading to sudden death from cardiac arrest during sports activities. *N Engl J Med* 333:337–342, Copyright 1995, Massachusetts Medical Society.)

Balanced Activation of Coagulation and Fibrinolysis After a 2-H Triathlon

Bartsch P, Welsch B, Albert M, Friedmann B, Levi M, Kruithof EKO (Univ of Heidelberg, Germany; Univ of Amsterdam, The Netherlands; Univ of Lausanne, Switzerland)

Med Sci Sports Exerc 27:1465–1470, 1995 6–10

Objective.—Physical exercise shortens coagulation and euglobulin clot lysis times (ECLT) and increases plasma levels of factor VIII and tissue plasminogen activator (t-PA). The effect of exercise on fibrinolysis is less clear. A recent immunoassay for plasmin-α2-antiplasmin (PAP) has been developed that allows the investigation of strenuous exercise on the formation of thrombin, fibrin, and plasmin in vivo.

Methods.—Thrombin-antithrombin (TAT) complexes, prothrombin fragment 1+2 (PTF1+2), fibrin monomers (FM), plasmin-antiplasmin

(PAP) complexes t−PA antigen, plasminogen activator inhibitor−1 (PAI−1), and fibrinopeptide A (FPA) levels were measured in venous blood drawn from 10 male athletes aged 19–38 years before, after, and at 2, 8, and 21 hours after a 128- to 163-minute triathlon.

Results.—Whereas fibrinogen levels did not change, t−PA, TAT complexes, and FPA increased significantly after exercise but returned to pre-exercise levels within 2 hours. PTF1+2, fibrin degradation products (FbDP), and PAP values increased by a factor of 1.5 to 2.0 after exercise but had returned to pre-exercise levels at 21 hours. There was an 85% shortening of the ECLT that was prolonged at 2 hours by 50% and at 21 hours by 30%. Plasminogen increased significantly 2 hours after exercise. Plasminogen activator antigen inhibitor-1 levels rose significantly after exercise and returned to baseline values after 8 hours. Levels of t-PA were highest immediately after exercise and returned to baseline levels after 21 hours.

Conclusion.—In healthy individuals, the hemostatic system is kept in balance after strenuous exercise. Exercise induces increases in thrombin and fibrin formation as well as activation of the fibrinolytic system. Plasmin production is mediated by an increase of PAI-1.

▶ Last year we reviewed articles showing that physical activity increases fibrinolysis acutely in proportion to effort and that active men may have more brisk basal fibrinolysis than do inactive men.[1, 2] It has long been known that running a marathon evokes a striking increase in fibrinolysis.[3] However, strenuous exercise can also be "prothrombotic," i.e., it can increase platelet count and activate coagulation. This report studies both edges of the sword during exercise: prothrombotic vs. fibrinolytic. It shows that a 2-hour triathlon does activate coagulation mildly, with low-grade formation of thrombin and fibrin, but that this prothrombotic action is outstripped by a brisk increase in fibrinolysis, so that the net immediate effect of exercise, at least in healthy people, is apt to be antithrombotic. In other words, this report supports the thesis that exercise is "nature's anticoagulant."[3]

E.R. Eichner, M.D.

References

1. 1995 Year Book of Sports Medicine, pp 451–453.
2. 1995 Year Book of Sports Medicine, pp 468–470.
3. 1991 Year Book of Sports Medicine, pp 90–91.

Moving?

I'd like to receive my ***Year Book of Sports Medicine*** without interruption.
Please note the following change of address, effective:

Name: ______________________________

New Address: ______________________________

____

City: ____________________ State: ________ Zip: ________

Old Address: ______________________________

____

City: ____________________ State: ________ Zip: ________

Reservation Card

Yes, I would like my own copy of ***Year Book of Sports Medicine.*** Please begin my subscription with the current edition according to the terms described below.* I understand that I will have 30 days to examine each annual edition. If satisfied, I will pay just $71.95 plus sales tax, postage and handling (price subject to change without notice).

Name: ______________________________

Address: ______________________________

City: ____________________ State: ________ Zip: ________

Method of Payment

❍ Visa ❍ Mastercard ❍ AmEx ❍ Bill me ❍ Check (in US dollars, payable to Mosby, Inc.)

Card number: ____________________ Exp date: ____________

Signature: ______________________________

LS-0909

*Your *Year Book* Service Guarantee:

When you subscribe to the *Year Book*, we'll send you an advance notice of future volumes about two months before they publish. This automatic notice system is designed to take up as little of your time as possible. If you do not want the *Year Book*, the advance notice makes it quick and easy for you to let us know your decision, and you will always have at least 20 days to decide. If we don't hear from you, we'll send you the new volume as soon as it's available. And, of course, the *Year Book* is yours to examine free of charge for 30 days (postage, handling and applicable sales tax are added to each shipment.).

NO POSTAGE
NECESSARY
IF MAILED
IN THE
UNITED STATES

BUSINESS REPLY MAIL

FIRST CLASS MAIL PERMIT No. 762 CHICAGO, IL

POSTAGE WILL BE PAID BY ADDRESSEE

Chris Hughes
Mosby-Year Book, Inc.
200 N. LaSalle Street
Suite 2600
Chicago, IL 60601-9981

NO POSTAGE
NECESSARY
IF MAILED
IN THE
UNITED STATES

BUSINESS REPLY MAIL

FIRST CLASS MAIL PERMIT No. 762 CHICAGO, IL

POSTAGE WILL BE PAID BY ADDRESSEE

Chris Hughes
Mosby-Year Book, Inc.
200 N. LaSalle Street
Suite 2600
Chicago, IL 60601-9981

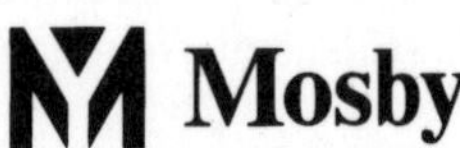

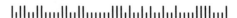

Dedicated to publishing excellence

Prognostic Value of Training-induced Change in Peak Exercise Capacity in Patients With Myocardial Infarcts and Patients With Coronary Bypass Surgery

Vanhees L, Fagard R, Thijs L, Amery A (Univ of Leuven, Belgium)
Am J Cardiol 76:1014–1019, 1995 6–11

Background.—Low exercise performance is known to predict cardiovascular mortality in patients with coronary artery disease, but the prognostic value of gain in exercise capacity after participation in a physical training program has not been studied previously. A group of patients who were referred for an outpatient cardiac rehabilitation program were fol-

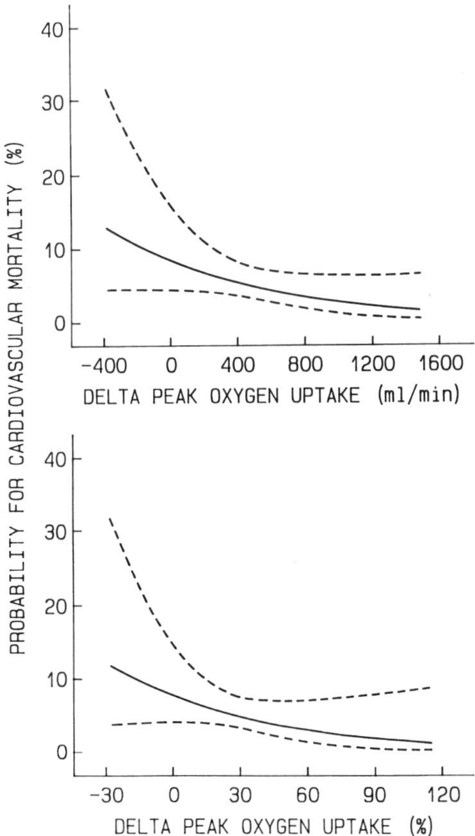

FIGURE 1.—Relation (*solid line*) between the absolute (**top**) and relative (**bottom**) change in peak oxygen uptake after exercise training and cardiovascular mortality with 95% confidence limits (*dotted lines*), from a study of 417 men with coronary artery disease. The relations were standardized to nonsmokers, aged 50 years, without history of hypertension or diabetes. (Reprinted by permission of Elsevier Science Inc. from Vanhees L, Fagard R, Thijs L, et al: Prognostic value of training-induced change in peak exercise capacity in patients with myocardial infarcts and patients with coronary bypass surgery. *Am J Cardiol* 76:1014–1019, Copyright 1995 by Excerpta Medica, Inc.)

lowed for an average of 6.2 years to determine the relationship between training-induced change in peak exercise capacity and cardiovascular mortality.

Methods.—The 417 patients who completed the exercise tests were all men. They had a history of acute myocardial infarction (235 patients, the AMI group), had undergone coronary bypass surgery (93 patients, the CBS group), or both (89 patients, the AMI + CBS group). Patients underwent a standard exercise test protocol, then entered a 3-month training program consisting of 75-minute exercise sessions 3 times weekly. The program was offered for a second 3-month period on a twice-weekly basis, after which the patients were advised to continue exercising through a sport club program for cardiac patients.

Results.—For the total group, peak oxygen uptake ($\dot{V}O_2$) increased 33% after the training program, and the heart rate at rest and during submaximal exercise was also decreased. Increases in peak $\dot{V}O_2$ were similar in the 3 subgroups. The cause of death was cardiovascular disease in 21 of the 37 patients who died during follow-up. The deaths occurred an average of 4.79 years after the second exercise test, administered at the end of the formal training program. The incidence of fatal events did not differ significantly between the AMI, CBS, and AMI + CBS groups. Significant risk indicators for all-cause mortality were age, systolic blood pressure, dyspnea in daily life, present smoking habits, and a history of diabetes. Cardiovascular mortality is lower for patients showing larger increases in peak $\dot{V}O_2$ after training (Fig 1). Even after adjusting for age and other significant covariates, the prognostic value of peak $\dot{V}O_2$ was higher after than before physical training.

Conclusion.—The magnitude of the gain in peak $\dot{V}O_2$ that occurs after a physical training program is an independent predictor of cardiovascular mortality in patients with cardiovascular disease. This is true for both patients with myocardial infarcts and for those who have undergone coronary bypass grafting. The relative hazard rate for the percent change in peak $\dot{V}O_2$ of 0.98 indicates that a 2% decrease in cardiovascular risk would accompany an additional 1% increase in peak $\dot{V}O_2$.

► Meta-analyses suggest that an appropriate exercise program reduces the risk of fatal reinfarction by about 25%. The present analysis suggests that a 12.5% increase of aerobic power (about the improvement in exercise tolerance commonly seen) would also yield a 25% decrease in risk. There have been suggestions that some of the poor response in cardiac patients is caused by advanced age, but in the present study the effect of training response was observed even after adjusting for age, smoking habits, a history of hypertension, and a history of diabetes. Moreover, and in contrast to a smaller earlier study,[1] the peak oxygen intake after training was still a significant predictor of prognosis even when account was taken of the initial aerobic power.

R.J. Shephard, M.D., Ph.D., D.P.E.

Reference

1. Fioretti P, Baardman T, Deckers J, et al: Social fate and long-term survival of patients with a recent myocardial infarction, after cardiac rehabilitation. *Eur Heart J* 9(suppl L):89–94, 1988.

Efficacy of High-intensity Exercise Training on Left Ventricular Ejection Fraction in Men With Coronary Artery Disease (The Training Level Comparison Study)

Oberman A, Fletcher GF, Lee J, Nanda N, Fletcher BJ, Jensen B, Caldwell ES
(Univ of Alabama, Birmingham; Emory Univ, Atlanta, Ga)

Am J Cardiol 76:643–647, 1995 6–12

Background.—Exercise training has long been advocated for patients with coronary artery disease (CAD). However, the direct effect of exercise training on the myocardium and left ventricular (LV) function is not well documented, especially in patients with depressed ventricular function. Determining whether such training can improve LV function without adverse events is important. The effects of high- and low-intensity exercise training on the change in echocardiographic LV ejection fraction (LVEF) from rest to peak exercise were compared.

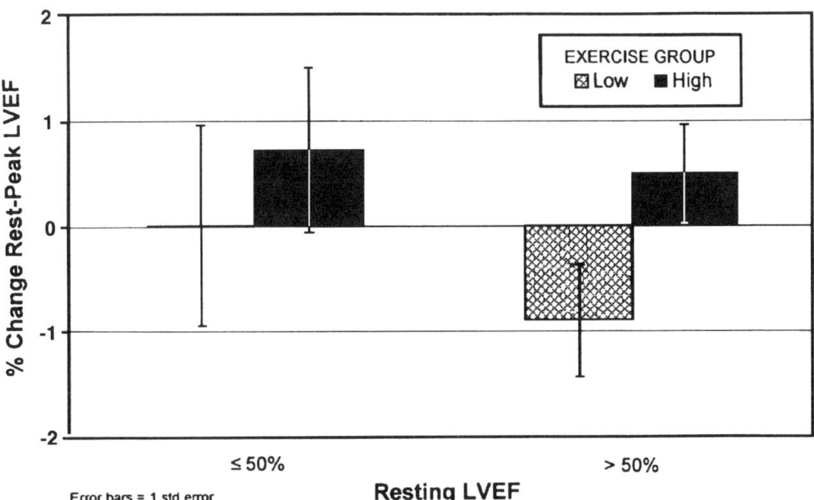

FIGURE 2.—Percent change in the difference between rest to peak exercise left ventricular ejection fraction (*LVEF*) over time, baseline to 1 year, in men with coronary artery disease. When the exercise groups are subdivided by initial resting LVEF ≤ 50% (n = 55) vs. > 50% (n = 123), the high-intensity exercise group showed a significantly (P = 0.05) greater increase in the rest-peak LVEF from baseline to 1 year, compared with the low-intensity exercise group, in those with the higher (> 50%) resting LVEF. (Reprinted by permission of Elsevier Science Inc. from Oberman A, Fletcher GF, Lee J, et al: Efficacy of high-intensity exercise training on left ventricular ejection fraction in men with coronary artery disease. [The Training Level Comparison Study] *Am J Cardiol* 76:643–647, Copyright 1995 by Excerpta Medica, Inc.)

Methods.—The study sample comprised sedentary men with CAD aged 30–70 years. By random assignment, 89 men participated in dynamic low-intensity exercise training, at 50% of their maximal oxygen consumption, and 111 participated in high-intensity exercise, at 85% of their maximal oxygen consumption. The patients were re-assessed at 6 and 12 months.

Findings.—In both groups, exercise capacity increased significantly, with no adverse events. However, the increase of function was greater in the high-intensity exercise group. In the high-intensity group, the mean increase of LVEF from rest to peak exercise increased from 6.2% at baseline to 6.5% at 6 months and to 6.7% at 12 months. By contrast, there was no improvement in the low-intensity group at 6 months, and at 12 months that value was decreased. In a multivariate analysis, high-intensity exercise significantly contributed to the change in rest-peak LVEF. When the patients were subgrouped by initial baseline LVEF of 50% or less and an LVEF exceeding 50%, men in the high-intensity group with the greater LVEF had more of an increase in the rest-peak LVEF between baseline and 1 year (Fig 2).

Conclusions.—During a 1-year period, exercise capacity increased in both high- and low-intensity exercise groups, though this increase was greater in the high-intensity group. No adverse events occurred in either group. Compared with patients in the low-intensity group, patients in the high-intensity group were more improved in the rest-peak LVEF, especially those with a greater LVEF at baseline.

► The main message of this study seems to be that training is of benefit for the patient with ischemic heart disease who has impaired LV function. The population sampled have only a minor level of impairment (average resting ejection fraction of 53%), and several other laboratories (including our own) have found benefit in those with stable cardiac failure and ejection fractions as low as 20%. Gains of function are here assessed by the somewhat bizarre measure of changes in the difference in ejection fraction between rest and peak exercise. Although benefit is ascribed to the adoption of a high-intensity exercise program, the initial, 6-month, and 12-month indices are not very different for either the high-intensity group (6.2, 6.5, and 6.7%) or the low-intensity group (6.6, 6.6, and 6.0%). It would have been more convincing had subjects been compared in terms of their maximal oxygen intake (which depends mainly on peak cardiac output). This measure showed gains in both the high-intensity group (25.3, 26.8, 28.0) and the low-intensity group (24.2, 26.0, 26.4), with little difference between the two regimens.

R.J. Shephard, M.D., Ph.D., D.P.E.

Profile of Mood States and Cardiac Rehabilitation After Acute Myocardial Infarction

Oldridge N, Streiner D, Hoffmann R, Guyatt G (Univ of Wisconsin, Milwaukee; McMaster Univ, Hamilton, Ont, Canada)

Med Sci Sports Exerc 27:900–905, 1995 6–13

Introduction.—Reactive anxiety and depression are not infrequent after acute myocardial infarction (AMI), and they may persist. It has been suggested that more disturbed patients are the most responsive to cardiac rehabilitation, but program-related improvements of psychological well-being have not been definitively documented.

Study Plan.—The Profile of Mood States (POMS), a well-validated adjective checklist, was used to monitor mood in 187 patients who had mild to moderate levels of anxiety and/or depression after AMI. Patients were randomized to usual care or to an 8-week cardiac rehabilitation program consisting of supervised low-level exercise as well as behavioral and risk factor counseling in a group setting. The Spielberger State Anxiety Inventory and Beck Depression Inventory were also used. Patients were followed for 1 year.

Results.—Anxiety improved significantly in those patients assigned to rehabilitation who initially had above-average anxiety scores (Table 3). No difference in depression scores was apparent at 8 weeks between the rehabilitated and control patients. Temporal trends in POMS scores suggested significant lessening of both anxiety and depression in both groups.

TABLE 3.—Changes in State Anxiety and Beck Depression (Mean ± SD) From Baseline to 8 Weeks and 12 Months in Patients Randomized to Rehabilitation (n = 93) or Usual Care

				Repeated Measures ANOVA		
	Baseline	8 wk	12 months	Treatment	Time	Interaction
State anxiety (N = 186)						
Rehabilitation	47 ± 9	42 ± 11*	42 ± 10	NS	<0.001	NS
Usual care	46 ± 9	45 ± 10	42 ± 10			
Above mean state anxiety						
Rehabilitation (N = 41)	55 ± 5	47 ± 9**	46 ± 10	NS	<0.001	NS
Usual care (N = 34)	55 ± 5	51 ± 8	49 ± 8			
Below mean state anxiety						
Rehabilitation (N = 52)	41 ± 6	39 ± 11	40 ± 10	NS	NS	NS
Usual care (N = 59)	41 ± 7	41 ± 9	39 ± 9			
Depression (N = 181)						
Rehabilitation	4.2 ± 4.1	3.4 ± 3.7	3.1 ± 3.4	NS	<0.005	NS
Usual care	3.9 ± 3.9	3.9 ± 4.5	2.9 ± 3.0			
Above mean depression						
Rehabilitation (N = 33)	8.3 ± 4.1	5.5 ± 4.5	4.0 ± 3.6	NS	<0.001	NS
Usual care (N = 27)	8.7 ± 4.1	7.5 ± 5.9	4.9 ± 3.6			
Below mean depression						
Rehabilitation (N = 57)	1.8 ± 1.3	2.3 ± 2.1	2.2 ± 2.5	NS	NS	NS
Usual care (N = 64)	1.9 ± 1.3	2.5 ± 2.9	2.0 ± 2.2			

Note: Baseline to 8 weeks (t test); *P < 0.05; ** P < 0.01.
Abbreviation: ANOVA, analysis of variance.
(Courtesy of Oldridge N, Streiner D, Hoffmann R, et al: Profile of mood states and cardiac rehabilitation after acute myocardial infarction. *Med Sci Sports Exerc* 27:900–905, 1995.)

At 8 weeks, patients with relatively high anxiety scores appeared to benefit more than control patients with respect to the POMS scales of tension-anxiety and depression-dejection.

Conclusion.—Patients who are mildly to moderately disturbed psychologically after AMI may benefit transiently from limited exercise rehabilitation, but most patients can be expected to improve in any case within a year after the event.

▶ We have previously noted that in the first few weeks after myocardial infarction, some patients show levels of depression that would raise serious concern if they were encountered in a psychiatric clinic.[1, 2] These dangerous trends are evident in responses to both the Minnesota Multiphasic Personality Inventory and the POMS questionnaires. In general, anxiety and depression scores return to normal over 12 months of rehabilitation, but as we have previously emphasized, this could reflect, at least in part, a natural recovery process rather than a direct outcome of rehabilitation. The present controlled study confirms that a cardiac rehabilitation program hastens the recovery of mood state, but even if such treatment is not provided, there is a gradual normalization of psychological function.

R.J. Shephard, M.D., Ph.D., D.P.E.

References

1. Kavanagh T, Shephard RJ, Tuck JA, et al: Depression following myocardial infarction: The effects of distance running. *Ann NY Acad Sci* 301:1029–1038, 1977.
2. Shephard RJ, Kavanagh T, Klavora P: Mood state during postcoronary cardiac rehabilitation. *J Cardiopulm Rehabil* 5:480–484, 1985.

Time Course of "Warm-up" in Stable Angina

Stewart RAH, Simmonds MB, Williams MJA (Univ of Otago, Dunedin, New Zealand)

Am J Cardiol 76:70–73, 1995 6–14

Purpose.—For patients with ischemic heart disease, angina may occur during an initial bout of exercise but fail to return after a period of rest or reduced level of physical activity. Knowledge of the time course of this "warm-up" effect would help in understanding the phenomenon and its mechanisms. The time course of warm-up was assessed in patients with stable exertional angina.

Methods.—Eighteen patients were studied, all with chronic stable exertional angina and a treadmill exercise test that was positive for ischemia (with at least a 1-mV flat or downsloping ST-segment depression). The patients completed sequential exercise tests, separated by a 10- or 30-minute rest. Comparisons of angina score, heart rate, blood pressure, and ST-segment depression were made for equivalent times during the first and second exercise bouts.

Results.—When the second exercise was performed after a 10-minute rest, times to 1-mV ST-segment depression and peak exercise were signifi-

TABLE 1.—Comparison of First and Second Exercises Separated by a 10-Minute Rest (n = 18)

	First Exercise	Second Exercise	*p* Value
1 mV ST depression			
Time (min)	5.69 ± 2.28	7.31 ± 2.31	<0.0001
Angina score	1.5 ± 1.8	1.4 ± 1.8	NS
Heart rate (beats/min)	117 ± 17	130 ± 19	<0.0001
Blood pressure (mm Hg)	191 ± 31	196 ± 22	NS
Heart rate·blood pressure (×1,000)	22.4 ± 5.2	25.6 ± 5.5	0.0002
Peak exercise			
Time (min)	7.32 ± 2.12	8.90 ± 2.32	<0.0001
ST depression (mV)	0.13 ± 0.06	0.13 ± 0.06	NS
Angina score	2.8 ± 2.1	2.7 ± 2.2	NS
Heart rate (beats/min)	130 ± 20	138 ± 20	NS
Blood pressure (mm Hg)	194 ± 25	191 ± 27	NS
Heart rate·blood pressure (×1,000)	25.4 ± 5.4	26.5 ± 6.1	NS
Equivalent submaximal stage			
Time (min)	6.56 ± 2.17		
ST depression (mV)	0.10 ± 0.04	0.03 ± 0.05	<0.0001
Angina score	2.0 ± 2.0	0.8 ± 1.3	0.0019
Heart rate (beats/min)	122 ± 17	121 ± 22	NS
Blood pressure (mm Hg)	187 ± 34	186 ± 24	NS
Heart rate·blood pressure (×1,000)	23.1 ± 6.0	22.8 ± 6.1	NS
Recovery			
ST depression (mV)	0.06 ± 0.05	0.04 ± 0.07	0.0080
Angina score at 1 minute	0.97 ± 1.33	0.83 ± 1.46	NS
Heart rate (beats/min)	86 ± 18	95 ± 20	<0.0001
Blood pressure (mm Hg)	163 ± 26	164 ± 31	NS
Heart rate·blood pressure (×1,000)	14.30 ± 4.30	16.10 ± 5.70	<0.0001

Note: Values are expressed as mean ± SD. $P > 0.05$ (NS).
(Reprinted by permission of Elsevier Science Inc. from Stewart RAH, Simmonds MB, Williams MJA: Time course of "warm-up" in stable angina. *Am J Cardiol* 76:70–73, Copyright 1995 by Excerpta Medica, Inc.)

cantly greater. Heart rate and rate-pressure product were higher at these times as well. At comparable stages of submaximal exercise, ST-segment depression and angina severity were also less during the second test, although there were no significant differences in heart rate and blood pressure. Ischemia seemed to resolve more rapidly after the second exercise bout, despite achievement of a greater work-rate (Table 1). Lesser, and usually nonsignificant, differences were observed when the 2 tests were separated by a 30-minute rest.

Conclusions.—In patients with stable angina, warm-up exercise followed by a 10-minute rest significantly reduces the severity of myocardial ischemia during a second exercise bout. The benefits of warm up are significantly lessened after a 30-minute rest. The mechanisms of this phenomenon warrant further investigation. The findings suggest a change in myocardial metabolism that is similar to ischemic preconditioning. Alternatively, there could be a sustained increase in myocardial perfusion to the ischemic territory, which has largely disappeared after 30 minutes of rest.

▶ The early descriptions of angina soon recognized that it was possible to "walk through" this disease, although the physiologic explanation of any clinical benefit from a preliminary warm-up has remained controversial.

Some authors have thought in terms of a peripheral vasodilatation, with a resulting reduction of the exercise-induced rise of blood pressure, lessening the work to be performed by the ischemic myocardium. However, in this study, the peak heart rate and blood pressure were actually higher during the second bout of exercise, so that the heart was working harder on the second occasion. Stewart and colleagues thus opted for a change in myocardial metabolism or a sustained dilatation of the coronary vessels induced by the first bout of exercise as a reasonable explanation of their findings. The last hypothesis seems the most plausible and is in keeping with some of our early work showing that a modified interval regimen provides an effective basis of training for the patient with angina.[1]

R.J. Shephard, M.D., Ph.D., D.P.E.

Reference

1. Kavanagh T, Shephard RJ: Conditioning of post-coronary patients. Comparison of continuous and interval training. *Arch Phys Med Rehabil* 56:72–76, 1975.

Dobutamine Stress-induced Angina in Patients With Denervated Cardiac Transplants: Clinical and Angiographic Correlates

Akosah K, Olsovsky M, Mohanty PK (Virginia Commonwealth Univ, Richmond)

Chest 108:695–700, 1995 6–15

Background.—In heart transplant recipients, ventricular sympathetic afferents are disconnected and the ability to sense cardiac pain is lost. Although angina has been reported in some transplant recipients, its clinical significance and relation to myocardial ischemia have not been investigated.

Methods.—To examine the relationship between angina and myocardial ischemia in heart transplant recipients, 82 heart transplant recipients were evaluated serially by dobutamine stress echocardiography (DSE). Patients who experienced angina during DSE were examined for stress-induced wall motion abnormalities. Coronary angiography was performed in 45 of these patients within 48 hours of DSE.

Results.—Of the 82 heart transplant patients in this study, 11 experienced typical angina during DSE. Diagnostic ECG changes were detected in 3 of these 11 patients. All 11 patients with angina had stress-induced regional wall motion abnormalities. Coronary angiographic data were available for 9 of the 11 patients, and significant coronary artery disease was detected in 8. There were no differences in peak heart rate, systolic blood pressure or rate pressure product after dobutamine between the group of patients with angina and the group without (Table 2). The mean time since transplant was significantly higher in the angina group.

Conclusions.—The occurrence of angina during a dobutamine stress test should be considered an important marker of allograft coronary artery disease and functional sympathetic reinnervation. Although further re-

TABLE 2.—Hemodynamic Responses to Dobutamine in 2 Groups (Angina vs. No Angina)

	Angina	No Angina	*P* Value
Baseline			
Heart rate	89 ± 4	88 ± 2	0.8(NS)
Systolic blood pressure	134 ± 7	131 ± 2	0.6(NS)
Diastolic blood pressure	86 ± 3	87 ± 1	0.8(NS)
Mean arterial pressure	102 ± 4	101 ± 1	0.9(NS)
Pulse pressure	48 ± 6	44 ± 2	0.9(NS)
Wall motion score	1.15 ± 0.05	1.19 ± 0.03	0.9(NS)
Peak			
Heart rate	141 ± 7	145 ± 3	0.7(NS)
Systolic blood pressure	154 ± 8	149 ± 3	0.6(NS)
Diastolic blood pressure	78 ± 3	81 ± 1	0.7(NS)
Mean arterial pressure	97 ± 4	96 ± 2	0.9(NS)
Pulse pressure	85 ± 6	79 ± 2	0.03
Rate pressure product	21,699 ± 1,490	21,650 ± 600	0.9(NS)
Peak wall motion score	1.74 ± 0.10	1.56 ± 0.05	0.05
Peak dobutamine dose, µg/kg/min	31 ± 2	37 ± 1	0.04

* All values expressed as the mean ± standard error of the mean.

(Courtesy of Akosah K, Olsovsky M, Mohanty PK: Dobutamine stress-induced angina in patients with denervated cardiac transplants: Clinical and angiographic correlates. *Chest* 108:695–700, 1995.)

search is required to demonstrate sympathetic reinnervation of graft tissue, periodic DSE examination may be of diagnostic use in the heart transplant population, which has a high prevalence of accelerated coronary artery disease.

► There is increasing evidence that a transplanted heart can undergo functional reinnervation over the course of 2–3 years, and the development of anginal pain is one obvious manifestation of this reinnervation. The authors' sample of patients had survived cardiac transplantation by an average of almost 5 years; in those with anginal pain, the survival period was even longer (7–8 years). Reinnervation is important not only for symptomatology, but also for exercise performance. The present group reached the quite respectable peak heart rate of 145 beats/min at an age of 53 years.

R.J. Shephard, M.D., Ph.D., D.P.E.

Exercise-induced Mitral Regurgitation Is a Predictor of Morbid Events in Subjects With Mitral Valve Prolapse

Stoddard MF, Prince CR, Dillon S, Longaker RA, Morris GT, Liddell NE (Univ of Louisville, Ky)

J Am Coll Cardiol 25:693–699, 1995 6–16

Introduction.—Serious complications leading to valve replacement, endocarditis, or sudden death can occur in patients with mitral valve prolapse (MVP) and regurgitation. Whereas mitral valve prolapse is a relatively common problem, only a small fraction of patients have regurgitation. This regurgitation can be intermittent and quite possibly undetected. A provocative test to reveal the regurgitation would be a great aid to cardiologists. Because dynamic exercise increases left ventricular pressure, it was expected that patients with MVP and no regurgitation at rest would experience regurgitation during exercise.

Methods.—A total of 94 patients with MVP and no regurgitation at rest met the inclusion criteria. The subjects were older than 18 years of age and had an MVP score of at least 3. The exercise test was a symptom-limited supine cycle ergometer task with 25-watt increments at 3-minute intervals. Blood pressure and 12-lead ECGs were collected. Echocardiography (m-mode, 2-dimensional and color Doppler) were obtained at rest, 2–3 minutes into each stage, at peak exercise, and every 5 minutes of recovery. The patients were followed for a minimum of 12 months for the outcomes of syncope, transient ischemic attacks, cerebrovascular accidents, endocarditis, congestive heart failure, or cardiac death.

Results.—Thirty-two percent of the patients showed exercise-induced mitral regurgitation. The regurgitation was resolved by 15 minutes of recovery. The two groups of subjects (regurgitation or no regurgitation) were not different on descriptive or cardiac variables. Syncope was more evident before the study in the group with regurgitation. Structurally, those patients with regurgitation had a significantly larger left atrial diameter and volume as well as a greater left ventricular end diastolic volume. The exercise duration was the same in both groups. Peak systolic pressure was greater in the group with regurgitation. There were significantly more morbid events in the group with regurgitation, including syncope, congestive heart failure, mitral valve replacement, and cardiovascular events (Table 3). The only predictors of a cardiovascular event were exercise-induced mitral regurgitation and a history of syncope. Exercise-induced regurgitation was also a predictor of poststudy syncope, congestive heart failure, and mitral valve prolapse score.

TABLE 3.—Morbid Events and Incidence of Mitral Valve Replacement in Subjects With Mitral Valve Prolapse During Follow-up

	Exer-MR (n = 30)	No-MR (n = 64)
Syncope	13 (43%)	3 (5%)*
TIA/CVA	2 (7%)	4 (6%)
Endocarditis	1 (3%)	0 (0%)
CHF	5 (17%)	0 (0%)†
MVR	3 (10%)	0 (0%)‡
Sudden death	1 (3%)	0 (0%)
CV event	16 (53%)	5 (8%)*

* $P < 0.0001$, † $P < 0.005$, ‡ $P < 0.05$ vs. subjects with exercise-induced mitral regurgitation (*Exer-MR*). Data presented are number (%) of subjects.

Abbreviations: No-MR, subjects with no exercise-induced mitral regurgitation; *CHF*, congestive heart failure; *CV*, cardiovascular; *CVA*, cerebrovascular accident; *MVR*, mitral valve replacement; *TIA*, transient ischemic attack.

(Reprinted with permission from the American College of Cardiology, Stoddard MF, Prince CR, Dillon S, et al: Exercise-induced mitral regurgitation is a predictor of morbid events in subjects with mitral valve prolapse. *J Am Coll Cardiol* 25:693–699, 1995.)

Conclusion.—Exercise was successfully used to induce mitral regurgitation in a subset of patients with MVP. Patients who had mitral regurgitation develop had an increased risk for future morbid events.

▶ Mitral valve prolapse is a fairly common finding at routine echocardiography. Estimates of prevalence in the general population range from 2.5 to 5.0%, [1, 2] but only 5% to 10% of these individuals have mitral regurgitation develop.[3] Detection of such individuals would be useful because they are at increased risk of a variety of cardiac events, and in a small proportion of cases a mitral valve replacement may be needed. However, the authors' data show that a history of syncope is just about as useful as an exercise echocardiogram in identifying those patients who are at increased risk. This emphasizes the important point that a careful clinical examination can often obviate the need for expensive laboratory testing.

R.J. Shephard, M.D., Ph.D., D.P.E.

References

1. Hickey AJ, Wolfers J, Wilcken DEL: Mitral valve prolapse: Prevalence in an Australian population. *Med J Aust* 1:31–33, 1981.
2. Savage DD, Garrison RJ, Devereux RB, et al: Mitral valve prolapse in the general population. I. Epidemiologic features: The Framingham study. *Am Heart J* 106: 571–576, 1983.
3. Devereux RB, Kramer-Fox R, Shear MK, et al: Diagnosis and classification of severity of mitral valve prolapse: Methodologic, biologic and prognostic considerations. *Am Heart J* 113:1265–1280, 1987.

Failure of "Effective" Treatment for Heart Failure to Improve Normal Customary Activity

Walsh JT, Andrews R, Evans A, Cowley AJ (Univ Hosp, Nottingham, England)

Br Heart J 70:373–376, 1995 6–17

Background.—Improving symptomatic well-being is important in the treatment of patients with chronic heart failure. However, the best way to assess such improvement is unclear. Whether an increase in exercise tolerance in laboratory-based tests parallels improvement in daily customary activity was investigated.

Methods.—Eighteen patients with mild to moderate chronic heart failure were assessed before and after 12 weeks of vasodilator drug therapy. Two types of treadmill exercise—one a ramp protocol and the other a fixed work rate—were used to measure exercise capacity. Corridor walk tests at 3 self-selected speeds were also performed, with measures of customary activity determined from pedometer scores. Findings from the patient group were compared with those of 10 age-matched, healthy control subjects.

Findings.—After 12 weeks of drug therapy, the patients had significantly increased exercise times compared with baseline values. The durations of

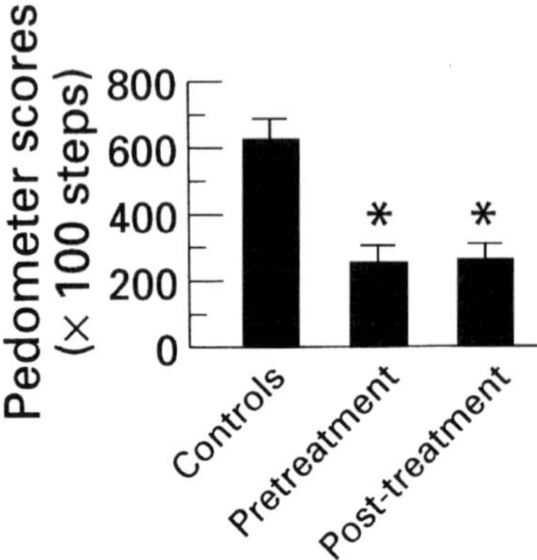

FIGURE 3.—Pedometer scores of patients with heart failure before and after treatment. Values are means (SEM). *P <0.001 vs. controls, Wilcoxon signed rank test. (Courtesy of Walsh JT, Andrews R, Evans A, et al: Failure of "effective" treatment for heart failure to improve normal customary activity. *Br Heart J* 70:373–376, 1995. Published by BMJ Publishing Group.)

treadmill exercise in the 2 protocols were positively correlated. Corridor walk tests of 100 m at a self-selected slow speed were also improved but uncorrelated with the changes in treadmill exercise time. Compared with control subjects, the patients had greatly decreased pedometer scores. After 12 weeks of treatment, these scores were unchanged (Fig 3).

Conclusions.—Different exercise protocols are needed to evaluate the benefits of drug therapy in patients with chronic heart failure. Treatments that appear to be effective according to conventional laboratory-based exercise tests may not improve the patient's ability to perform daily activities. The failure of seemingly effective treatment should be considered in the interpretation of clinical trials.

► This is not the first time that laboratory findings have failed to match what occurs in "real life." There are various possible explanations. One is that termination of the laboratory test depends largely on the confidence of the patient and the examining physician in the laboratory setting. This confidence is liable to increase as contacts with the laboratory personnel are repeated. The poor correlation between treadmill times and corridor walking suggests that instability of the treadmill criterion may have been a factor in the present results. Another difficulty is that the pedometer measures only walking distance. It does not measure other daily activities, nor does it consider whether it is necessary for the patient to rest when walking. Finally, some patients have decided that they are invalids and have arranged their lives to cope with such a decision, irrespective of any changes in functional status that can be achieved by the physician.

R.J. Shephard, M.D., Ph.D., D.P.E.

Prolonged Kinetics of Recovery of Oxygen Consumption After Maximal Graded Exercise in Patients With Chronic Heart Failure: Analysis With Gas Exchange Measurements and NMR Spectroscopy

Cohen-Solal A, Laperche T, Morvan D, Geneves M, Caviezel B, Gourgon R (Hôpital Beaujon, Clichy, France; Hôpital Cochin, Paris)

Circulation 91:2924–2932, 1995 6–18

Background.—Prolonged dyspnea often follows exercise in patients with chronic heart failure (CHF). The determinants of oxygen consumption after exercise have not been established in this patient population. It was hypothesized that the kinetics of oxygen consumption recovery after graded exercise would be prolonged in parallel with the slow recovery of muscle energy stores but would be unaffected by exercise level and thus could be used in evaluation of the circulatory response to exercise.

Methods and Findings.—Seventy-two patients with CHF and 13 healthy subjects performed maximal upright cycle ergometer exercise with breath-by-breath respiratory gas analysis. The time to reach 50% of peak oxygen consumption ($T_{1/2}$) increased with the severity of CHF. Similarly, CO_2 production and ventilation increased as CHF worsened. $T_{1/2}$ oxygen consumption showed a reproducible negative association with the individual's peak oxygen consumption. A second graded exercise test at 75% and/or 50% of peak work rate was performed by some of the subjects to char-

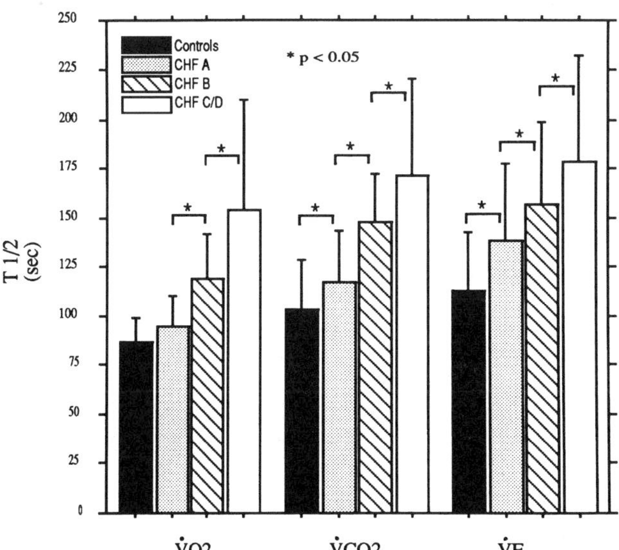

FIGURE 2.—Bar graph showing the mean values of the half-times of recovery of oxygen consumption ($T_{1/2}$ $\dot{V}O_2$), CO_2 production ($T_{1/2}$ $\dot{V}CO_2$), and minute ventilation ($T_{1/2}\dot{V}E$) in the 4 groups of subjects (in seconds). *$P < 0.05$. *Abbreviation: CHF,* chronic heart failure. (Courtesy of Cohen-Solal A, Laperche T, Morvan D, et al: Prolonged kinetics of recovery of oxygen consumption after maximal graded exercise in patients with chronic heart failure: Analysis with gas exchange measurements and NMR spectroscopy. *Circulation* 91:2924–2932, Copyright 1995, American Heart Association.

acterize the relationship between $T_{1/2}$ oxygen consumption and exercise duration. At 50% of peak work rate, $T_{1/2}$ oxygen consumption was shortened minimally. In 19 patients undergoing phosphorus-31 nuclear MR spectroscopy of the anterior compartment of the leg during exercise, the half-time of recovery of the ratio of inorganic phosphate to creatinine phosphate (reflecting the involvement of oxidative metabolism in the restoration of phosphagen stores after exercise), was linearly associated with the half-time of oxygen consumption recovery (Fig 2).

Conclusions.—Postexercise $T_{1/2}$ oxygen consumption rises as CHF worsens, possibly in part because of the slower kinetics of recovery of muscle phosphagen stores. The time course of oxygen consumption recovery may be a useful criterion for determining impairment of the circulatory response to exercise in CHF, even when exercise is submaximal.

► Recent research has demonstrated the effects of cardiac transplantation in slowing the rate of increase of oxygen consumption following cardiac transplantation.[1] In this situation, the primary problem is a loss of the normal sympathetic innervation of the heart, with the associated chronotropic and inotropic responses to exercise. In CHF, the sympathetic innervation of the heart remains intact, but cardiac output again increases relatively slowly during exercise because of an underlying deterioration in performance of the ventricular muscle. As the present paper demonstrates, the recovery process is also prolonged in CHF, in part because a larger oxygen deficit has been accumulated at the beginning of exercise. The slow recovery process can be observed after exercising at as little as 50% of maximal oxygen intake. It seems to be relatively independent of exercise intensity over the range of 50% to 75% of maximal aerobic effort, thus offering the possibility of developing a simple test of cardiac function with a low demand on a disabled patient. Success of the test plainly depends on the availability of an oxygen consumption measuring system that can make measurements over a short time interval (e.g., 15 seconds), and there is also a need to explore further whether such a test might be invalidated if a patient has an irregular breathing pattern.

R.J. Shephard, M.D., Ph.D., D.P.E.

References

1. Shephard RJ, Kavanagh T, Mertens D, et al: Kinetics of the transplanted heart: Implications for the choice of field test protocol. *J Cardiopulm Rehabil* 15:288–296, 1995.

Perfusion/Ventilation Mismatch During Exercise in Chronic Heart Failure: An Investigation of Circulatory Determinants

Banning AP, Lewis NP, Northridge DB, Elborn JS, Henderson AH (Univ of Wales, Cardiff)

Br Heart J 74:27–33, 1995 6–19

Background.—During exercise, the ventilatory cost of eliminating CO_2 is increased in patients with chronic heart failure (CHF), in part because mismatching of perfusion with ventilation causes an increased physiologic dead space. In addition, production of CO_2 is increased by bicarbonate that buffers the lactic acid resulting from anaerobic metabolism of exercising muscle. Whether perfusion-ventilation mismatching relates directly to limited pulmonary flow during exercise or whether it is a persistent feature of CHF was investigated.

Study Plan.—Forty-five clinically stable patients with CHF (resting left ventricular ejection fraction less than 40%) were studied, along with 23 patients having coronary artery disease and exercise-induced myocardial ischemia, and 15 normal individuals. Thirty-six of the patients with CHF had ischemic heart disease and 9 had dilated cardiomyopathy. An additional 13 patients had been maintained by rate-responsive cardiac pacing for longer than 2 years. Maximal symptom-limited treadmill exercise testing was carried out.

Findings.—The slope of minute ventilation to minute CO_2 production was significantly steeper in patients with CHF than in normal persons (Fig 1). All subjects exercised at close to peak levels, as indicated by a respiratory exchange ratio exceeding unity. The arterial $PaCO_2$ remained constant during exercise. The exercise ventilation response remained normal in patients with coronary disease but normal ventricular function. Fixed-rate

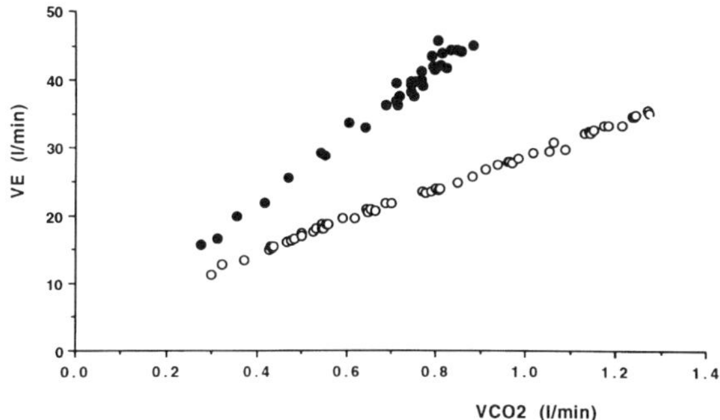

FIGURE 1.—Representative examples showing a steeper minute ventilation/minute carbon dioxide production ($\dot{V}E/\dot{V}CO_2$) linear relation in a patient with chronic heart failure (*closed circles*) than in a normal control (*open circles*). (Courtesy of Banning AP, Lewis NP, Northridge DB, et al: Perfusion/ventilation mismatch during exercise in chronic heart failure: An investigation of circulatory determinants. *Br Heart J* 74:27–33, 1995. Published by BMJ Publishing Group.)

cardiac pacing in the pacemaker-dependent patients lowered exercise capacity and peak oxygen uptake compared to rate-responsive pacing. In patients with CHF, the ventilatory cost of eliminating CO_2 was increased during fixed-rate pacing.

Conclusions.—Mismatching of perfusion and ventilation during exercise in patients with CHF is a consequence of the syndrome itself rather than a direct result of limited pulmonary blood flow. The basic defect may be a dysfunction of the pulmonary resistance arteries.

▶ It is generally agreed that one of the causes of dyspnea in the patient with congestive heart failure is that ventilation for a given oxygen consumption or power output is greater than in a normal person. Various explanations of this phenomenon have their advocates. Because peak cardiac output is impaired and the rate of increase of cardiac output at the beginning of exercise is slower than normal, a greater accumulation of lactate is likely, which will increase ventilation (although not necessarily the ratio of ventilation to carbon dioxide elimination). There is some evidence of reflex peripheral vascular spasm in patients with congestive failure, and this could further increase the production of lactate at a given power output.[1] A second factor that increases ventilation is a mismatching of alveolar ventilation and pulmonary blood flow that leads to an increase in the physiologic dead space. Banning and associates suggest that there may also be some dysfunction of the pulmonary resistance arteries, but another important factor is probably a change in pulmonary compliance associated with congestion of the dependent part of the lungs; this would encourage a ventilation of the apices of the lungs, a region that is poorly perfused unless cardiac output is large.

R.J. Shephard, M.D., Ph.D., D.P.E.

Reference

1. Wilson JR, Martin JL, Schwartz D, et al: Exercise tolerance in patients with chronic heart failure: Role of impaired nutritive flow to skeletal muscle. *Circulation* 69:1079–1087, 1984.

Dissociation Between Exertional Symptoms and Circulatory Function in Patients With Heart Failure

Wilson JR, Rayos G, Yeoh TK, Gothard P, Bak K (Vanderbilt Univ, Nashville, Tenn)

Circulation 92:47–53, 1995 6–20

Objective.—Although exercise intolerance in patients with heart failure is usually attributed to circulatory dysfunction, there is evidence that exercise training can improve exertional symptoms in these patients without modifying hemodynamic function. The results of a study investigating the relationship between exertional symptoms and circulatory function

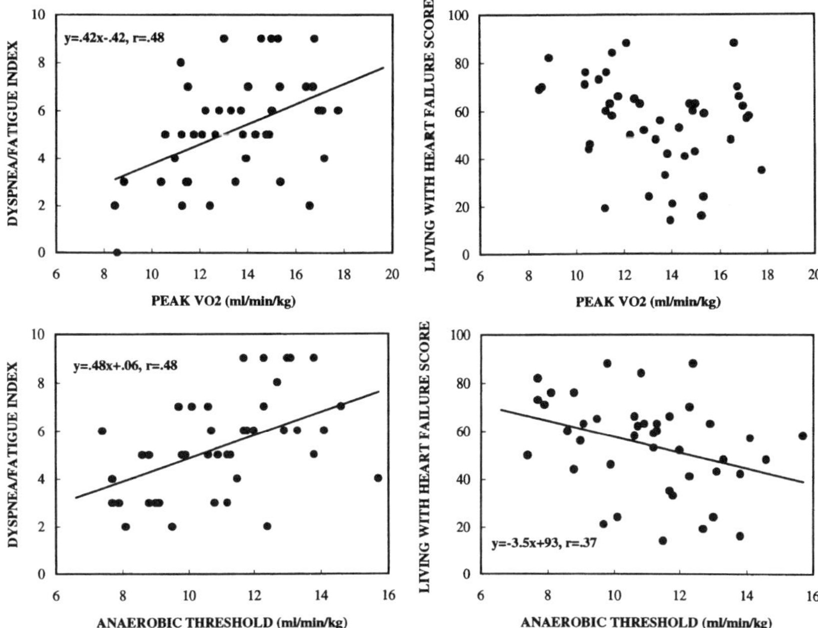

FIGURE 5.—Plots showing relationship between questionnaire results and peak exercise oxygen consumption and the anaerobic threshold during maximal treadmill exercise testing. (Courtesy of Wilson JR, Rayos G, Yeoh TK, et al: Dissociation between exertional symptoms and circulatory function in patients with heart failure. *Circulation* 92:47–53. Reproduced with permission [*Circulation*]. Copyright 1995, American Heart Association.)

and between hemodynamic function and perceived functional intolerance in ambulatory heart failure patients were presented.

Methods.—A total of 52 patients with heart failure (14 women) aged 26–67 years underwent hemodynamic monitoring during treadmill exercise testing. The severity of dyspnea and fatigue was determined. Perceived functional limitations were assessed using the Minnesota "Living With Heart Failure" Questionnaire and the Yale Dyspnea-Fatigue Index.

Results.—The average pulmonary wedge pressure increased to 28 mm Hg, lactate concentration to 34.5 mg/dL, and oxygen consumption per unit of time ($\dot{V}O_2$) increased to 13.4 mL/kg per minute during peak exercise. Mild hemodynamic dysfunction was observed in 11 patients; it was moderate in 22 and severe in 19. Mean dyspnea and fatigue scores increased to 15.7 and 14.8, respectively. Pulmonary artery hemoglobin oxygen saturation decreased to a mean of 30%. There was a small but significant correlation between peak exercise $\dot{V}O_2$ and the Dyspnea-Fatigue Index (Fig 5). Both the Living With Heart Failure Questionnaire and the Dyspnea-Fatigue Index were weakly correlated with the anaerobic threshold.

Conclusion.—Exercise intolerance is not correlated with circulatory, ventilatory, or metabolic dysfunction. Patients' reports of exercise intolerance should be compared with objective measures of hemodynamic parameters to determine possible circulatory dysfunction.

► A recent study of patients with congestive heart failure has demonstrated a substantial parallel between the subjective improvement over 12 months of progressive rehabilitation and physiologic data such as peak oxygen intake.[1] However, there are wide interindividual differences in patients' perceptions of disability on any given day, and this accounts for the weakness of the relationship demonstrated in this cross-sectional study. Although the systems in some patients may have little objective circulatory basis, they are, nevertheless, real to the patient and will require treatment before effective rehabilitation can be undertaken.

R.J. Shephard, M.D., Ph.D., D.P.E.

Reference

1. Myers MG, Baigrie RS, et al: Quality of life and cardiorespiratory function in chronic heart failure: Effects of 12 months' aerobic training. *Heart* 76:42–49, 1996.

Role of Beta-adrenergic Receptor Downregulation in the Peak Exercise Response in Patients With Heart Failure Due to Idiopathic Dilated Cardiomyopathy

White M, Yanowitz F, Gilbert EM, Larrabee P, O'Connell JB, Anderson JL, Renlund D, Mealey P, Abraham WT, Bristow MR (Montreal Heart Inst; Univ of Utah, Salt Lake City; Univ of Mississippi, Jackson; et al)

Am J Cardiol 76:1271–1276, 1995 6–21

Rationale.—Patients with heart failure characteristically are intolerant of exercise. One reason may be that a peak exercise response depends on cardiac output being rapidly augmented by mechanisms that may be minimally operative in the resting state. Downregulation of myocardial β_1-adrenergic receptors plays a key role in the decreased chronotropic and inotropic response to stimulation by β-agonists, and it might help explain the blunted exercise response of the failing heart.

Objective and Methods.—The relationship between the density of β-adrenergic receptors (Bmax) in the myocardium and exercise performance was studied in 72 patients with symptomatic heart failure secondary to idiopathic dilated cardiomyopathy. All had a left ventricular ejection fraction of 40% or less. Maximal exercise testing was done using a treadmill or a cycle ergometer. Right heart catheterization was performed and an endomyocardial biopsy obtained to measure Bmax by ^{125}I-iodocyanopindolol binding. Receptor density was also estimated in peripheral lymphocytes.

Results.—Myocardial Bmax was markedly reduced and was significantly less than values for lymphocytes. Exercise variables correlated significantly with receptor density values in endomyocardial biopsy tissue but

TABLE 4.—Results of Stepwise Linear Regression Analysis for the Significant Independent Variables Versus Biopsy Tissue β-Receptor Density

Variable	Coefficient	Standard Error	Standard Coefficient	*t* Value	*P* Value (2-tailed)
Constant (no variables)	−5.9	8.46	0.000	−0.701	0.48
Δ Heart rate x systolic blood pressure	0.005	0.002	0.351	3.08	<0.003
Left ventricular ejection fraction	0.697	0.243	0.265	2.87	0.006
VO_2max	1.34	0.529	0.562	2.53	0.014

Abbreviation: VO_2max, peak oxygen uptake.

(Reprinted by permission of Elsevier Science Inc., from White M, Yanowitz F, Gilbert EM, et al: Role of beta-adrenergic receptor downregulation in the peak exercise response in patients with heart failure due to idiopathic dilated cardiomyopathy. *Am J Cardiol* 76:1271–1276, Copyright 1995 by Excerpta Medica, Inc.)

not with lymphocyte values. The closest correlation was with peak oxygen consumption during exercise. On regression analysis, peak oxygen uptake, change in the heart rate–systolic pressure product, and ejection fraction all correlated independently with Bmax (Table 4).

Conclusion.—These findings suggest that downregulation of cardiac β-adrenergic receptors does have a role in the inadequate exercise response typically seen in patients with chronic heart failure.

► Because they do not have the opportunity of undertaking ventricular biopsies, many investigators have assessed the density and/or sensitivity of β-adrenoreceptors on peripheral blood lymphocytes. One important finding in this report is the lack of parallelism between data obtained on peripheral blood lymphocytes and biopsy samples taken from the right interventricular septum. There is good evidence of a downregulation of the β-receptors in the latter site, and the authors deduce that this change may be limiting the chronotropic response of the sinoatrial node and, thus, peak oxygen transport in patients with dilated cardiomyopathy. Although this is a reasonable inference, it is now necessary to find some way of extending observations from the ventricular septum to the region of the sinoatrial pacemaker, as there can also be substantial divergence of changes in Bmax between different regions of the heart.[1]

R.J. Shephard, M.D., Ph.D., D.P.E.

Reference

1. Beau SL, Tolley TK, Saffitz JE: Transmural distribution of β-adrenergic receptor subtypes in normal and failing human hearts. *Circulation* 88:2501–2509, 1993.

Dissection of the External Iliac Artery in Highly Trained Athletes

Cook PS, Erdoes LS, Selzer PM, Rivera FJ, Palmaz JC (Saint Joseph Hosp, Denver; Univ of Arizona, Tucson; Meriter/Madison Gen Hosp, Madison, Wis; et al)

J Vasc Surg 22:173–177, 1995 6–22

Objective.—Three patients, all highly trained athletes, experienced acute external iliac artery dissection after intense athletic events. This complication of ultraendurance events appears to be a variant of the previously reported iliac occlusive syndromes in athletes. Diagnostic and treatment modalities were presented.

Patients.—The patients were a 45-year-old man who competed in the Ironman Triathlon in Hawaii, a 50-year-old woman marathoner, and a 50-year-old man who had recently increased his running mileage and started to practice calisthenics and use a rowing machine. Arteriography confirmed dissection of the external iliac artery in all 3 patients, and 1—the 50-year-old man—was found to have bilateral lesions.

Treatment and Outcome.—The patient with bilateral involvement was treated conservatively with low-dose aspirin and close follow-up. He is now able to exercise regularly without claudication. Treatment in the 2 remaining cases was initiated with percutaneous transluminal angioplasty. The 45-year-old man had a successful result. He is being maintained on low-dose aspirin and is training again for athletic events. The woman required operative repair and placement of a graft. She continues to run 6–9 miles a week. With a mean follow-up of 32 months, all 3 patients have normal resting hemodynamics.

Discussion.—The complication reported here contrasts with the previously reported syndromes of nonatherosclerotic vascular disease in young, highly trained athletes. Local hemodynamic factors appear to be important in both acute dissection and chronic stenosis, and long-term repetitive trauma is also suspected of being a factor. Dissection of the artery may be a result of the adaptive hypertension of vigorous exercise. Conservative treatment and endovascular or surgical therapy can achieve a successful outcome.

▶ This is a newly described syndrome in the "aging warrior" that should interest sports medicine physicians. In 1991, we reviewed stenotic intimal thickening of the external iliac artery in competitive cyclists, which causes acute, severe claudication pain in the buttock or thigh, followed by numbness, and occurs during peak effort, as in a sprint or when riding uphill. The responsible lesion is intimal fibrosis without atherosclerosis and seems to occur from repeated trauma. In the aerodynamic cycling position, the thigh is strongly flexed and the external iliac artery is abnormally sinuous; the lesion occurs in the greatest curve of arterial bending.[1] This "new" syndrome is seen in athletes 45 years of age or older soon after a long race or workout, with short-distance claudication and weak femoral and distal pulses. It also involves the external iliac artery, but the lesion is *dissection* of a normal (if "aging") artery, presumably from local exertional hemodynamic factors and/or repeated local trauma. The ideal treatment is unclear; each athlete here was treated differently.

E.R. Eichner, M.D.

Reference

1. 1991 Year Book of Sports Medicine, pp 280–281.

Exercise Rehabilitation Programs for the Treatment of Claudication Pain: A Meta-analysis

Gardner AW, Poehlman ET (Univ of Maryland, Baltimore, Md; Baltimore Veterans Affairs Med Ctr, Md)

JAMA 274:975–980, 1995 6–23

Introduction.—Intermittent claudication occurs at an annual incidence of 20 per 1,000 individuals 65 years of age or older. Disabling symptoms are expected to occur in 1.3 million elderly United States citizens every 2 years over the next 50 years. Treatment for claudication consists of drug therapy, which is expensive and minimally effective, and surgery, which has risks of cardiovascular complications. Exercise rehabilitation is a noninvasive, inexpensive, and effective method of treating symptoms of intermittent claudication. A meta-analysis was conducted to identify which components of exercise rehabilitation programs were the most effective in decreasing claudicant pain.

Methods.—A search of the English-language literature was conducted to locate studies on exercise rehabilitation programs for patients with intermittent claudication. To be considered for inclusion, studies had to use treadmill testing before and after an exercise program as part of the assessment. Studies were excluded if times or distances walked before the onset of pain and maximal pain were not reported. Duration and mode of exercise, program length, pain end point used during the exercise session, and level of supervision were recorded for each study. Patient characteristics, walking times and distances to onset of pain, and treadmill protocol intensity were also noted.

Results.—Twenty-one studies met the criteria for study inclusion; 18 were noncontrolled and nonrandomized and 3 were randomized trials. The mean duration of exercise and program length were 39.1 minutes per session (3.1 sessions per week) and 21.8 weeks, respectively, for the 18 noncontrolled trials. For the three randomized trials, the mean duration of exercise was 30 minutes per session (3 sessions per week) for 30.3 weeks. In the nonrandomized trials, there was a significant increase from baseline values in the distance walked to onset of pain and the distance to maximal pain (Table 2). Exercised patients in the randomized trials also experienced significant increases in distance to onset of pain and to onset of maximal pain as compared with control patients. Individual components of the exercise programs were evaluated for their independent effects on claudi-

TABLE 2.—Claudication Pain Distance, Maximal Pain Distance, and Effect Size for Patients With Peripheral Arterial Disease in 21 Exercise Rehabilitation Studies

Studies on Exercise Rehabilitation Programs for Patients With PAD, Source, y	No. of Subjects	Claudication Pain Distance			Maximal Pain Distance		
		Pretest, m	Posttest, m	Effect Size	Pretest, m	Posttest, m	Effect Size
Larsen and Lassen, 1966	7	105.2 ± 33.4	268.3 ± 104.5	9.15*	226.9 ± 112.8	626.5 ± 423.1	6.65
Skinner and Strandness, 1967	5	97.1 ± 34.9	171.9 ± 88.9	4.80	288.4 ± 231.5	2495.3 ± 285.2	11.23
Alpert et al, 1969	19	111.9 ± 48.3	224.6 ± 164.1	10.17	209.3 ± 79.0	361.9 ± 187.1	8.42
Ericsson et al, 1970	7	186.0 ± 163.0	380.0 ± 366.0	3.15	273.0 ± 196.0	537.0 ± 370.0	3.56
Zetterquist, 1970	9	191.0 ± 18.0	331.0 ± 20.0	3.89	320.0 ± 21.0	> 400.0	...
Holm et al, 1973	6	100.0 ± 26.7	346.7 ± 193.3	9.15	320.0 ± 106.7	693.3 ± 200.0	6.17
Dahllof et al, 1974	10	91.0 ± 34.8	265.0 ± 103.0	10.54	296.0 ± 167.6	650.0 ± 104.3	4.45
Dahllof et al, 1976	23	127.0 ± 21.0	345.4	4.35	318.0 ± 37.0	725.0	11.18
Ekroth et al, 1978	129	108.0 ± 33.0	392.0±75.0	3.36	283.0 ± 42.0	720.0 ± 67.0	3.20
Clifford et al, 1980	20	...	...	...	299.4 ± 30.0	535.1 ± 46.4	5.24
Lepantalo et al, 1984	12	75.0 ± 34.6	173.0 ± 152.4	9.81	...	...	...
Ruell et al, 1984	14	67.0 ± 59.5	402.5 ± 267.2	8.33	283.0 ± 193.2	795.5 ± 149.5	5.87
Rosetzsky et al, 1985	79	...	...	...	133.0 ± 190.5	401.0 ± 112.1	12.51
Emst et al, 1987	22	59.0 ± 37.0	120.0 ± 52.0	7.73	127.0 ± 59.0	281.0 ± 91.0	12.24
Jonason and Ringqvist, 1987	63	114.0 ± 74.0	197.0 ± 125.0	8.90	430.0 ± 213.0	717.0 ± 304.0	10.70
Carter et al, 1989	56	240.0 ± 200.0	430.0 ± 50.0	7.11	590.0 ± 30.0	1000.0 ± 70.0	13.67
Lundgren et al, 1989	21	67.0 ± 35.0	187.0	8.83	183.0 ± 110.0	459.0	6.46
Mannarino et al, 1989	8	40.0 ± 17.0	75.0 ± 27.6	5.82	76.4 ± 18.7	127.4 ± 26.3	7.74
Rosfors et al, 1989	25	111.0 ± 105.0	270.0 ± 340.0	7.57	575.0 ± 345.0	924.0 ± 460.0	5.06
Mannarino et al, 1991	10	50.4 ± 22.5	95.3 ± 30.9	6.31	80.8 ± 33.6	150.3 ± 35.3	6.54
Feinberg et al, 1992	19	96.5 ± 56.6	816.6 ± 894.2	9.64	205.1 ± 94.3	1351.6 ± 718.9	6.98

Note: Pretest and posttest values are shown as mean ± standard deviation, except in cases where no standard deviation is available. *Ellipses* indicate data were not given in the source study.

* Posttest distance − pretest distance/standard deviation.

Abbreviation: PAD, peripheral arterial disease.

(Courtesy of Gardner AW, Poehlman ET: Exercise rehabilitation programs for the treatment of claudication pain: A meta-analysis. *JAMA* 274:975–980, Copyright 1995, American Medical Association.)

cant pain. An exercise duration of 30 minutes or longer, an exercise frequency of 3 sessions or more per week, programs of 26 weeks or longer, walking as the exercise used, and near-maximal pain as an end point for each training session each resulted in significantly greater improvements in distance to onset of pain and distance to maximal pain. A large percentage of the variance in increases in distance to onset and to maximal pain could be explained by the use of pain as an end point during exercise, program length, and type of exercise used. Age was found to correlate with improvement in walking ability, with older patients experiencing greater gains than younger patients.

Conclusion.—Participation in exercise rehabilitation programs resulted in increases of 120% to 180% in distances to onset of and to maximal claudicant pain in patients with peripheral vascular disease. Use of near-maximal pain as an end point during exercise sessions, a program duration of 6 months or more, and the use of walking as the exercise were the components of the rehabilitation program responsible for most of the patients' improvements in walking ability.

► Most of the studies of exercise and intermittent claudication, although encouraging, have been quite small in scale; indeed, the grouping of the 18 uncontrolled investigations reported here still yielded a subject pool of only 548 patients, and the 3 randomized trials contributed only a further 23 cases. Plainly, there is still scope for randomized tests on a larger group of patients, and the present analysis may be enough to spur funding for such a development.

R.J. Shephard, M.D., Ph.D., D.P.E.

Lung-heart Interaction as a Substrate for the Improvement in Exercise Capacity After Body Fluid Volume Depletion in Moderate Congestive Heart Failure

Agostoni PG, Marenzi GC, Sganzerla P, Assanelli E, Guazzi M, Perego GB, Lauri G, Doria E, Pepi M, Guazzi MD (Università di Milano, Italy)

Am J Cardiol 76:793–798, 1995 6–24

Background.—Patients with moderate congestive heart failure (CHF) benefit from body fluid volume depletion with isolated ultrafiltration. In addition to improving clinical condition and exercise performance, ultrafiltration influences circulating norepinephrine in a manner consistent with decreased disease severity. Exercise capacity after fluid depletion was investigated in patients with moderate CHF.

Methods.—Ultrafiltration was performed in 21 patients. Before and 3 months after ultrafiltration, patients underwent echocardiography, pulmonary function tests, and cardiopulmonary exercise testing with hemodynamic and esophageal pressure monitoring. Noninvasive testing was repeated 4 and 30 days after ultrafiltration. Another 21 patients who did not have ultrafiltration served as a control group. Nine patients who had

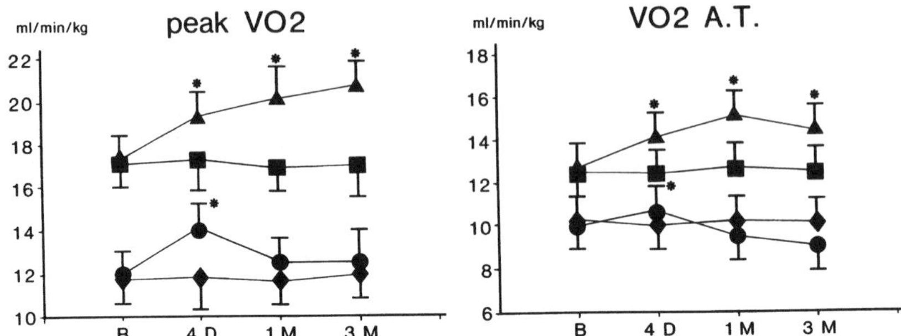

FIGURE 1.—Mean oxygen consumption ($\dot{V}O_2$) at peak exercise (**left panel**) and at anaerobic threshold (*AT*) (**right panel**) at baseline (*B*), 4 days (*4D*), 1 month (*1M*), and 3 months (*3M*) for all groups. Patients with congestive heart failure who underwent ultrafiltration and increased peak $\dot{V}O_2$ by > 10% at the 3-month evaluation were separated from those who did not. Control patients did not undergo ultrafiltration and were matched according to peak VO_2 at baseline to group A1 (control B1) or group A2 (control B2). *Vertical bars* represent standard error of the mean; *triangle*, group A1; *square*, group A 2; *circle*, group B1; *diamond*, group B2; *asterisk*, $P < 0.01$ vs. baseline and controls of the same step of the study. (Reprinted by permission of Elsevier Science Inc., from Agostoni PG, Marenzi GC, Sganzerla P, et al: Lung-heart interaction as a substrate for the improvement in exercise capacity after body fluid volume depletion in moderate congestive heart failure. *Am J Cardiol* 76:793–798, Copyright 1995 by Excerpta Medica, Inc.)

ultrafiltration had an increase in peak oxygen consumption of more than 10% at 3 months; this group (A1) were analyzed separately from the 8 patients in the intervention group who did not have such increases in oxygen consumption and who were designated as group A2.

Findings.—Four days after the procedure, the peak oxygen consumption per unit of time of group A1 increased from a mean of 17.3 to 19.3 mL/kg per minute and that of group A2 increased from 11.9 to 14.1 mL/kg per minute. In group A2, plasma norepinephrine and pulmonary function indicated CHF of greater severity. In group A1, the relationship of filling pressure to cardiac index of the right and left ventricles was shifted upward at 3 months. In addition, the esophageal pressure swing for a given tidal volume was lower, and peak exercise dynamic lung compliance increased from 0.1 to 0.14 L/mm Hg. None of these changes occurred in group A2 or the control group (Fig 1).

Conclusion.—In patients with moderate CHF, variations in lung mechanics and cardiac hemodynamics with body fluid volume withdrawal contribute to the amelioration of exercise performance. The duration of the benefit is inversely associated with CHF severity.

▶ Bring on the leeches! A decrease of blood volume has been a mainstay of treatment in CHF for many years, whether achieved by high-technology ultrafiltration or the more simple (but probably equally cost-effective approach) of salt and fluid restriction plus diuretics. This study provides a nice illustration of the immediate effect of decreasing blood volume upon cardiac performance. It is interesting that the benefit is less persistent in those with more severe disease; possibly, the myocardium of these patients has deteriorated to the point at which it is less able to benefit from a temporary respite.

R.J. Shephard, M.D., Ph.D., D.P.E.

Do the Competition Rules of Synchronized Swimming Encourage Undesirable Levels of Hypoxia?

Davies BN, Donaldson GC, Joels N (Queen Mary and Westfield College, London)

Br J Sports Med 29:16–19, 1995 6–25

Introduction.—Although synchronized swimming is not a hazardous sport, the extended breath-holding periods can lead to a rapid development of hypoxia. The rules require the swimmer to perform 4 set figures "slowly" followed by a 3.5-minute free program. The program is usually begun with an underwater sequence that can last up to 45 seconds. Although no synchronized swimmer has ever had a sustained loss of consciousness, there are complaints of dizziness, disorientation, and brief blackouts. These symptoms occur around the underwater segments of a program. The purpose of this study was to determine alveolar gas fractions during selected underwater figures during synchronized swimming.

Methods.—Nine members of the national team of Great Britain (average age, 19 years) volunteered for the study. The underwater time of 4 figures (spiral, castle, albatross, and barracuda) was determined, as well as the time underwater during the opening of the free program. All swimmers practiced the use of the Haldane alveolar gas-sampling tube. They performed the maneuvers (spiral and albatross) or the initial portion of their free program, then swam to the edge of the pool without taking a breath and delivered an alveolar gas sample. This was subsequently analyzed for oxygen and carbon dioxide.

Results.—Competitions showed an inverse relationship between breath-holding time and eventual placing. Consciously or unconsciously, judges seem to place considerable importance on breath-holding. This was true for the required figures as well as for the free program. The longer the breath-holding time for the studied figures, the lower the alveolar oxygen tension (Fig 3). After the free program, the swimmers were somewhat cyanosed and mildly confused, but their alveolar oxygen tension was related to the time spent underwater. Three swimmers lowered their oxygen tension to below 4 kPa.

Conclusion.—Synchronized swimmers can be exposed to undesirable levels of hypoxia. Because there appears to be a judging bias in favor of long periods of breath-holding, the swimmer must withstand such hypoxia. Less importance should be placed on extended periods of breath-holding. Underwater sequences should be limited to 40–45 seconds.

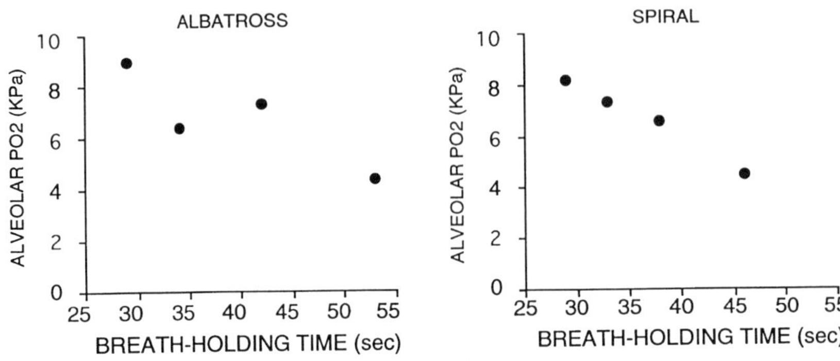

FIGURE 3.—Duration of breath-holding and alveolar partial pressure of oxygen on completion of spiral and albatross figures. (Courtesy of Davies BN, Donaldson GC, Joels N: Do the competition rules of synchronized swimming encourage undesirable levels of hypoxia? *Br J Sports Med* 29:16–19, 1995.)

▶ Loss of consciousness underwater is very common during breath-hold diving, and it can occasionally lead to fatalities. The usual reason for loss of consciousness is a preliminary period of hyperventilation. This eliminates the normal carbon dioxide drive to ventilation. The subject then remains underwater until the partial pressure of oxygen has fallen to a critical level. During the ascent to the surface, the reduction of pressure in the lungs leads to a further rapid drop in the partial pressure of oxygen, so that consciousness can no longer be sustained.

In synchronized swimming events, the depth of submersion is limited, so pressure changes on surfacing are relatively small, and even if consciousness were to be lost, this would rapidly be noticed by other team members. Nevertheless, if judging is predicated on the period of submersion, there will be a temptation to extend the underwater time by preliminary hyperventilation, with a potential for the type of accident that occurs in divers. The alveolar CO_2 levels seen by Davies and associates are not particularly low, but oxygen pressure of 4 kPa is plainly not compatible with sustained consciousness.

R.J. Shephard, M.D., Ph.D., D.P.E.

Pulmonary Oedema and Haemoptysis Induced by Strenuous Swimming

Weiler-Ravell D, Shupak A, Goldenberg I, Halpern P, Shoshani O, Hirschhorn G, Margulis A (Israel Naval Med Inst, Haifa)

BMJ 311:361–362, 1995 6–26

Background.—Pulmonary hemorrhage is known to develop in racehorses after exercising, ostensibly because a marked rise in pulmonary blood flow and pressure leads to pulmonary capillary rupture. Pulmonary edema has been described in swimmers and divers immersed in very cold water, even in the absence of great exertion.

Series.—Thirty young men engaged in a military fitness training program took part in a time trial involving a 2.4 km-swim in temperate seawater (23°C). Each subject drank approximately 5 liters of water within 2 hours before the swim.

Observations.—Eight of the 30 swimmers became markedly short of breath within 45 minutes, and 5 ended the swim prematurely. All of them received oxygen, and those in the most distress were given 20 mg of IV frusemide. In no individual did hypertension or other cardiovascular abnormalities develop. The disorder had resolved spontaneously by the next day. Two of the 8 affected individuals had recurrent pulmonary edema and/or hemoptysis when attempting the swim again.

Conclusion.—The pulmonary edema and hemoptysis occasionally associated with immersion is attributable to either cold-induced vasoconstriction or—as in these cases—a combination of exercise and excessive fluid intake.

▶ Various reports over the years have suggested that prolonged exercise can give rise to pulmonary edema. Typically, the evidence has been something such as a small decrease of lung volume or pulmonary diffusing capacity after a marathon run, and in such circumstances it has been difficult to separate the effects of the prolonged activity from the consequences of exposure to air pollutants.

This report describes a situation in which a gross excess of fluid was ingested, and it shows that, at least when the central blood volume is boosted by a combination of a cold skin and fluid ingestion, edema is a real possibility. A water temperature of 23°C is no more than thermally neutral, even when a person is swimming hard, and at this temperature, considerable cutaneous vasoconstriction would be anticipated.

R.J. Shephard M.D., Ph.D., D.P.E.

Exercise-induced Laryngomalacia

Smith RJH, Bauman NM, Bent JP, Kramer M, Smits WL, Ahrens RC (Univ of Iowa, Iowa City)

Ann Otol Rhinol Laryngol 104:537–541, 1995 6–27

Introduction.—Exercise-induced laryngomalacia (EIL), a syndrome characterized by wheezing, stridor, and dyspnea, can be misdiagnosed as exercise-induced asthma. The typical symptoms of EIL and the diagnostic methods undertaken were described.

> *Case Report.*—Girl, 10 years, was seen at a pediatric otolaryngology clinic because of exercise-induced dyspnea of 18 months' duration. Her breathing had become noisy after she started to compete in track and soccer. The patient had previously undergone tonsillectomy and adenoidectomy but had no early history of wheezing or chronic cough; allergy skin testing and pulmonary

function tests yielded normal results. Flexible fiberoptic laryngoscopy during maximal exercise on a stationary bicycle revealed abnormal motion of the arytenoid region. Vibration of the corniculate cartilages resulted in inspiratory stridor and coincided with anterior prolapse of the arytenoid region. The patient was successfully treated by laser epiglottoplasty to remove the corniculate cartilages. Follow-up laryngoscopy during exercise confirmed resolution of EIL.

Discussion.—Dynamic collapse of the upper airways can result from negative transmural pressure gradients that occur during inhalation. This condition usually resolves spontaneously when present in infants but can persist indefinitely in individuals with certain neurologic impairments. In some cases, laryngomalacia occurs only with strenuous exercise. The clinical syndrome of exercise-induced asthma is suggested by the association of upper respiratory tract dysfunction and poor athletic performance. Diagnosis can be confirmed by flexible fiberoptic laryngoscopy before, during, and after exercise. Laser epiglottoplasty effectively alleviates symptoms and improves the airway.

▶ This report is a practical tip for the sports medicine physician: Some cases that may mimic exercise-induced asthma are really EIL. As the rate of airflow increases, the relative contribution of the upper airway to total pulmonary resistance increases. At very high flow rates, as during all-out exercise, the laryngeal component of resistance approaches 66%. Telltale clues to EIL (or dynamic, inspiratory collaspe of the arytenoid region anteriorly, toward the epiglottis, encroaching on the airway) are loud inspiratory stridor, only mild wheezing, severe dyspnea that resolves quickly as exercise is decreased, and failure to respond to the usual asthma regimens. Diagnosis hinges on laryngoscopy during exercise.

E.R. Eichner, M.D.

Effects of Combined Inspiratory Muscle and Cycle Ergometer Training on Exercise Performance in Patients With COPD

Wanke Th, Formanek D, Lahrmann H, Brath H, Wild M, Wagner Ch, Zwick H
(Lainz Hosp, Vienna; Technical Univ, Vienna)

Eur Respir J 7:2205–2211, 1994 6–28

Introduction.—A primary goal of rehabilitation of patients with chronic obstructive pulmonary disease (COPD) is the improvement of physical capacity. Work tolerance should be increased and dyspnea decreased. The use of inspiratory muscle training (IMT) has been proposed because of the poor exercise tolerance of the COPD patient. Although IMT might increase work capacity, there are 3 reasons to doubt its effectiveness, depending on whether the respiratory muscles are weak, chronically fatigued, or normal. First, IMT can be hazardous to patients with neuromuscular disease, in which the muscle fibers are more susceptible to damage and splitting. Second, if the muscles are fatigued, rest, rather than IMT should be the treatment of choice. Finally, IMT will not have much effect on the respiratory muscles if their function is well preserved. The purpose of this study was to determine whether addition of IMT to an exercise program would enhance exercise tolerance or whether it would be hazardous by causing the muscles to be overworked.

Methods.—Sixty patients with COPD served as subjects. Their impairment was mild to severe. The patients were divided into two groups: one received cycle exercise training (CET) alone; the other received CET and IMT. Chronic medications such as aminophylline or β-adrenergic agents were used by all subjects. Lung function was assessed by spirometry and plethysmography. Symptom-limited graded exercise tests were performed on a cycle ergometer. Work load increments were based on measurements of forced expiratory volume in 1 second. Inspiratory muscle and diaphragmatic strength were assessed respectively, from esophageal and transdiaphragmatic pressure during sniffing. Inspiratory muscle endurance was determined by having the patient inhale through a 2-way valve, with the inspiratory side of the valve connected to a chamber and plunger to which weights could be added. The duration of time that the patient could inhale against a resistance was used as a measure of endurance. The subjects trained on the cycle ergometer 4 days a week for 8 weeks. The daily duration was 20 minutes for the first 3 weeks, 25 minutes for the next 3 weeks, and 30 minutes for the last 2 weeks. The training intensity was 60% of heart rate reserve. Half of the patients also received inspiratory muscle training. The strength training consisted of 12 static inspiratory efforts from residual volume against a nearly totally occluded airway to

TABLE 3.—Maximal Exercise Data in the 2 Study Groups

		Group 1 CET + IMT		Group 2 CET	
		Pre*	Post*	Pre*	Post*
$\dot{V}O_2max$	$l\cdot min^{-1}$	1.09 ± 0.37	1.32 ± 0.41	1.14 ± 0.28	1.24 ± 0.35
	% pred	63 ± 12	76 ± 14	66 ± 11	73 ± 14
Wmax	W	80.4 ± 31.6	98.8 ± 37.9	83.2 ± 27.1	92.8 ± 32.7
	% pred	58 ± 13	73 ± 15	60 ± 12	67 ± 12
HRmax	$beats\cdot min^{-1}$	135 ± 13	146 ± 13	138 ± 15	136 ± 13
	% pred	77 ± 7	83 ± 9	80 ± 8	78 ± 8
$\dot{V}Emax$	$l\cdot min^{-1}$	47.6 ± 15.3	54.8 ± 16.9	48.5 ± 11.9	48.4 ± 0.5
$\dot{V}Tmax$	l	1.41 ± 0.39	1.60 ± 0.44	1.42 ± 0.41	1.43 ± 0.5
PaO_2	kPa	8.7 ± 1.2	8.8 ± 1.2	8.9 ± 1.2	8.9 ± 1.3
$PaCO_2$	kPa	5.3 ± 0.8	5.0 ± 1.0	5.2 ± 0.8	5.1 ± 1.0

Note: Data are presented as mean ± standard deviation.

* Pretraining and posttraining values.

Abbreviations: CET, cycle ergometer training; *IMT,* inspiratory muscle training; *$\dot{V}O_2max$,* maximal oxygen uptake; *Wmax,* maximal power output; *HRmax,* maximal heart rate; *$\dot{V}Emax$,* maximal minute ventilation; *VTmax,* maximal tidal volume; *PaO_2,* arterial oxygen tension; *$PaCO_2$,* arterial carbon dioxide tension.

(Courtesy of Wanke Th, Formanek D, Lahrmann H, et al: Effects of combined inspiratory muscle and cycle ergometer training on exercise performance in patients with COPD. *Eur Respir J* 7:2205–2211, 1994.)

80% to their predetermined maximal pressure. Daily endurance training for the respiratory muscles consisted of 10 minutes at 70% of the maximum transdiaphragmatic pressure.

Results.—Forty-two of the patients completed the program. Baseline inspiratory muscle function was similar in both groups. Inspiratory muscle function improved in the group that performed cycle training plus IMT. However, there was no significant improvement in the group that performed only the CET. Maximal exercise data—such as oxygen consumption, work output, maximal heart rate, ventilation, and tidal volume—improved in the CET plus IMT group, but in the CET only group, only oxygen consumption and work output increased (Table 3).

Conclusion.—Exercise training alone improves peak oxygen consumption and exercise tolerance but not inspiratory muscle function. By adding IMT, the training effects are intensified and maximal performance, as well as inspiratory muscle function, is improved. Inspiratory muscle training should be included in the rehabilitation of patients with COPD.

▶ There is continuing controversy regarding the value of IMT in patients with COPD, and many studies have shown little physiologic improvement in response to either local or general training. The observations in this paper show a substantial 21% improvement in peak aerobic power in the group who received the combined therapy, compared with 9% in the group who received CET alone. The peak power output shows a corresponding differential improvement (23% vs. 11.5%). The larger gains of function with the combined therapy seem linked to a greater peak ventilation and peak heart rate. The probable reason for benefit is that stronger chest muscles allow a faster inspiration and, thus, a slower expiration; this, in turn, avoids expiratory collapse of the airways.

R.J. Shephard, M.D., Ph.D., D.P.E.

Exhaustive Treadmill Exercise Does Not Reduce Twitch Transdiaphragmatic Pressure in Patients With COPD

Polkey MI, Kyroussis D, Keilty SEJ, Hamnegard CH, Mills GH, Green M, Moxham J (Kings College School of Medicine and Dentistry, London; Royal Brompton Hosp, London)

Am J Respir Crit Care Med 152:959–964, 1995 6–29

Background.—Respiratory muscle fatigue during exercise might be expected to cause problems for patients with chronic obstructive pulmonary disease (COPD). The finding of reduced diaphragmatic contractility after whole-body endurance exercise is an indicator of low frequency fatigue, but its clinical relevance remains unclear. The effects of exhaustive exercise on diaphragmatic contractility in patients with COPD were assessed.

Methods.—The controlled study included 6 patients with severe COPD (mean forced expiratory volume in 1 second, 0.71, or 27% of predicted). After a brief control treadmill walk, the patients rested, then walked to the

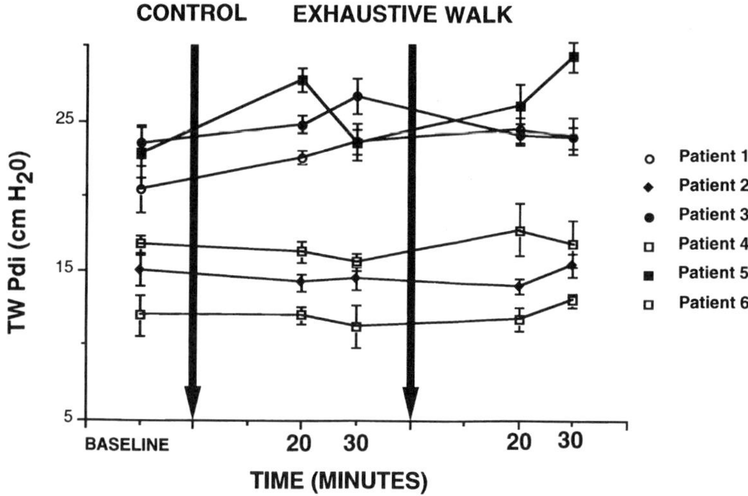

FIGURE 4.—Mean twitch transdiaphragmatic pressure (with standard deviation) for all patients. (Total number of twitches, 147.) (Courtesy of Polkey MI, Kyroussis D, Keilty SEJ, et al: Exhaustive treadmill exercise does not reduce twitch transdiaphragmatic pressure in patients with COPD. *Am J Respir Crit Care Med* 152:959–964, 1995.)

point of severe dyspnea. The study used cervical magnetic stimulation of the phrenic nerve roots—which is less painful but otherwise comparable to electrode stimulation—to detect diaphragmatic fatigue. Cervical magnetic stimulation was performed at the beginning of the study and 20 and 30 minutes after each bout of walking exercise.

Results.—Twitch transdiaphragmatic pressure (Tw Pdi) was a reproducible parameter, with a mean coefficient of variation of about 5%. Mean values for Tw Pdi were 18.4 cm of H_2O at baseline, 19.6 cm of H_2O 20 minutes after the control walk, and 19.2 cm of H_2O 30 minutes after the control walk. After the exhaustive walk, mean Tw Pdi was 19.6 and 20.4 cm of H_2O at 20 and 30 minutes, respectively. Thus, treadmill walking to exhaustion did not significantly reduce Tw Pdi (Fig 4).

Conclusion.—Patients with severe COPD who exercise to severe dyspnea do not experience a significant reduction in Tw Pdi and, thus, do not have low-frequency fatigue of the diaphragm. The findings support the notion that these patients' perception of muscle loading limits their exercise performance before they reach the point of overt contractile failure of the respiratory muscles.

► There are a number of theoretical reasons why the respiratory muscles might become fatigued in COPD: Hyperinflation causes the chest muscles to work at a severe mechanical disadvantage, and metabolism is impeded by a combination of hypoxia and acidosis. There is some empirical evidence supporting a hypothesis of respiratory muscle fatigue, including a fall in the high/low frequency electromyographic ratio[1] and a rightward shift of the force/frequency curve for the sternomastoid muscle.[2]

Polkey and associates argue that a reduced response to electrical stimulation of the phrenic nerve is not observed after a bout of exhaustive exercise because symptoms cause the patient to stop the activity before the respiratory muscles are substantially fatigued. Although their findings are essentially negative, the authors do not entirely exclude the possibility of respiratory fatigue. Measurements were made only on the diaphragmatic muscles, and a substantial (20-minute) recovery period was allowed after the walk to exhaustion.

R.J. Shephard, M.D., Ph.D., D.P.E.

References

1. Bye PT, Esau SA, Levy RD, et al: Ventilatory muscle function during exercise in air and oxygen in patients with chronic air-flow limitation. *Am Rev Respir Dis* 132:236–240, 1985.
2. Wilson S, Cooke N, Moxham J, et al: Sternomastoid muscle function and fatigue in normal subjects and patients with chronic obstructive pulmonary disease. *Am Rev Respir Dis* 129:460–464, 1984.

Lack of Effect of Inhaled Morphine on Exercise-induced Breathlessness in Chronic Obstructive Pulmonary Disease

Masood AR, Reed JW, Thomas SHL (Univ of Newcastle, Newcastle upon Tyne, England)

Thorax 50:629–634, 1995 6–30

Background.—Controlled trials investigating the ability of inhaled nebulized morphine to decrease breathlessness in patients with lung disease have yielded conflicting results. Some authorities have postulated that morphine acts directly on the lung. The efficacy of nebulized morphine in decreasing exercise-induced breathlessness in patients with chronic obstructive pulmonary disease (COPD) was investigated.

Methods.—Twelve men with COPD were enrolled in a double-blind, randomized, crossover study comparing the effects of nebulized morphine, 10 and 25 mg; equivalent IV doses, 1 and 2.5 mg; and placebo. Measures of breathlessness, ventilation, gas exchange, and exercise endurance were obtained during graded cycle ergometer exercise.

Findings.—Breathlessness, ventilation, and gas exchange at rest or at any time during exercise were not affected by any of the treatments. Exercise endurance was also unchanged. At peak exercise, mean changes in ventilation from placebo were −0.8 L/min for the highest IV dose and −0.4 L/min for the highest nebulized dose. The respective values for breathlessness were 2 and 1 mm, respectively, on a visual analogue scale.

Conclusion.—These doses of nebulized morphine had no effect on exercise-induced breathlessness. Thus, intrapulmonary opiates apparently do not modulate the sensation of breathlessness in patients with COPD (Figure).

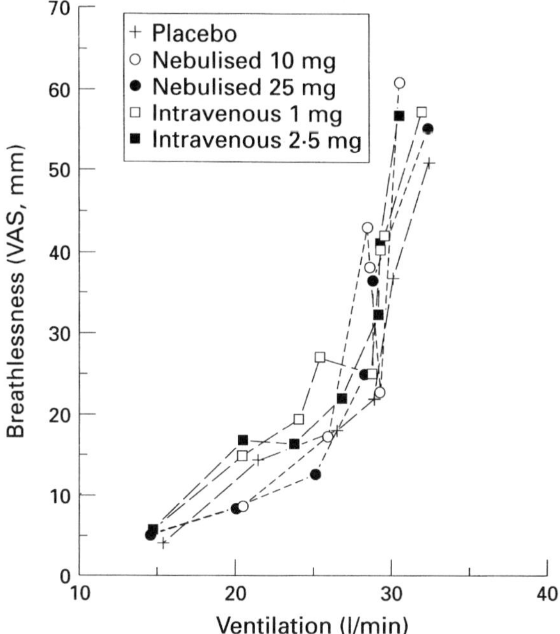

FIGURE.—Effects of nebulized and IV morphine on the relationship between ventilation and breathlessness. Mean values for 12 patients at rest, 50% and 80% of maximum workload, oxygen uptake values of 0.5 and 0.75 L/min, highest equivalent workload, and peak exercise. (Courtesy of Masood AR, Reed JW, Thomas SHL: Lack of effect of inhaled morphine on exercise-induced breathlessness in chronic obstructive pulmonary disease. *Thorax* 50:629–634, 1995.)

► Morphine has been used successfully in controlling breathlessness in patients with certain forms of cancer,[1, 2] but in such a situation, life expectancy is short and complications of opiate therapy are not a major issue. In chronic obstructive lung disease, the disease is protracted, and there is, thus, substantial interest in the possibility of minimizing the complications of opiate therapy (both drowsiness and addiction) by inhalation rather than systemic administration of the drug.

These data show little benefit at doses of up to 25 mg. Given that some other authors have reported modest benefits,[3] there may be merit in repeating observations with a larger dosage, a more potent opiate, or one that is retained in the lungs for a longer period.

R.J. Shephard, M.D., Ph.D., D.P.E.

References

1. Ahmedzai S: Respiratory distress in the terminally ill patient. *Resp Dis Practice* Oct/Nov:20–29, 1988.
2. Farncombe M, Chater S: Case studies outlining use of nebulised morphine for patients with end-stage chronic lung and cardiac disease. *J Pain Symptom Management* 8:221–225, 1993.

3. Young JH, Daviskas E, Keena VA: Effect of low dose nebulised morphine on exercise endurance in patients with chronic lung disease. *Thorax* 44:387–390, 1989.

A Comparison of Outpatient Cardiac and Pulmonary Rehabilitation Patients

Reardon JZ, Levine S, Peske G, Elnaggar A, Normandin E, Clark B, ZuWallack RL (Yale Univ, New Haven, Conn; Saint Francis Hosp, Hartford, Conn; Pulmonary Therapy Group, Greensburg, Pa; et al)
J Cardiopulmon Rehabil 15:277–282, 1995 6–31

Rationale.—The realms of cardiac and pulmonary rehabilitation frequently are considered together in the form of "cardiopulmonary" programs. This likely reflects a number of similarities in the patients served, but differences between the 2 populations have not been sufficiently taken into account.

Objective.—Clinical and therapeutic aspects were compared in 55 patients who completed phase II cardiac rehabilitation (CR) and 47 others who completed outpatient pulmonary rehabilitation (PR) in the same period. Most CR patients were referred by a cardiologist after myocardial infarction or coronary bypass surgery. Patients exercised 3 times a week for 6–12 weeks and were educated in cardiovascular risk modification. The PR patients had similar sessions twice a week for 6 weeks.

Demographics.—Men predominated in the CR group. These patients were about 7 years younger, on average, than the PR patients (Table 1). The CR patients had significantly higher body mass indices. The number of pack-years of cigarettes consumed was twice that of the CR group.

TABLE 1.—Patient Characteristics (χ ± Standard Deviation)

Variable	Cardiac†	Pulmonary‡	*P*
Percent male	80	49	.004
Age (years)	59.0 ± 11.0	66.2 ± 11.8	.002
Cigarette use (pack/years)	20.0 ± 24.1	50.7 ± 27.7	.0001
BMI (kg/m^2)	27.3 ± 5.2	23.3 ± 5.1	.0005
Functional status*	1.3 ± 1.4	3.2 ± 0.8	.0001
Employed (%)	60.8	7.1	.0001
Total number of diagnoses	2.2 ± 1.0	3.1 ± 1.4	.0006
Number of nonprincipal diagnoses	1.1 ± 1.0	2.0 ± 1.4	.0001
Number of medications	3.6 ± 1.8	5.3 ± 2.3	.0001
Number of nonprincipal medications	1.1 ± 1.1	2.1 ± 1.7	.001
Number of hospital admissions previous year	1.4 ± 0.7	0.6 ± 0.7	.0001
Number of hospital days previous year	11.6 ± 6.2	4.8 ± 7.4	.0001

* Functional status: 1 = uncompromised; 2 = slightly compromised; 3 = moderately compromised; 4 = severely compromised.
† *n* = 55.
‡ *n* = 47.
Abbreviation: BMI, body mass index.
(Courtesy of Reardon JZ, Levine S, Peske G, et al: A comparison of outpatient cardiac and pulmonary rehabilitation patients. *J Cardiopulmon Rehabil* 15:277–282, 1995.)

Diagnoses.—A majority of both groups had 1 or more significant but unrelated medical problems, but these were more numerous in the PR group. Hypertension and hyperlipidemia were the most common secondary diagnoses in the CR group. Seventeen percent of PR patients but no CR patients had a history of cancer.

Management.—The CR patients used fewer medications than the PR patients. Psychotropic drugs, in particular, were used less often in CR patients. Nearly one third of the PR patients were taking regular oral steroids.

Function.—The CR patients had a much higher functional status than those in the PR group, as assessed by New York Heart Association scoring. Most PR patients were moderately to severely limited. Fully 61% of CR patients but only 7% of the PR group were employed. The CR patients had spent significantly more time in hospital in the year before rehabilitation.

Implication.—Patients undergoing cardiac and pulmonary rehabilitation are distinct populations that require different approaches to management.

► We noted a number of years ago that it was much more difficult to persuade chest patients to exercise than those who had sustained a myocardial infarction[1]; we suggested that the poorer motivation of the chest group reflected the unpleasant nature of the dyspnea encountered during exercise, together with a lack of the critical incident that often encourages a change of lifestyle among "postcoronary" patients. This paper by Reardon and associates highlights a number of other important differences between chronic obstructive lung disease and "postcoronary" patients. Although smoking is a risk factor for coronary vascular disease, it is more dominant in the chest patient, as shown by the greater average pack-years of cigarettes consumed. The chest patients are also older; this, in itself, reduces their initial working capacity and increases the likelihood that serious secondary disorders have developed with associated medication. Given these differences, it is important to arrange separate classes for the rehabilitation of cardiac and chest patients.

R.J. Shephard, M.D., Ph.D., D.P.E.

Reference

1. Mertens DJ, Shephard RJ, Kavanagh T: Long-term exercise therapy for chronic obstructive lung disease. *Respiration* 35:96–107, 1978.

Long Term Benefits of Rehabilitation at Home on Quality of Life and Exercise Tolerance in Patients With Chronic Obstructive Pulmonary Disease

Wijkstra PJ, Ten Vergert EM, van Altena R, Otten V, Kraan J, Postma DS, Koëter GH (Rehabilitation Centre Beatrixoord, Haren, The Netherlands; Univ Hosp, Groningen, The Netherlands)

Thorax 50:824–828, 1995 6–32

Objective.—The quality of life and exercise tolerance after rehabilitation has not been previously evaluated for patients with chronic obstructive pulmonary disease (COPD). To determine whether rehabilitation improves quality of life and exercise tolerance for such patients, monthly physiotherapy sessions were compared with weekly home-based physiotherapy sessions.

Methods.—After the first 12 weeks of an 18-month home-based physiotherapy program, 11 patients (group A) received a weekly physiotherapy session, and 12 patients (group B) received monthly sessions. Thirteen COPD patients (group C) served as controls. Total lung capacity, residual volume, forced expiratory volume in 1 second (FEV_1), inspiratory vital capacity (IVC), and transfer factor for carbon monoxide were measured at

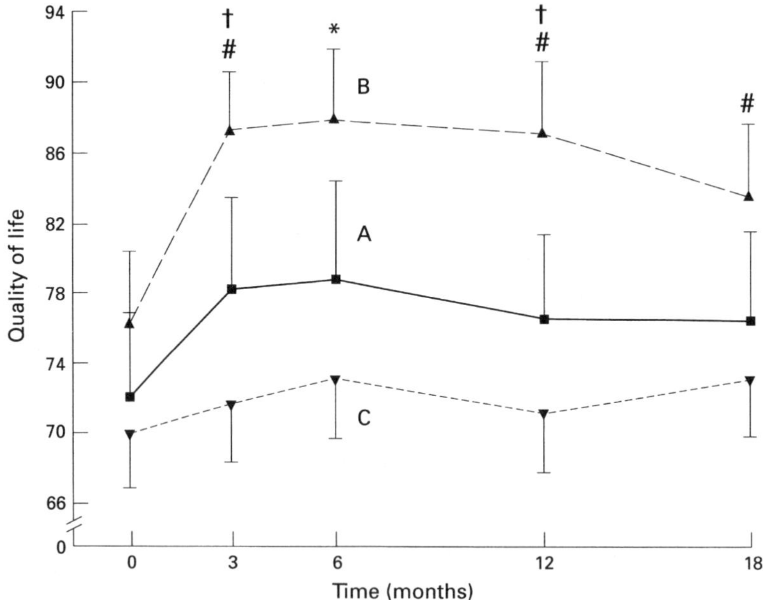

FIGURE 1.—Quality of life (sum score). *Solid line* represents group A (during first 12 months, $n = 11$; at 18 months, $n = 10$). *Broken line* represents group B (during first 12 months, $n = 12$; at 18 months, $n = 11$). *Dotted line* represents group C (during first 12 months, $n = 13$; at 18 months, $n = 12$). *Asterisk,* $P < 0.05$; *number symbol,* $P < 0.01$ compared with baseline; *single dagger,* $P < 0.05$ compared with control group C. (Courtesy of Wijkstra PJ, Ten Vergert EM, van Altena R, et al: Long term benefits of rehabilitation at home on quality of life and exercise tolerance in patients with chronic obstructive pulmonary disease. *Thorax* 50:824–828, 1995.)

baseline and at 18 months. At 3, 6, and 12 months, quality of life was assessed using the Chronic Respiratory Questionnaire, exercise tolerance as measured by distance walked in 6 minutes, and lung function as measured by FEV_1 and IVC.

Results.—Thirty-six patients completed the study, 23 of whom received home physiotherapy. Forced expiratory volume in 1 second, IVC values, and 6-minute walking distance did not differ significantly among groups. Quality-of-life scores were higher at all time points for groups A and B than for group C, and differences were significant for group B at all time points. (Fig 1).

Conclusion.—Twelve weeks of home-based rehabilitation followed by monthly physiotherapy sessions improved the quality of life over 18 months for COPD patients. The quality-of-life improvement was not associated with improved exercise tolerance. There was a significant decrease in the 6-minute walking distance and IVC in control patients.

▶ The general consensus is that although exercise programs improve subjective reactions in COPD, objective data show few changes. The absence of change in lung function in the study by Wijkstra et al. supports this view. Some investigators have argued that a part of the subjective benefit comes from an exercise rehabilitation program because patients learn to walk in a mechanically more efficient manner. However, the lack of change in 6-minute walking distance in this study speaks against this hypothesis. We are left with the probability that much of the apparent response to exercise is a placebo effect, and this viewpoint is supported here by the finding of at least equal benefit from monthly, as opposed to weekly, treatment.

R.J. Shephard, M.D., Ph.D., D.P.E.

7 Nutrition and Viscera, Metabolism, Body Composition

Eating Disorder Symptoms in Female College Gymnasts
O'Connor PJ, Lewis RD, Kirchner EM (Univ of Georgia, Athens)
Med Sci Sports Exerc 27:550–555, 1995 7–1

Objectives.—Because athletes engaging in sports that place a premium on being lean may be at increased risk of having eating disorders develop, a study was undertaken among college gymnasts to learn how a strong drive to be thin might affect health. Another goal was to check the validity of the Eating Disorders Inventory-2 (EDI-2), which measures a number of constructs theoretically related to eating disorders.

Can Questionnaire Responses Be Faked?—Twenty-one college women averaging 20 years of age completed the EDI-2 on 2 occasions, first when given the usual instructions and immediately afterward after being instructed to fake the test by presenting themselves as being as mentally healthy as possible. Scores on the 2 tests differed significantly, particularly with respect to body dissatisfaction. Under the standard condition, all participants expressed some dissatisfaction with the shape and size of their bodies; all expressed satisfaction when faking the test.

Validation.—A fake profile derived from the first study was used to screen for symptoms of eating disorder in 25 college gymnasts and 25 controls matched with the athletes for age, height, and body weight. Twelve percent of the entire study group had EDI-2 scores matching the fake profile. After eliminating these individuals, no significant subscale differences were found between the gymnasts and the controls (Table 1). Both gymnasts and controls had an increased drive for thinness when their data were compared with normative data for female college students. The gymnasts had lower energy intakes than controls (1,401 vs. 1,688 kcal/day) and higher bone mineral density. More of the gymnasts described menstrual irregularity; amenorrhea was most frequently reported by those

TABLE 1.—Eating Disorders Inventory-2 Subscale Means (± Standard Deviation) for Norms, Gymnasts, and Controls

	Norms (n = 205)*		Gymnasts (n = 23)		Controls (n = 21)	
Variables	Mean	SD	Mean	SD	Mean	SD
Drive for thinness	5.5	5.5	9.0	6.7	9.2	7.0
Bulimia	1.2	1.9	1.4	3.2	1.7	2.3
Body dissatisfaction	12.2	8.3	11.5	9.4	17.7	7.5
Ineffectiveness	2.3	3.6	0.9	1.8	3.3	5.6
Perfectionism	6.2	3.9	5.9	4.4	5.6	4.3
Interpersonal distrust	2.0	3.1	2.2	3.8	2.2	4.1
Interoceptive awareness	3.0	3.9	3.1	4.3	4.0	5.0
Maturity fears	2.7	2.9	1.5	1.5	1.7	2.1
Asceticism	3.4	2.2	4.2	3.0	4.1	2.8
Impulse regulation	2.3	3.6	1.7	2.3	1.8	3.2
Social insecurity	3.3	3.3	2.4	2.4	3.0	2.5

* College female norms are courtesy of Garner DM: *Eating Disorders Inventory–2.* Odessa, Fla, Psychological Assessment Resources, 1991, Tables 10 and 11, pp 1–70.

(Courtesy of O'Connor PJ, Lewis RD, Kirchner EM: Eating disorder symptoms in female college gymnasts. *Med Sci Sports Exerc* 27:550–555, 1995.)

with elevated drive-for-thinness scores. No significant differences were found in reported binge eating, purging, or the use of laxatives, diet pills, or diuretics.

Conclusion.—Women preoccupied with remaining thin may limit their dietary intake, and menstrual irregularity may develop. The ED1-2 can be easily faked.

Eating Disorder Characteristics and Psychiatric Symptomatology of Eumenorrheic and Amenorrheic Runners

Klock SC, DeSouza MJ (Harvard Med School, Boston; Univ of Connecticut)
Int J Eat Disord 17:161–166, 1995 7–2

Background.—It has been suggested that obligatory runners—men who feel impelled to run 80–120 km each week—are psychologically similar to anorexic women. Both are intensely preoccupied with regulating their physical state, and in both cases adaptation is compromised. If this comparison is valid, anorexic individuals and amenorrheic runners should be similar psychologically, and both should differ from eumenorrheic runners and controls.

Objective and Methods.—In the course of a study of endocrine function, psychological status was compared in 7 runners who had been amenorrheic for at least 3 months, 9 others who were eumenorrheic, and 6 sedentary women with normal menstrual function. All participants were 18 to 45 years of age and in good general health. The Beck Depression Inventory and a modified 10-item version of the Body Image Questionnaire were administered, along with the Symptom Checklist-90 and the Eating Disorders Inventory.

TABLE 3.—Group Scores for the Body Image Questionnaire, Beck Depression Inventory, Symptom Checklist-90, and the Eating Disorder Inventory

	Eumenorrheic Controls (n = 6)	Eumenorrheic Runners (n = 9)	Amenorrheic Runners (n = 7)
BIQ	29.3 ± 5.3	31.0 ± 4.8	30.4 ± 5.8
BDI	3.0 ± 3.5	3.8 ± 3.73	8.3 ± 6.2
SCL-90	49.7 ± 33.5	57.2 ± 25.5	65.7 ± 27.7
EDI (total score)	17.8 ± 10.4	28.0 ± 19.6	31.4 ± 20.1
Drive for Thinness	2.0 ± 2.2	4.5 ± 4.8	4.7 ± 4.6
Interoceptive Awareness	0.5 ± 0.8	3.4 ± 4.6	2.7 ± 3.5
Bulimia	0.0 ± .0	0.5 ± 1.3	0.2 ± 0.4
Body Dissatisfaction	7.0 ± 7.5	8.4 ± 7.6	8.1 ± 5.4
Ineffectiveness	1.3 ± 1.2	2.0 ± 2.4	3.4 ± 4.6
Maturity Fears	1.0 ± 1.2	2.7 ± 2.7	1.7 ± 2.0
Perfectionism	4.1 ± 3.5	4.2 ± 3.3	6.8 ± 4.4
Interpersonal Distrust	1.8 ± 2.6	2.0 ± 3.2	3.5 ± 4.2

Note: Values are means ± standard deviation.

Abbreviations: BIQ, Body Image Questionnaire; *BDI*, Beck Depression Inventory; *SCL-90*, Symptom Checklist-90; *EDI*, Eating Disorder Inventory.

(Courtesy of Klock SC, DeSouza MJ: Eating disorder characteristics and psychiatric symptomatology of eumenorrheic and amenorrheic runners. *Int J Eat Disord* 17:161–166, Copyright 1995. Reprinted by permission of John Wiley & Sons, Inc.)

Findings.—The amenorrheic runners weighed significantly less than the other women, but no significant group differences were found in reproductive age or percentage of body fat. The amenorrheic women were older at menarche. Body satisfaction, as reflected by Body Image Questionnaire scores, was comparable in all groups (Table 3). The women in general were "somewhat satisfied" with their appearance. Depression scores were substantially higher in the amenorrheic runners, 3 of whom were clinically depressed. Eating Disorders Inventory scores did not differ significantly, although the amenorrheic women did have scores indicating a clinically significant eating disorder.

Conclusion.—The suggestion that the amenorrhea found in both obligatory runners and anorexic individuals reflects a common underlying factor was not supported.

▶ The selection of an appropriate instrument to detect eating disorders among female athletes is limited by the number of validated instruments available and whether the instrument has been validated for athletes (see the 2 preceding abstracts). Although it might appear reasonable to expect the average college woman and the female athlete with an eating disorder to have similar symptoms, there are a number of external pressures on the athlete that the average woman is not subjected to that might influence the response to the Eating Disorders Inventory. Taking this difference into account, it would have been interesting to see whether athletes provided the same "fake profile" that nonathletes did in the O'Connor et al. study (Abstract 7–1). Using an instrument that can easily be faked does not lead to confidence in the results of studies using that instrument.

The Klock and DeSouza study (Abstract 7–2) also found no difference between athletes and controls in the Eating Disorders Inventory scores. In this study the small number of research subjects, suggesting a low power to detect differences among groups, may explain the lack of a significant difference because the scores for the amenorrheic runners were double those of the controls in 5 of the subscales. It is apparent that the present techniques for identifying women at risk of an eating disorder are not entirely satisfactory when used with athletes.

B.L. Drinkwater, Ph.D.

The Effects of Estrogen Administration on Trabecular Bone Loss in Young Women With Anorexia Nervosa

Klibanski A, Biller BMK, Schoenfeld DA, Herzog DB, Saxe VC (Gen Clinical Research Ctr, Boston; Massachusetts Gen Hosp, Boston; Harvard Med School, Boston)

J Clin Endocrinol Metab 80:898–904, 1995 7–3

Introduction.—Anorexia nervosa is common in young women, and the severe restrictive eating pattern is associated with profound metabolic complications of malnutrition, including prolonged amenorrhea. Severe osteopenia occurs in these women, and clinical fractures at multiple sites have been documented in women in their 20s. To analyze the effects of

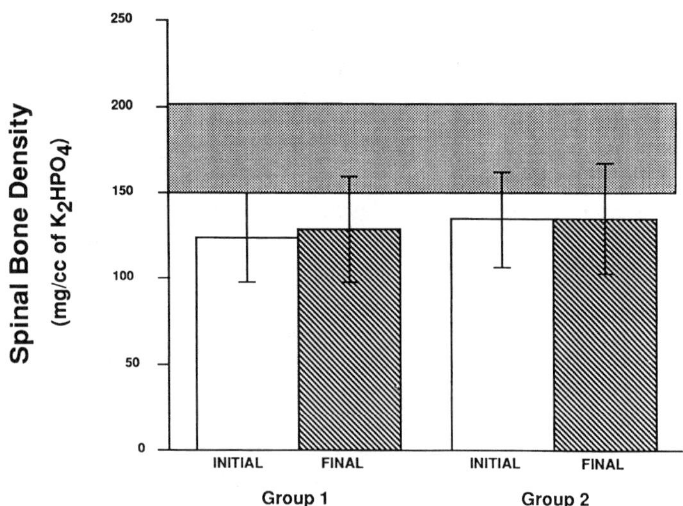

FIGURE 1—Initial and final trabecular bone densities in patients treated with estrogen and controls. No significant difference was found in initial and final bone densities in either group. The *shaded areas* indicate the normal mean bone density ± 1 standard deviation. (Courtesy of Klibanski A, Biller BMK, Schoenfeld DA, et al: The effects of estrogen administration on trabecular bone loss in young women with anorexia nervosa. *J Clin Endocrinol Metab* 80:898–904, Copyright 1995, The Endocrine Society.)

TABLE 3.—Percentage Change in Bone Density by Patient Subgroup

Estrogen group			Control group		
2.8 ± 11.0 (n = 19)			−5.4 ± 22.6 (n = 25)		
% IBW <70 4.0 ± 8.8 (n = 6)	% IBW >70 2.2 ± 12.0 (n = 13)		% IBW <70 −20.1 ± 16.2 (n = 10)	% IBW > 70 4.3 ± 21.2 (n = 15)	
	No recovery 1.2 ± 12.5 (n = 11)	Recovery 7.5 ± 12 (n = 2)		No recovery −5.7 ± 17.1 (n = 9)	Recovery 19.3 18.4 (n = 6)

Abbreviation: IBW, ideal body weight.

(Courtesy of Klibanski A, Biller BMK, Schoenfeld DA, et al: The effects of estrogen administration on trabecular bone loss in young women with anorexia nervosa. *J Clin Endocrinol Metab* 80:898–904, Copyright 1995, The Endocrine Society.)

prolonged anorexia nervosa on bone density and to determine whether estrogen administration prevents bone loss in women with this disorder, a prospective study was conducted.

Study Design.—Forty-eight amenorrheic women with anorexia nervosa (mean age, 24.9 years) randomly received either estrogen and progestin replacement or no replacement. Initially, mean bone density (BD) was significantly lower than normal (130 vs. 176 mg K_2HPO_4/cm^3) in all 48 women and more than 2 standard deviations below normal in 21 women. Clinical data, biochemical indices, and spinal BD measured by dual-energy techniques were obtained every 6 months for a mean of 1.5 years.

Results.—Nineteen women in the estrogen group and 25 women who did not receive replacement therapy completed the study. The initial BD did not differ between the 2 groups. Final BD was also comparable between the estrogen group and the control group, but the effect of estrogen replacement was highly dependent on initial percent ideal body weight (Fig 1). Women with an initial ideal body weight of less than 70% had a 4.0% increase in mean BD during estrogen replacement, whereas controls with comparably low initial ideal body weight had a 20.1% decrease in BD. Six controls, all with initial ideal body weight greater than 70%, recovered from anorexia nervosa with spontaneous resumption of menses and had a 19.3% increase in bone mass (Table 3). In contrast, bone mass decreased by 13.3% in 19 control women who remained amenorrheic.

Conclusion.—This is the first study to show progressive trabecular bone loss in adult women with chronic anorexia nervosa and prolonged amenorrhea and the first prospective study of estrogen replacement in these women with premenopausal osteoporosis. In contrast to the beneficial effects of estrogen in menopausal women, estrogen and progestin administration does not reverse the profound osteopenia in these young women. However, a subset of women may improve with estrogen and progestin administration, depending on initial body weight. Recovery from anorexia nervosa and resumption of normal menses is associated with significant improvement in bone mass.

► This article should be of interest to sports medicine professionals who deal with the issue of disordered eating among female athletes. Although "disordered eating," a subclinical form of anorexia or bulimia, may not meet all the *Diagnostic and Statistical Manual of Mental Disorders, ed IV-R* criteria for an eating disorder, amenorrhea is a frequent by-product, with resulting reduced levels of bone mineral density. Contrary to the author's expectation, hormone replacement therapy for postmenopausal women does not markedly increase bone mass. There is an apparent increase in BD as estrogen slows bone resorption while previous resorption sites benefit from bone formation. If bone loss in young women is irreversible, intervention must occur early to prevent significant loss of bone.

B.L. Drinkwater, Ph.D.

Effects of Weight Gain and Resumption of Menses on Reduced Bone Density in Patients With Anorexia Nervosa

Iketani T, Kiriike N, Nakanishi S, Nakasuji T (Osaka City Univ, Japan)

Biol Psychiatry 37:521–527, 1995 7–4

Background.—Although osteoporosis is highly unusual in young adults, it has been found in adolescents and adults with anorexia. Several factors have been implicated in the reduced bone density in these patients, including malnutrition, low calcium intake, weight loss, estrogen deficiency, and glucocorticoid excess. However, the relative contribution of these factors has not been determined. The relationships between these factors and bone density were analyzed in both a cross-section and a longitudinal sample of patients undergoing treatment for anorexia nervosa, bulimia nervosa, or both.

Methods.—In the cross-section study, bone mineral density (BMD) was measured with dual-photon absorptiometry in the lumbar vertebrae and in the whole body in 45 female patients with anorexia nervosa (23 of whom also had bulimia nervosa), 10 female patients with bulimia nervosa and a history of anorexia nervosa, and 10 age-matched healthy women. In the longitudinal study, repeated BMD measurements were obtained before and after weight gain in 17 anorexic patients (of whom 12 also had bulimia nervosa) and 4 amenorrheic patients with bulimia nervosa and a history of anorexia nervosa. Bone mineral density was measured after weight normalization and after menses resumed.

Results.—The cross-section series showed that lumbar BMD, but not whole-body BMD, was significantly reduced in patients with anorexia nervosa with or without bulimia nervosa, compared with controls. Patients with bulimia nervosa alone had lumbar BMD midway between the anorexia nervosa group and the controls. Lumbar BMD correlated negatively with the duration of anorexia and of amenorrhea and was not influenced by age or age at menarche. However, BMD was significantly lower in patients in whom amenorrhea began when they were younger than 18 years of age than in those in whom amenorrhea began when they were older than 18 years of age.

All patients in the longitudinal study gained weight during treatment. In addition, 4 patients with both anorexia and bulimia nervosa and 2 patients with bulimia nervosa resumed regular menses. Lumbar BMD increased with weight gain, with greater BMD in those with normal weight gain than in those with subnormal weight gain. Bone mineral density was higher in the normal-weight patients with resumption of menses than in those without resumption of menses.

Conclusions.—The age of onset of amenorrhea has a greater influence on bone loss than the age of onset of anorexia nervosa, and recovery of BMD requires both weight gain and resumption of menses.

▶ Contradictions abound in the literature concerning the effect of anorexia nervosa and the recovery from the disease on bone density. Some investigators have reported that physical activity confers some protection against bone loss; others find no effect. Several studies have concluded that weight gain is the primary factor responsible for an increase in the bone density of recovering patients with anorexia; others believe a return of menses, signaling an increased level of endogenous estrogen, is necessary for optimal recovery.

Although identification of the variables responsible for the reversal of bone loss in patients with anorexia is essential, preventing bone loss is even more important. Obviously, the sooner the condition is diagnosed the greater the probability that bone loss can be minimized by initiating treatment. Whether the treatment should include estrogen supplementation, however, also is controversial. There are no long-term prospective studies demonstrating the efficacy of either oral contraceptives or hormone replacement therapy in preventing bone loss or increasing bone density in patients with anorexia.

B.L. Drinkwater, Ph.D.

A Multivariate Analysis of Kinanthropometric Profiles of Elite Female Orienteers

Creagh U, Reilly T (Liverpool John Moores Univ, England)

J Sports Med Phys Fitness 35:59–66, 1995 7–5

Introduction.—In orienteering, a timed cross-country event, competitors face difficult physical conditions while simultaneously navigating their way around a series of checkpoints. The activity has a substantial cognitive component.

Objective.—The influence of various kinanthropometic characteristics on orienteering performance was studied in 12 women who participated successfully in the Student World Orienteering Championships and in 11 others who were less successful. Twenty women in their early 20s who were not orienteers also were studied.

Methods.—Five skinfold thicknesses, 2 limb girths, 2 bone breadths, and 3 proportional body lengths were measured during the week of the competition. In addition, grip strength, back-leg strength, and flexibility were estimated. Adiposity, somatotype, and various anthropometric indices were derived from these measurements.

Results.—Competitive performance correlated significantly with both age and measures of adiposity. Discriminant function analysis using these variables correctly distinguished the successful competitors from those who were less successful. In general, measures of proportionality and physical test results were similar in the orienteers and the reference individuals. Adiposity was greater in the latter individuals.

Conclusion.—The older—and presumably more experienced athletes—had a better finishing time and placed higher among those finishing the event. The more successful orienteers also had lower levels of adiposity, which also correlated significantly with performance.

► It is unfortunate that orienteering is not more popular in this country, for it challenges both the physical and cognitive capabilities of the participants in a unique fashion. As an endurance event, it demands many of the same physiologic attributes as distance running, so it is no surprise that body composition was a factor in orienteering success. However, it is important to note that the average percentage of body fat for the top orienteers in this study was 20.4%. These women were lean—but not unusually so—and the correlation of the 2 performance measures with percentage of body fat explained only 16% to 23% of the variance in performance.

Too much emphasis on body weight, percentage of body fat, or both has led many athletes to adopt poor nutritional habits and has even led to serious eating disorders. This article does not presume to identify which variables are most important for success—only that kinanthropometric variables in general are not a deciding factor.

B.L. Drinkwater, Ph.D.

Physical Activity, Obesity, and Risk for Colon Cancer and Adenoma in Men

Giovannucci E, Ascherio A, Rimm EB, Colditz GA, Stampfer MJ, Willett WC (Harvard Univ, Cambridge, Mass)

Ann Intern Med 122:327–334, 1995 7–6

Introduction.—Colon cancer, the second leading cause of malignant death in the United States, seems to be a result of westernization or industrialization. Risk factors include a diet high in red meat and animal fat and low in fruits and vegetables. There also is an inverse relationship between physical activity, either occupational alone or in combination with recreational exercise, and colon cancer, especially in men. Abdominal adiposity and height in men seem to be further risk factors. The association between physical activity, obesity, and height on the risk of colon cancer was studied.

Methods.—In 1986, the Health Professionals Follow-up Study received questionnaires from 51,529 male dentists, optometrists, osteopaths, podiatrists, pharmacists, and veterinarians. They ranged in age from 40 to 75 years. The men reported on leisure activity (metabolic equivalents), current weight, weight at age 21 years, height, personal and family medical and cancer history, medications, and food and alcohol intake. Exposure information was updated in 1988, 1990, and 1992. Only adenomas detected during colonoscopy or sigmoidoscopy were recorded. Waist and hip circumferences were requested in 1987, with 65% of research subjects responding. Deaths were reported by family members or ascertained from the National Death Index. Research subjects who did not give information about their physical activity, had previous cancer, implausibly high or low food intake, or left 70 or more items on the questionnaire blank were excluded, leaving 47,723 eligible individuals.

TABLE 2.—Relative Risk for Colon Cancer by Level of Physical Activity and Body Mass Index

Variable	Category					*P* Value for Trend
	1	2	3	4	5	
Median total MET-hours*	0.9	4.8	11.3	22.6	46.8	
Cases/person-years	55/51 660	41/52 391	47/52 548	37/53 411	23/53 544	
Relative risk† (95% CI)	1.0	0.69 (0.46–1.02)	0.83 (0.56–1.23)	0.67 (0.44–1.02)	0.44 (0.27–0.71)	0.002
Multivariate relative risk (95% CI)‡	1.0	0.73 (0.48–1.10)	0.94 (0.63–1.39)	0.78 (0.51–1.20)	0.53 (0.32–0.88)	0.03
Body mass index, *kg/m²*	<22	22–24.9	25–26.9	27–28.9	≥29	
Cases/person-years	34/52 904	38/72 721	60/69 865	38/37 311	33/30 664	
Relative risk* (95% CI)	1.0	0.84 (0.52–1.33)	1.33 (0.88–2.03)	1.62 (1.03–2.55)	1.82 (1.14–2.91)	<0.001
Multivariate relative risk† (95% CI)	1.0	0.87 (0.54–1.39)	1.31 (0.85–2.02)	1.48 (0.89–2.56)	1.48 (0.89–2.46)	0.02
Height, *in*	≤68	69	70–71	72	≥73	
Cases/person-years	49/70 118	28/31 523	57/80 527	30/35 980	39/45 188	
Relative risk† (95% CI)	1.0	1.44 (0.91–2.28)	1.26 (0.86–1.84)	1.65 (1.04–2.61)	1.96 (1.28–3.01)	0.002
Multivariate relative risk§ (95% CI)	1.0	1.37 (0.86–2.19)	1.19 (0.81–1.76)	1.54 (0.96–2.46)	1.76 (1.13–2.74)	0.02

* MET-hours are the sum of the average time per week spent in each activity × MET value of each activity.

$$\text{MET value} = \frac{\text{caloric need per kg of body weight per hour of activity}}{\text{caloric need per kg of body weight per hour at rest}}$$

† Relative risk adjusted for age.

‡ From proportional hazards model that included body mass index, physical activity, age, history of endoscopic screening or polyp diagnosis, parental history of colorectal cancer, pack-years of smoking, aspirin use, and intake of folate, methione, alcohol, dietary fiber, red meat, and total energy.

§ From proportional hazards model that included height, physical activity, age, history of endoscopic screening or polyp diagnosis, parental history of colorectal cancer, pack-years of smoking, aspirin use, and intake of folate, methione, alcohol, dietary fiber, red meat, and total energy.

Abbreviation: MET, metabolic equivalents.

(Courtesy of Giovannucci E, Ascherio A, Rimm EB, et al: Physical activity, obesity, and risk for colon cancer and adenoma in men. *Ann Intern Med* 122:327–334, 1995.)

Results.—The data were categorized into quintiles and grouped according to tumor size. An inverse relationship was found between colon cancer and physical activity (Table 2). After controlling for age; polyp history; previous endoscopy; family history; smoking; body mass; aspirin intake; and red meat, fiber, folate, and alcohol intake, the relative risk was 0.53. Body mass was directly associated with colon cancer risk. Waist circumference and waist-to-hip ratio were strong risk factors. If the ratio was 0.99 or greater vs. 0.90 or less, the relative risk was 3.41. If the waist circumference was greater than 109 cm vs. 86 cm or less, the relative risk was 2.56. Height also was associated with colon cancer risk. A height of 185 cm vs. 173 cm carried a relative risk of 1.76.

Conclusion.—An inverse association was found between the risk of colon cancer and physical activity. Furthermore, height and obesity, abdominal obesity in particular, increase the risk of colon cancer. Additional work on other populations, especially women, is warranted.

▶ There have been sufficient studies of physical activity and colon cancer to be fairly certain that a sedentary lifestyle is associated with an increased risk of this condition. The effect is particularly striking for tumors of the horizontal and descending colons.[1] Although moderate activity stimulates some aspects of immune function, most authors are inclined to attribute the reduction of cancer risk to other factors associated with vigorous physical activity; these could include the ingestion of increased quantities of aspirin, an increase of colonic motility or segmentation, a lesser risk of obesity, and a health consciousness that encourages an increased consumption of dietary fiber and antioxidants.

To date, the association of colon cancer with inactivity seems stronger in occupational studies than in surveys of leisure behavior. This could result from the long-term nature of the carcinogenic process; occupational activity may be more stable than leisure activity. It also could reflect difficulties in assessing leisure activity accurately. In this article, the authors claim that obesity had an adverse effect on cancer risk even after control of their data for habitual physical activity; they may be correct, although this observation could again reflect unmeasured variance in physical activity patterns.

R.J. Shephard, M.D., Ph.D., D.P.E.

Reference

1. Shephard RJ: Exercise in the prevention and treatment of cancer: An update. *Sports Med* 15:258–280, 1993.

Impact of Intensive Physical Exercise and Low-fat Diet on Collateral Vessel Formation in Stable Angina Pectoris and Angiographically Confirmed Coronary Artery Disease

Niebauer J, Hambrecht R, Marburger C, Hauer K, Velich T, von Hodenberg E, Schlierf G, Kübler W, Schuler G (Medizinische Universitätsklinik Heidelberg, Germany; Herzzentrum der Universität Leipzig, Germany)
Am J Cardiol 76:771–775, 1995 7–7

Background.—Although animal studies have shown that chronic intensive physical exercise increases capillary growth in the myocardium and causes enlargement or even growth of epicardial coronary arteries, clinical studies of human beings have not confirmed these findings. In previous research, the authors demonstrated that a low-fat diet and 3 hours of intensive physical exercise a week significantly retard coronary artery disease. To determine the impact of this intervention on the formation of coronary collateral arteries, coronary angiograms of these patients were assessed.

Methods.—Fifty-six unselected patients with coronary artery disease were placed on a low-fat diet and performed more than 3 hours of physical exercise per week. Fifty-seven patients receiving standard care by their

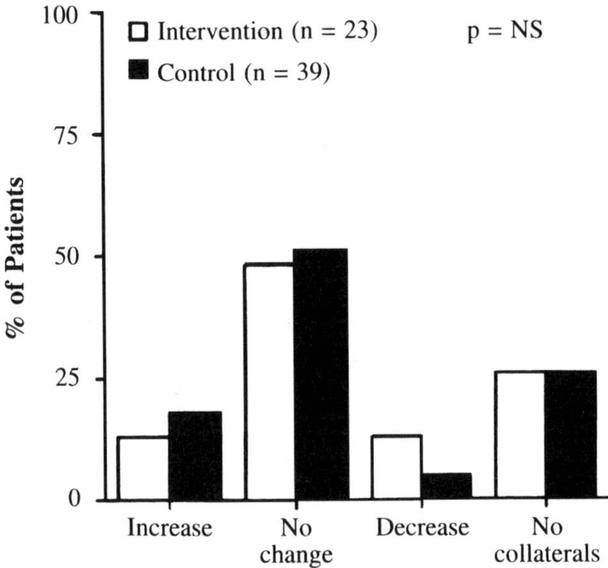

FIGURE 2.—Collateral formation in patients with previous myocardial infarction. In patients with myocardial infarction before the beginning of the study, no significant difference was found between patients in the intervention group and control group with respect to changes in collateral formation. (Reprinted by permission of Elsevier Science Inc., from Niebauer J, Hambrecht R, Marburger C, et al: Impact of intensive physical exercise and low-fat diet on collateral vessel formation in stable angina pectoris and angiographically confirmed coronary artery disease. *Am J Cardiol* 76:771–775, Copyright 1995 by Excerpta Medica, Inc.)

private physicans comprised a control group. Quantitative coronary angiography was performed at the beginning of the study and, in 92 patients, after 1 year.

Findings.—At 1 year, the progression of coronary artery disease was significantly retarded in the intervention group, compared with the control group. However, the groups did not differ in collateral formation. Changes in hemodynamic and metabolic factors and in leisure time activity were not associated with changes in collateral formation. Although disease progression was significantly correlated with an increase in collateral formation, regression was significantly associated with a reduction in collateral formation (Fig 2).

Conclusions.—Although the current intervention significantly retarded coronary artery disease progression, the intervention and control groups did not differ significantly in collateral formation after 1 year. It is questionable whether an exercise program within the safety tolerance of patients would be able to induce coronary collateralization when coronary artery disease is regressing.

▶ Various authors have attempted to demonstrate that an exercise program for human patients with cardiac disease can induce the formation of collateral vessels. All such investigators have had a notable lack of success. This report shows collateral vessels actually *decreasing* despite a very substantial 10 megajoules (2,500 kcal) of leisure activity per week. Plainly, the patient with cardiac disease cannot do much more than this! On the other hand, this article offers some encouragement in showing a regression of coronary vascular disease with the combination of exercise and a low-fat diet, although, as in other work from the same laboratory,[1] 5–6 hours of exercise per week seem to be needed to achieve this objective.

R.J. Shephard, M.D., Ph.D., D.P.E.

Reference

1. Hambrecht R, Niebauer J, Marburger C, et al: Various intensities of leisure time physical activity in patients with coronary artery disease: Effects on cardiorespiratory fitness and progression of coronary atherosclerotic lesions. *J Am Coll Cardiol* 22:468–477, 1993.

Gastro-oesophageal Reflux and Exercise: Important Pathology to Consider in the Athletic Population

Shawdon A (Alphington Sports Medicine Clinic, Northcote, Australia)

Sports Med 20:109–116, 1995 7–8

Background.—Recently, gastroesophageal reflux (GOR) has been found to occur more often during exercise than at rest. The pathophysiologic features and assessment of GOR disease were reviewed.

Pathophysiology.—In GOR, the esophagus is abnormally exposed to gastric juices. The main factors resulting in excessive exposure of the esophagus to gastric contents are an abnormally high rate of reflux episodes and an abnormally slow clearance of the refluxate back into the stomach. The latter occurs in about half of the patients. The nature of the refluxate, the degree to which it irritates the esophageal mucosa, and the ability of the mucosa to withstand injurious effects are additional variables.

Assessment.—The diagnosis of exercise-induced GOR can be confirmed by ambulatory pH monitoring. When exercise-induced reflux is identified in patients with negative angiographic findings, the management of a patient with angina-like chest pains is completely altered. Athletes with exertional chest pain need to be evaluated thoroughly to exclude cardiac abnormalities and establish a definitive diagnosis.

Treatment.—Persons prone to GOR should avoid exercising just after eating. Foods and drinks to be avoided include fatty foods, chocolate and mint, caffeine, and alcohol. Large meals tend to increase reflux. Certain types of sport and exercise may predispose to reflux.

Conclusions.—A substantial number of athletes report exertional upper gastrointestinal symptoms and exercise-induced chest pain. Management can involve simple measures, such as changes in diet, timing of meals, and nature of exercise. However, pharmacologic treatments may be indicated in some athletes. A more comprehensive understanding of GOR will likely lead to reductions in morbidity associated with cardiac origins of exercise-induced pain.

▶ Very little research has been done on exercise and the esophagus, and this review article is thus particularly welcome. Gastroesophageal reflux is frequently confounded with myocardial ischemia, and it is thus important to recognize that such reflux is increased by exercise and is a problem in a substantial number of athletes.

R.J. Shephard, M.D., Ph.D., D.P.E.

Exercise-induced Gastric Mucosal Acidosis

Nielsen HB, Svendsen LB, Jensen TH, Secher NH (Univ of Copenhagen)

Med Sci Sports Exerc 27:1003–1006, 1995 7–9

Introduction.—Celiac and mesenteric arterial blood flow have been shown to be reduced during periods of exercise. Reductions in splanchnic blood flow may be more pronounced during rowing, because higher plasma catecholamine concentrations occur with rowing as compared with some other types of exercise. Assessment of gastric intramucosal pH was used to determine the effect of rowing on splanchnic blood flow.

Methods.—Gastric tonometry was used to assess gastric mucosal acidosis in 6 male rowers during 30 minutes of ergometer rowing. A single dose of omeprazole 40 mg was administered on the morning of the study. Blood samples also were obtained to determine arterial bicarbonate, carbon dioxide tension, arterial oxygen tension, arterial pH, oxygen satura-

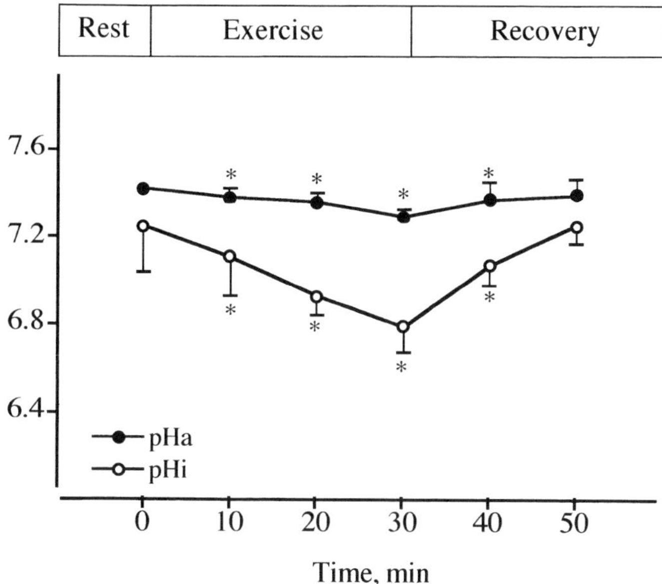

FIGURE 1.—The calculated pH of the gastric mucosal tissue (*pHi*) and pH of arterial blood in response to 30-minute ergometer rowing for 6 oarsmen. Values are mean ± standard deviation. Compared to rest, $*P < 0.05$. (Courtesy of Nielsen HB, Svendsen LB, Jensen TH, et al: Exercise-induced gastric mucosal acidosis. *Med Sci Sports Exerc* 27:1003–1006, 1995.)

tion, and serum lactate. Measurements were taken before rowing, every 10 minutes during rowing, and at 10 and 20 minutes after rowing.

Results.—As compared with arterial blood pH, gastric mucosal tissue pH was found to decrease significantly to 6.8 from 7.25 during the 30 minutes of rowing (Fig 1). During that same time, arterial blood pH decreased to 7.29. Ten minutes after exercise, both arterial blood and gastric tissue pH returned to baseline values. Arterial oxygen tension and saturation also decreased during rowing, but both values had returned to normal after 30 minutes of rowing.

Conclusion.—The gastric mucosal tissue pH found during exercise (6.8) is similar to the value found in patients with minimal mesenteric blood flow (7.0). Splanchnic blood flow seems to have been reduced in these indivduals during 30 minutes of ergometer rowing.

► The determination of gastric mucosal pH after administration of an antacid (omeprazole) is an interesting way of looking at the influence of exercise on gastric blood flow, and it should be tried during other forms of exercise. One difficulty is that up to half an hour may be required for complete equilibration of gas pressures between the tonometer and the mucosa. The values observed in this experiment were even lower than in patients with vascular obstruction, suggesting that there may have been virtually a complete occlusion of the mesenteric vessels during rowing exercise.

R.J. Shephard, M.D., Ph.D., D.P.E.

Physical Activity and the Risk of Progression of Retinopathy or the Development of Proliferative Retinopathy

Cruickshanks KJ, Moss SE, Klein R, Klein BEK (Univ of Wisconsin, Madison)

Ophthalmology 102:1177–1182, 1995 7–10

Introduction.—Patients with insulin-dependent diabetes who exercise are at reduced risk of dying or having macrovascular complications develop. The association between physical activity level and retinopathy is, however, less certain.

Objective and Methods.—Levels of physical activity were correlated with the course of retinopathy in 606 patients with diabetes enrolled in a longitudinal study of retinopathy. The patients, who were younger than 30 years when found to be diabetic, were free of proliferative changes when initially examined from 1984 to 1986, and they were followed up for 6 years. The severity of retinopathy was determined by examining stereoscopic fundus photos, and level of physical activity was estimated using a questionnaire.

Findings.—Those participants who initially reported being regularly active enough to work up a sweat were more likely than others to continue exercising to the time of follow-up. After adjusting for age and sex, the physical activity level did not correlate significantly with glycemia. In men, only the distance walked each day was related to the risk of proliferative change, and then only marginally. No such association was found in women. Similar findings were obtained when only patients who initially had moderate-to-marked nonproliferative retinopathy were analyzed.

Conclusion.—No convincing evidence was found that regular physical activity will lessen the risk of proliferative retinopathy developing in patients with insulin-dependent diabetes.

▶ Retinopathy is an important complication of diabetes mellitus, and sometimes vigorous physical activity can exacerbate damage to the retina in the patient with diabetes. It is encouraging that in this group of patients the retinopathy was no more marked among those who were exercising vigorously, but the sample was a relatively young group, and it will be important to repeat such observations on an older group. It would be particularly interesting to test the value of exercise as a means of preventing retinopathy in those with type II (maturity-onset) diabetes mellitus.

R.J. Shephard, M.D., Ph.D., D.P.E.

Splanchnic and Muscle Metabolism During Exercise in NIDDM Patients

Martin IK, Katz A, Wahren J (Karolinska Inst, Stockholm; Victoria Univ, Australia)

Am J Physiol 269:E583–E590, 1995 7–11

Background.—Exercise training is known to produce long-term improvements in glycemic control in patients with non–insulin-dependent

TABLE 5.—Contribution of Gluconeogenic Substrates to Splanchnic Glucose Output at Rest and During Exercise

	NIDDM			Controls		
	Rest	10 min Ex	40 min Ex	Rest	10 min Ex	40 min Ex
Splanchnic glucose output, mmol/min	0.52 ± 0.06	1.74 ± 0.33	2.37 ± 0.26	0.79 ± 0.12	1.42 ± 0.20	2.44 ± 0.38
Splanchnic uptake, mmol/min						
Lactate	0.16 ± 0.04	0.33 ± 0.07	0.39 ± 0.08	0.11 ± 0.02	0.22 ± 0.13	0.32 ± 0.08
Pyruvate	0.002 ± 0.006	0.00	0.00	0.01 ± 0.01	0.00	0.01 ± 0.003
Glycerol	0.03 ± 0.01	0.04 ± 0.01	0.06 ± 0.01	0.03 ± 0.01	0.04 ± 0.01	0.08 ± 0.01
Amino acids	0.10 ± 0.02	0.06 ± 0.03	0.08 ± 0.01	0.14 ± 0.03	0.09 ± 0.03	0.08 ± 0.02
Total	0.29	0.43	0.53	0.29	0.35	0.48
Total uptake/glucose output, %	56	25	22	37	25	20

Note: Values are means ± standard error. Splanchnic uptake values are expressed as glucose equivalents; amino acid values are the sum of splanchnic uptake of glycogenic amino acids (Ala, Gly, Val, Ile, Phe, Tyr, Arg, His, Ser, Thr, Met, Asn, Gln, Glu).

Abbreviation: NIDDM, non–insulin-dependent diabetes mellitus.

(Courtesy of Martin IK, Katz A, Wahren J: Splanchnic and muscle metabolism during exercise in NIDDM patients. *Am J Physiol* 269:E583–E590, 1995.)

diabetes mellitus (NIDDM). Insulin sensitivity and glucose tolerance are enhanced. However, little is known about the metabolic changes occurring in NIDDM during an acute exercise bout. The metabolic response of patients with NIDDM to moderate exercise was determined by measuring exchange of glucose and other energy substrates across the leg and splanchnic bed.

Methods.—Eight nonobese men with NIDDM and 7 healthy controls exercised on a cycle ergometer for 40 minutes at 60% of maximal oxygen intake. Biopsy specimens were taken from the quadriceps femoris muscle at rest and just after exercise.

Findings.—At the end of exercise, arterial glucose concentration had declined by 10% in the patients with NIDDM and increased by 21% in the healthy individuals. Leg glucose uptake increased from a mean of 0.19 mmol/min at rest to 2.25 mmol/min at the end of exercise in the NIDDM group and from 0.13 to 1.17 mmol/min in the control group. Splanchnic glucose output rose from 0.52 to 2.37 mmol/min in the patients with NIDDM and from 0.79 to 2.44 mmol/min in the healthy individuals (Table 5). In the patients with NIDDM, leg lactate output during exercise was 2 times greater. At rest, the muscle contents of lactate and glycogen were similar in the 2 groups. After exercise, however, lactate tended to be higher and glycogen lower in the patients with NIDDM. The patients had a higher whole-body respiratory exchange ratio during exercise. Exercise-induced changes in other muscle metabolites were comparable in the 2 groups.

Conclusions.—In nonobese patients with NIDDM, moderate exercise produces a gradual decrease in blood glucose levels, a result of the increase in peripheral glucose utilization exceeding a normal rise in splanchnic glucose output. Patients with NIDDM have more stimulation of muscle carbohydrate utilization than controls do. Otherwise, the metabolic profiles of the muscle in patients and healthy individuals immediately after exercise are similar.

▶ These are interesting data. The only limitation on generalization of the findings is that both groups had very high maximal oxygen intakes for people in the sixth decade of life (3.63 L/min for the patients and 3.53 L/min for the controls).

R.J. Shephard, M.D., Ph.D., D.P.E.

Runner With Gout and an Aortic Valve Nodule

Moore GE, Anderson AL (Univ of Pittsburgh, Pa; Presbyterian Hosp, Dallas)
Med Sci Sports Exerc 27:626–628, 1995 7–12

Introduction.—Nearly all joint pain in athletes results from acute or chronic overuse injuries. One case report suggests that drinking beer after exercising in warm weather can precipitate acute gouty arthritis.

Case Report.—Man, 33, was a 2:50 marathoner who regularly ran 80–90 miles per week and often consumed 6 beers a day. He frequently took aspirin or indomethacin for relief of chronic musculoskeletal back and groin pain. After completing a 10-mile run and drinking several beers, the patient noted that his knee and his ankle became painful and swollen, and he experienced fever and night sweats. He sought medical attention 6 days later after failing to respond to some leftover antibiotics.

A cardiac examination identified a 2/6 systolic murmur in the aortic area, with a 1/6 diastolic murmur radiating from the aortic area to the apex. Laboratory data showed normal electrolyte and creatinine levels but an abnormal white blood cell count, hemoglobin level, and uric acid value. Borderline cardiomegaly was noted at chest x-ray examination and left ventricular hypertrophy at ECG. An echocardiogram revealed an aortic valve nodule and mild mitral valve thickening. A small amount of purulent material was aspirated from the left knee.

The patient was given nafcillin for presumed endocarditis with septic arthritis. On the second hospital day, analysis of synovial fluid from the right knee showed acute gout. The patient was then switched to IV colchicine and orally administered indomethacin, which brought about rapid improvement. The patient was advised to follow a low-purine diet, moderate his alcohol intake, and avoid dehydration during exercise. Allopurinol failed to resorb the unexplained valvular nodule.

Discussion.—Athletes who exercise in warm weather and then drink cold beer may be at risk of acute gout. Gout can lead to multiple joint involvement, and acute gout can mimic infectious endocarditis. Undertreated gout can progress to visceral gout, a rare cause of valvular heart nodules.

► Last year we reviewed an article emphasizing that occasionally rheumatologic diseases—when they cause pain or fatigue in athletes—can be sports injury look-alikes or can mimic overuse syndrome. That article highlighted a rower (aged 33 years) with sore shoulders as the harbinger of acute rheumatoid arthritis; a black female runner (aged 21 years) with knee pain and fatigue not from overtraining but from lupus; and a heavyset, beer-drinking, recreational basketball player (aged 39 years) with ankle pain that was not from a basketball injury but from gout.[1] This report reinforces this lesson; the runner aged 33 years precipitated acute gout (in his knee and ankle) by running in warm weather and quaffing beer afterward. It is not certain that the aortic valve nodule here was a gouty tophus, but this case serves to suggest that "sports medicine" is a microcosm of internal medicine.

E.R. Eichner, M.D.

Reference

1. 1995 Year Book of Sports Medicine, pp 506–508.

Patterns of Splenic Injuries Seen in Skiers

Sartorelli KH, Pilcher DB, Rogers FB (Med Ctr Hosp of Vermont, Burlington; Univ of Vermont, Burlington)

Injury 26:43–46, 1995 7–13

Objective.—The spleen is the most frequently injured abdominal organ in blunt trauma, but splenic injuries in skiing accidents appear to be rare. To gain insight into the epidemiology of splenic injuries resulting from ski accidents, all ski-related injuries over a 12-year period were retrospectively reviewed.

Patients.—Between 1979 and 1992, 18 patients were seen in a university hospital for splenic injuries secondary to skiing accidents. All were men.

Findings.—Splenic injuries secondary to ski trauma fell into 2 distinct patterns related to the mechanism of injury. Twelve skiers sustained splenic injuries during low-speed falls on moguls or the ski trail or low-speed impact with a trailside object (stump or rock). The other 6 skiers sustained splenic injuries during high-speed collisions with trees, lift towers, or other solid objects. All skiers who sustained low-speed falls had isolated splenic injuries and had no other significant concomitant injuries other than minor renal contusions (in 5 skiers). Eight skied down the mountain without assistance, and 6 of these skiers sought medical attention after an average delay of 3.75 hours; 2 of these skiers sought medical attention because of hematuria. In contrast, all skiers who had high-speed collisions were transported down the mountain by toboggan, had significant multisystem trauma in addition to their splenic injuries, and had higher morbidity from complications.

The operative rate was similar in both groups of skiers, although the splenic salvage rate was higher in the those who sustained low-speed falls (68%) than in those who sustained high-energy collisions (17%). Overall, concomitant renal injuries occurred in 10 of 18 patients, a rate higher than previously reported. The length of stay in the hospital or ICU, transfusion requirements, and complications were similar in both groups.

Implication.—Skiers who ski down a mountain after a low-speed collision may seek medical care after a delay and still have serious abdominal injury. An underlying splenic injury, particularly in someone with gross or microscopic hematuria, should be highly suspected. A potentially higher rate of spleen salvage may be expected in skiers who sustain low-impact falls.

▶ This report should help sports medicine physicians who cover ski resorts. It outlines 2 general patterns of spleen injury in skiers. The first is major trauma, from high-speed impacts with trees or the like; this usually requires splenectomy. In this regard, a recent report noted that 6 of 9 skier deaths in Colorado in 1990 were from collisions with trees.[1] The second and more subtle presentation is spleen injury (sometimes with renal contusion) from low-speed falls, as on moguls. Skiers with the latter injury tend to get up, ski down the mountain and wait before seeing a physician, sometimes because they see gross hematuria. With careful CT evaluation and close monitoring, these skiers, who tend to have minor spleen injury, may not need splenectomy. See also Abstract 7–14.

E.R. Eichner, M.D.

Reference

1. 1995 Year Book of Sports Medicine, pp 28–29.

Splenic Injury From Blunt Abdominal Trauma in Children: Follow-up Evaluation With CT

Benya EC, Bulas DI, Eichelberger MR, Sivit CJ (Children's Natl Med Ctr, Washington, DC; George Washington Univ, Washington, DC)

Radiology 195:685–688, 1995 7–14

Objective.—Most children with hemodynamically stable splenic injuries after blunt abdominal trauma can be treated successfully without surgery. This is the first study to evaluate the time course of splenic healing with follow-up CT in these children. To determine whether the initial CT grade of splenic injury could help predict rate of healing, 37 children were studied.

Methods.—The children, aged 12 months to 16 years, with splenic injury graded at emergent CT, were prospectively followed up with non-enhanced and contrast material–enhanced CT at 2 weeks to 11 months after injury. Using a modified classification of Mirvis et al., initial CT was classified as grade 1 in 3 patients with superficial laceration or subcapsular hematoma less than 1 cm in diameter; grade 2 in 12 patients with parenchymal lacerations 1–3 cm deep or central or subcapsular hematoma less than 3 cm in diameter; grade 3 in 11 patients with lacerations greater than 3 cm deep or central or subcapsular hematoma greater than 3 cm in diameter; and grade 4 in 11 patients with 3 or more lacerations greater than 3 cm deep or foci of devascularized spleen. All children were managed nonoperatively.

Outcome.—All 15 grade 1 and 2 splenic injuries healed at follow-up, including 8 in patients who underwent follow-up within 4 months after injury. All but 1 grade 3 splenic injuries healed by 6 months. In all grade 4 splenic injuries, residual lesions were evident within 4 months, and complete healing occurred up to 11 months. Contrast-enhanced CT scans allowed clear visualization of 5 of 9 residual splenic injuries, including 4

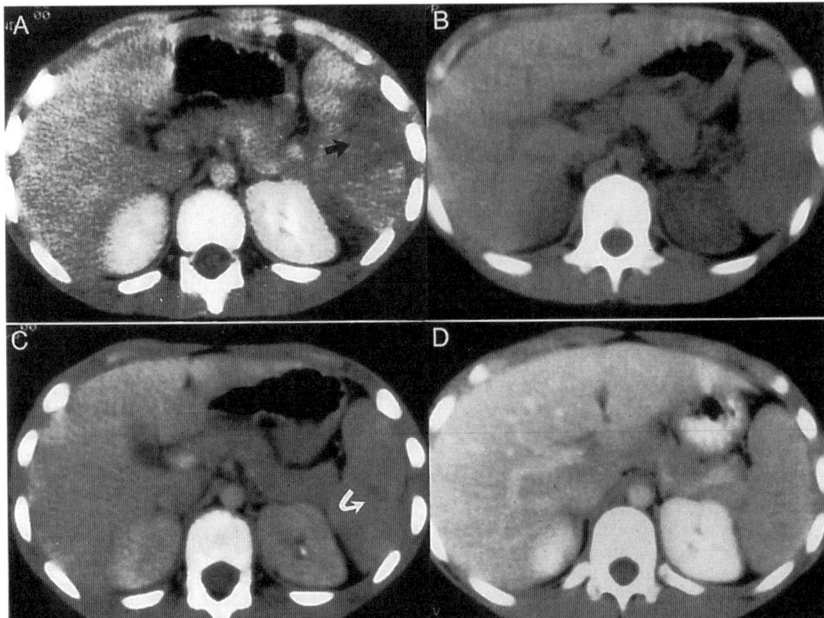

FIGURE 1.—Computed tomography scans of a boy 11 years of age injured in a bicycle accident. **A**, initial CT scan shows a grade 3 splenic injury *(arrow)* with splenic hematoma measuring more than 3 cm in diameter. Nonenhanced (**B**) and contrast-enhanced (**C**) follow-up CT scans obtained 4 months after injury. The nonenhanced image fails to show any intrasplenic hematoma. After IV administration of contrast material, a small residual area of intrasplenic hematoma *(arrow* C) is identified. **D**, second follow-up CT scan obtained 6 months after injury shows complete healing of the spleen. (Courtesy of Benya EC, Bulas DI, Eichelberger MR, et al: Splenic injury from blunt abdominal trauma in children: Follow-up evaluation with CT. *Radiology* 195:685–688, 1995, Radiological Society of North America.)

that were depicted as healed injuries on nonenhanced CT scans (Fig 1). Splenic calcification was evident in a child with persistent abdominal pain (Fig 2).

Recommendations.—The optimal time for follow-up CT scanning of splenic injury should be based on the grade of splenic injury established at initial CT. Grade 1 and 2 splenic injuries may be scanned at 2 months, grade 3 at 3 months, and grade 4 at 6 months. If unhealed, follow-up CT may be performed at 4 months for grade 1 and 2 injuries; 6 months, for grade 3; and 9 months, for grade 4.

▶ In 1993, we reviewed 2 practical articles on how to classify splenic trauma (via diagnostic imaging, especially the CT scan) and when to operate.[1] In general, grades I and 2 splenic injuries (e.g., subcapsular hematomas, localized capsular ruptures, or lacerations not involving the hilum or major vessels) are treated nonsurgically, whereas grades 3 and 4 injuries often need surgery. This article offers practical guidelines to personal and team physicians on how fast such splenic injuries can be expected to heal, based on serial CT imaging. In general, mild splenic injuries (grades 1 and 2) seem to heal by CT within 4 months, whereas grade 3 injuries take up to 6

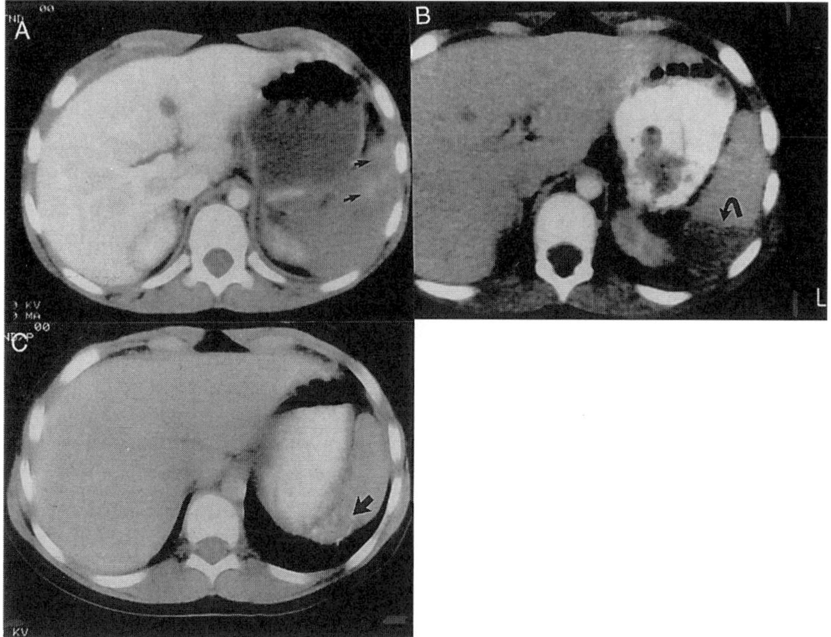

FIGURE 2.—Computed tomography scans of a boy 10 years of age with left-sided abdominal pain after a fall. **A,** initial CT scan shows a grade 4 splenic injury with devascularization of most of the spleen and 2 small foci (*arrows*) of enhancing splenic tissue. **B,** follow-up CT scan obtained 6 months after injury shows healing with persistent area of splenic injury posteriorly (*arrow*). **C,** second follow-up CT scan obtained 11 months after injury shows that the spleen has healed with calcification posteriorly (*arrow*). (Courtesy of Benya EC, Bulas DI, Eichelberger MR, et al: Splenic injury from blunt abdominal traumas in children: Follow-up evaluation with CT. *Radiology* 195:685–688, 1995, Radiological Society of North America.)

months and grade 4 injuries nearly a year to heal. The incidence, settings, features, and management of splenic rupture in infectious mononucleosis have also recently been reviewed.[2] See also Abstract 7–13.

E.R. Eichner, M.D.

References

1. 1993 YEAR BOOK OF SPORTS MEDICINE, pp 4–7.
2. Eichner ER: Infectious mononucleosis: Recognizing the condition, reactivating the patient. *Physician Sportsmed* 24:49, 1996.

Evaluation of Body Composition by Dual Energy X-ray Absorptiometry and Two Different Software Packages

van Loan MD, Keim NL, Berg K, Mayclin PL (Western Human Nutrition Research Ctr, San Francisco; Univ of Bonn, Germany)
Med Sci Sports Exerc 27:587–591, 1995 7–15

Background.—Assessing body composition is important for following the development of children, the course of disease, and recovery from illness. Various techniques are used to assess body composition; most use basic assumptions about the constancy of body compartments, which lead to inherent inaccuracies. Dual-energy x-ray absorptiometry can measure body composition, but changes in software may affect the data.

Objectives.—The purpose of this study was to examine the differences in body composition results from dual-energy x-ray absorptiometry using 2 software versions and to compare this method with hydrodensitometry in evaluating total body fat and fat-free mass.

Methods.—In 15 healthy women aged 20 to 40 years, whole-body density, body fat, and fat-free mass were measured densitometrically. Whole-body density was corrected for variations in bone mineral content. Fat and fat-free values were used as the criterion variable to compare the dual-energy x-ray absorptiometry results of Lunar software versions 3.4 and 3.6R. Bone mineral content and bone mineral density were evaluated using dual-energy x-ray absorptiometry. Total body and regional soft tissue also were assessed.

Results.—Analysis of pixel data showed a significant decrease of 5.5% in bone mineral content and a decrease of 1.8% in bone mineral density for total body from version 3.4 to version 3.6R. For the arm, bone mineral content increased 9.2% and bone mineral density increased 5.2%. For the leg, bone mineral content decreased 2.1% and bone mineral density increased 0.4%. The sum of bone mineral content and total soft tissue was comparable to body weight. The percentage total weight as fat was 39.9% for version 3.4 and 41.9% for version 3.6R. Results of body composition from version 3.6R and from densitometry were statistically different. Version 3.6R significantly underestimated fat-free mass compared with the criterion technique, by an average of 2.7% to 5.5%. Statistical differences were found between the 2 software versions for amount of fat tissue in the legs, trunk, and total body; version 3.6R had higher values. Version 3.6R had significantly lower values for fat tissue in the arms (Table 3).

TABLE 3.—Comparison of Soft-tissue Composition From Software Versions 3.4 and 3.6R

	Fat, g		
	Version 3.4	Version 3.6R	% Change
Arms	4,805 ± 2,503	3,610 ± 1,243*	24.9 ± 50.3
Legs	12,104 ± 3,135	12,673 ± 4,310*	4.7 ± 37.5
Trunk	11,763 ± 2,625	14,512 ± 4,012*	23.4 ± 52.8
Total	30,569 ± 8,193	32,061 ± 8,969*	4.9 ± 9.5
	Lean, g		
	Version 3.4	Version 3.6R	
Arms	5,427 ± 1,264	5,184 ± 728	4.5 ± 42.4
Legs	15,792 ± 2,000	14,602 ± 1,779*	7.5 ± 11.1
Trunk	19,631 ± 1,784	19,306 ± 1,630	1.7 ± 8.6
Total	42,865 ± 4,019	41,751 ± 3,739*	2.6 ± 7.0

* Denotes a significant difference ($P < 0.01$).

(Courtesy of van Loan MD, Keim NL, Berg K, et al: Evaluation of body composition by dual energy x-ray absorptiometry and two different software packages. *Med Sci Sports Exerc* 27:587–591, 1995.)

Discussion.—Significant differences were found between the body composition results from these 2 software packages. For overweight individuals, results of soft-tissue analysis from version 3.6R may not be as accurate as densitometry. The influence of tissue thickness on results of the dual-energy x-ray absorptiometry method needs further research. There is evidence that error increases with increasing depth of soft tissue. When comparing studies and results from different software versions, caution is recommended.

▶ The ease with which body composition can be assessed by dual-energy x-ray absorptiometry has led many investigators to select this technique as the method of choice for measuring the percentage of body fat without a thorough understanding of the factors that can influence the validity and reliability of the measurement. Van Loan et al. described 2 common problems that may influence the accuracy of the dual-energy x-ray absorptiometry measurement: the effect tissue thickness has on dual-energy x-ray absorptiometry results, and the effect a change in software can have on the measurement of body composition. Those who plan on using dual-energy x-ray absorptiometry in assessing changes in body composition over time would be wise not to change software during the course of the study.

B.L. Drinkwater, Ph.D.

Regular Exercise Dissociates Fat Mass and Bone Density in Premenopausal Women

Reid IR, Legge M, Stapleton JP, Evans MC, Grey AB (Univ of Auckland, New Zealand)

J Clin Endocrinol Metab 80:1764–1768, 1995 7–16

Background.—Body weight is a main determinant of bone density and fracture frequency, and weight loss has been found to be associated with decreased bone density. Study results differ regarding the contributions of the lean and fat components of body weight to bone density. The inconsistencies may result from using different methods of assessing body composition, using indices of bone density that are dependent on body size, or pooling data from different populations. Both body composition and bone density also are influenced by physical activity, which may affect the relationship. The objective of this study was to re-evaluate the dependence of bone density on body composition in physically active and sedentary premenopausal women.

Methods.—The study included 36 women with a mean age of 36 years who were not physically active, and 63 women with a mean age of 33 years who were physically active. Areal bone mineral density was measured in the lumbar spine, proximal femur, and total body. Body fat and lean mass were also measured for the total body. The effect of exercise on the relationships between these variables was determined. Patients reported their calcium intake in a questionnaire.

Results.—For inactive patients, bone mineral density was significantly weight dependent; both fat and lean tissues contributed to this relationship. A positive correlation was found between percentages of fat and bone mineral density/height throughout the skeleton. For active women, there was a weaker dependence of bone mineral density on weight; no dependence was noted in the proximal femur. Lean mass was related to bone mineral density, but there was a weaker relation of fat mass to bone mineral density. Fat mass was inversely related to bone mineral density in the proximal femur. Weight, fat mass, and lean mass were unrelated to bone mineral density/height. In the proximal femur, a positive correlation was found between the percentage of lean mass and bone mineral density/height.

Discussion.—The correlation between fat mass and bone density in physically inactive premenopausal women was confirmed. Customary levels of exercise can strongly affect this relationship. Re-evaluation of current literature and further research must take this effect into account.

▶ Any number of studies have examined the relationship of bone density to body composition using dual-energy x-ray absorptiometry technology. Unfortunately, there has been no consistent result. Some investigators have reported that the percentage of fat is the best predictor of bone mineral density; others, the percentage of lean body mass. Reid et al. suggested several reasons for the discrepancies, including differences between dual-energy x-ray absorptiometry instruments, and then add another potential confounding factor—physical activity. Obviously, the purpose of these studies is not to predict bone mineral density as that is actually measured by dual-energy x-ray absorptiometry but to examine the mechanisms responsible for the relationship. At this time, the variability in results makes any conclusion regarding mechanisms premature.

B.L. Drinkwater, Ph.D.

Differential Effects of Swimming Versus Weight-bearing Activity on Bone Mineral Status of Eumenorrheic Athletes

Taaffe DR, Snow-Harter C, Connolly DA, Robinson TL, Brown MD, Marcus R
(Stanford Univ, Calif; Oregon State Univ, Corvallis)

J Bone Miner Res 10:586–593, 1995 7–17

Introduction.—Physical activity appears to improve bone mass, but there are few data on what type, intensity, duration, and frequency of exercise are optimal for bone mineral accretion. In addition to weight-bearing forces, pull on the skeleton during muscular contraction could be an important osteogenic stimulus. Studies of bone mineral density (BMD) in swimmers, who perform forceful muscular contractions in the absence of weight bearing, have given conflicting results. The skeletal effects of loading patterns and repetitive muscular contraction were assessed in eumenorrheic women trained in high-impact weight-bearing vs. non–weight-bearing sports.

Methods.—Thirty-nine Division I college women athletes—26 swimmers and 13 gymnasts—and 19 nonathlete controls provided detailed information on their health, exercise, nutrition, and menstrual history. All of the women had had at least 10 menstrual cycles per year for at least the 2 previous years. For the athletes, calculation of training hours included not only sport-specific activity but also supplementary training.

Dual-energy x-ray absorptiometry was performed to measure BMD at the lumbar spine, femoral neck, trochanter, and whole body. Regional analyses of the arms, legs, ribs, thoracic and lumbar spine, and pelvis were performed using the whole-body scans. Bone-free lean mass (LM), fat mass, percentage of body fat, and regional fat distribution were assessed.

Results.—The swimmers were taller and heavier and had greater lean body mass than the gymnasts and controls. However, the difference between the 2 groups of athletes disappeared after adjustment for body surface area. Fat mass was lower for gymnasts, but there were no differences in body fat distribution. Although the gymnasts were older at menarche than the other 2 groups, there were no differences in menstrual history during the last year. The athletic groups trained a similar number of hours per week.

TABLE 2.—Bone Mineral Density, Bone Mineral Apparent Density, Bone Mineral Density Relative to Body Weight, and Percentage of Normative Database for the Lumbar Spine, Femoral Neck, Trochanter, and Whole Body

	Swimmers (n = 26)	Gymnasts (n = 13)	Controls (n = 19)	
Lumbar spine				
BMD	1.114 ± 0.095	1.199 ± 0.167	1.111 ± 0.110	
BMAD	0.168 ± 0.026	0.182 ± 0.023	0.167 ± 0.016	
BMD/Wt	0.017 ± 0.002	0.021 ± 0.002	0.019 ± 0.001	G > C, S*
BMD % norm	103.5 ± 9.2	112.0 ± 16.1	103.4 ± 10.3	
Femoral neck				
BMD	0.875 ± 0.105	1.117 ± 0.110	0.974 ± 0.105	G > C > S*
BMAD	0.189 ± 0.040	0.247 ± 0.028	0.228 ± 0.054	G, C > S†
BMD/Wt	0.013 ± 0.002	0.019 ± 0.002	0.016 ± 0.002	G > C > S*
BMD % norm	97.4 ± 10.8	124.2 ± 12.9	108.8 ± 11.5	G > C > S*
Trochanter				
BMD	0.748 ± 0.085	0.898 ± 0.130	0.784 ± 0.097	G > C, S†
BMD/Wt	0.012 ± 0.002	0.016 ± 0.001	0.013 ± 0.002	G > C > S*
BMD % norm	104.0 ± 12.0	125.2 ± 18.2	109.0 ± 13.3	G > C, S†
Whole body				
BMD	1.076 ± 0.066	1.127 ± 0.092	1.092 ± 0.064	
BMAD	0.085 ± 0.004	0.090 ± 0.004	0.087 ± 0.003	G > S‡
BMD/Wt	0.017 ± 0.002	0.020 ± 0.001	0.018 ± 0.001	G, C > S*
BMD % norm	97.6 ± 6.0	102.2 ± 8.5	99.2 ± 5.9	

Note: Values are mean ± standard deviation. Bone mineral density relative to body weight is measured in kilograms.
* $P < 0.0001$.
† $P < 0.001$.
‡ $P < 0.005$.
Abbreviations: BMD (g/cm^2), bone mineral density; *BMAD* (g/cm^3), bone mineral apparent density; *% norm*, percentage of normative database.

(Courtesy of Taaffe DR, Snow-Harter C, Connolly DA, et al: Differential effects of swimming versus weight-bearing activity on bone mineral status of eumenorrheic athletes. *J Bone Miner Res* 10:586–593, 1995. Reprinted by permission of Blackwell Science, Inc.)

Bone mineral density values for the lumbar spine and the whole body were not significantly different between groups. However, femoral neck BMD was greater in gymnasts than in controls and greater in controls than in swimmers. Trochanter BMD was greater in gymnasts than in controls and swimmers. Gymnasts had greater lumbar spine BMD after adjustment for body weight. On subregion analyses, the gymnasts had greater arm BMD than the swimmers and controls and greater leg BMD than the swimmers. No difference was found in thoracic spine BMD, but lumbar spine and pelvis BMD from the whole-body scan were greater in gymnasts than in swimmers and controls (Table 2). For gymnasts and controls, LM was an independent predictor of BMD at the femoral neck, trochanter, and whole body. Lumbar spine BMD was predicted by LM and menarcheal age in controls, but only by menarcheal age in gymnasts. Thirty-eight percent of the variance in whole-body BMD in swimmers was explained by body weight and height.

Conclusions.—In college gymnasts with normal menstruation, BMD is greater at both the axial and appendicular sites than in nonathletic controls. In contrast, the BMD of college swimmers is not significantly different from that of controls. Where there is a difference—at the femoral neck—BMD is lower in swimmers than in controls. High-impact loading of the type encountered in gymnastics appears to be a powerful osteogenic stimulus. In contrast, swimming—which is characterized by powerful muscular contractions in the absence of weight bearing—has no significant benefit in terms of BMD. Skeletal responsiveness to high-impact loading should be assessed in an intervention study.

► Evidence has been accumulating that swimming is not an activity that encourages increases in bone density. What is puzzling is that here is another group in which additional training in the form of running or cycling and resistance training did not provide swimmers with any advantage in bone density compared with sedentary controls. Once again, details related to the non–sport-specific training are missing, so one cannot compare the training regimen with that of the previous study.

In addition to the impact loading of gymnastic routines, the gymnasts may have benefited from beginning their training at a younger age. Animal studies suggest that young animals not only respond more quickly to bone-loading activities but that the adaptive response is greater. Although studies of children and adolescents are few in number, some evidence indicates that the same response occurs in boys and girls.

B.L. Drinkwater, Ph.D.

Bone Mineral Density in Female Athletes Representing Sports With Different Loading Characteristics of the Skeleton

Heinonen A, Oja P, Kannus P, Sievänen H, Haapasalo H, Mänttäri A, Vuori I (UKK Inst, Tampere, Finland; Tampere Research Station of Sport Medicine, Finland)

Bone 17:197–203, 1995 7–18

Background.—The osteogenic effects of physical loading may increase with increasing peak forces and strain rates. To test this hypothesis, a cross-section study evaluated the bone mineral density (BMD) of squash players, aerobic dancers, speed skaters, and their controls.

Participants and Methods.—Fifty-nine competitive Finnish female athletes were studied: 18 squash players, 27 aerobic dancers, and 14 speed skaters; as well as 25 physically active referents reporting an average of 5 various types of exercise sessions per week and 25 healthy sedentary referents reporting 2 exercise sessions per week. None of the participants were amenorrheic. Twenty-one of the athletes reported oral contraceptive use. Calcium intake was estimated using a 7-day intake diary. Directly evaluated maximal oxygen uptake served as the measure of cardiorespiratory fitness. A strain gauge dynamometer was used to determine maximal isometric strength of the trunk extensors and flexors and dominant forearm flexors, and an isometric leg press dynamometer was used to measure maximal strength of leg extensors. Dual-energy x-ray absorptiometry was used to determine bone mineral density (BMD) at the lumbar spine (L2–L4), femoral neck, distal femur, patella, proximal tibia, calcaneus, and distal radius of the dominant extremity.

Results.—No significant differences in BMD were observed at any skeletal site among participants with different calcium intakes. Athletes were found to have a higher maximal oxygen uptake compared with the physi-

TABLE 2.—Bone Mineral Density of the Athlete Groups, the Physically Active Reference Group, and Sedentary Reference Group, Mean (Standard Deviations)

	BMD (g/cm^2)				
Skeletal Site	Squash players n = 18	Aerobic dancers n = 27	Speed skaters n = 14	Physically active reference n = 25	Sedentary reference n = 25
Lumbar spine (L2–4)	1.216 (0.131)‡	1.092 (0.111)	1.138 (0.129)	1.071 (0.103)	1.059 (0.106)
Femoral neck	1.155 (0.117)‡	1.041 (0.107)†	1.031 (0.107)	0.983 (0.114)	0.971 (0.128)
Distal femur	1.405 (0.094)†	1.291 (0.124)	1.357 (0.105)*	1.261 (0.118)	1.248 (0.125)
Patella	1.127 (0.080)*	1.063 (0.084)	1.116 (0.115)	1.057 (0.109)	1.045 (0.107)
Proximal tibia	1.220 (0.085)†	1.120 (0.099)*	1.151 (0.123)	1.104 (0.105)	1.071 (0.106)
Calcaneus	0.760 (0.081)‡	0.709 (0.062)‡	0.661 (0.070)	0.671 (0.083)	0.631 (0.064)
Distal radius	0.409 (0.055)†	0.334 (0.040)†	0.352 (0.032)	0.350 (0.046)	0.368 (0.044)

* Significant mean difference between sedentary reference group and the given group: $P < 0.05$.
† Significant mean difference between sedentary reference group and the given group: $P < 0.01$.
‡ Significant mean difference between sedentary reference group and the given group: $P < 0.001$.

cally active and sedentary referents. The highest weight-adjusted BMD values were noted among the squash players at all measured skeletal sites (Table 2). Significantly higher BMD values also were noted for aerobic dancers and speed skaters at the loaded sites, compared with the sedentary reference group. Between-group differences ranged between 5.3% and 13.5%. No differences in BMD values were observed between the physically active and the sedentary referent groups at any site.

Conclusions.—Both high strain rates in versatile movements and high peak forces have a greater effect on bone formation than does training with a large number of low-force repetitions.

▶ Although weight-bearing activity is considered essential in maintaining bone density, there are still unanswered questions as to the type of activity and the intensity, frequency, and duration that are most effective as an osteogenic stimulus. Cross-section studies such as this one provide data to stimulate hypotheses that can be tested in carefully designed prospective studies. Of particular interest in this study is that the bone density of the physically active women did not differ significantly from that of the sedentary controls. This observation reinforces that of Mazess and Barden,[1] who reported no difference in the bone density of the spine, femoral neck, or radius between college women grouped by quartiles of physical activity.

In this study, 5 hours of activity per week did not benefit the bones—at least as reflected by BMD. In recommending exercise as a means of decreasing the risk of osteoporosis, we have to take into account the likelihood that most women are willing or able to take up those activities that have been shown to be effective in increasing bone density. Fortunately, aerobic dance appears to have a slight but positive effect on bone density at most sites, for not many women will have the opportunity to add squash or speed skating to their activity program.

B.L. Drinkwater, Ph.D.

Reference

1. Mazess RB, Barden H: Bone density in premenopausal women: Effect of age, dietary intake, physical activity, smoking, and birth-control pills. *Am J Clin Nutr* 53:132–142, 1991.

A Comparison of Bone Mineral Densities Among Female Athletes in Impact Loading and Active Loading Sports

Fehling PC, Alekel L, Clasey J, Rector A, Stillman RJ (Skidmore College, Saratoga Springs, NY; Univ of Illinois, Urbana)

Bone 17:205–210, 1995 7–19

Background.—Evidence suggests that children who take part in impact-loading sports—for example, running, gymnastics, and tumbling—have greater bone mineral density (BMD) at the femoral neck than children participating in active, nongravitational activities, such as swimming. The purpose of this study was to compare BMDs in female college athletes in impact-loading vs. active-loading sports.

Methods.—Forty-five healthy white women competing at the Division I level and 17 nonathletic controls were studied. Twenty-one women were in impact-loading sports—that is, volleyball and gymnastics—and 7 were in swimming, an active-loading sport. Most women were eumenorrheic, except for the gymnasts, most of whom were oligomenorrheic. Fifteen women were current or former users of oral contraceptives. All 3 groups underwent dual-energy x-ray absorptiometry for measurement of total-body and regional bone mass. Body density was assessed by hydrostatic weighing and used to calculate the percentage of body fat.

Results.—The volleyball players were taller and heavier than the other groups, and the swimmers were taller than the gymnasts and controls and heavier than the gymnasts. However, no significant differences were found in body mass index. The gymnasts were significantly older at menarche than those in any of the other activity groups (Table 2).

At most sites, the volleyball players had significantly greater BMD than the swimmers or controls. In addition, the volleyball players had significantly greater total-body and left- and right-leg BMD than the gymnasts. Torso BMD was not significantly different between groups. On correction for height and weight differences by analysis of covariance, the volleyball players and gymnasts had significantly increased BMD at the lumbar spine, femoral neck, Ward's triangle, total body, right leg, and pelvis, compared with the swimmers and the controls. The gymnasts had significantly greater right- and left-arm BMD than all other groups. The swimmers and controls were similar in BMD at all sites (Table 3).

TABLE 2.—Descriptive Characteristics (Mean ± Standard Deviation) of Patients Grouped by Physical Activity

	Physical activity			
Measurement	Volleyball (n = 8)	Swimming (n = 7)	Gymnastics (n = 13)	Control (n = 17)
Age (years)	19.5 ± 1.3	20.1 ± 0.8	19.6 ± 1.0	20.8 ± 1.2
Height (cm)	181.6 ± 4.5*	170.9 ± 5.3†	161.4 ± 4.5	162.6 ± 5.4
Weight (kg)	76.3 ± 7.1*	65.6 ± 5.7‡	55.6 ± 4.8	58.6 ± 10.5
BMI (kg/m^2)	23.2	22.5	21.3	22.2
Body fat (%)	24.2 ± 2.7	23.9 ± 3.9	19.0 ± 3.9‖	27.5 ± 5.8
Lean body mass (kg)	57.8 ± 5.2*	49.9 ± 5.0§	45.0 ± 3.9	42.1 ± 5.0
Menarche (age)	13.7 ± 0.9	13.9 ± 1.9	15.7 ± 1.4¶	12.7 ± 1.0
Training onset (age)	11.7 ± 1.8	7.8 ± 7.9	9.9 ± 2.2	
Years competing	8.0 ± 2.8	12.3 ± 3.0	9.8 ± 2.3	

* $P < 0.05$; volleyball greater than swimming, gymnastic, and control.
† $P < 0.05$; swimming greater than gymnastic and control.
‡ $P < 0.05$; swimming greater than gymnastic.
§ $P < 0.05$; swimming greater than control.
‖ $P < 0.05$; gymnastic less than control.
¶ $P < 0.05$; gymnastic greater than volleyball, swimming, and control.

TABLE 3.—Mean (Mean ± Standard Deviation) Bone Mineral Densities (g/cm²) Grouped by Physical Activity

Skeletal Site	Physical Activity			
	Volleyball	Swimming	Gymnastic	Control
Lumbar spine (L1–4)	1.22 ± 0.11*	1.05 ± 0.07	1.17 ± 0.12*	1.02 ± 0.07
Femoral neck	1.12 ± 0.09*	0.92 ± 0.05	1.06 ± 0.10*	0.91 ± 0.07
Ward's triangle	1.05 ± 0.12*	0.83 ± 0.04	0.95 ± 0.11*	0.80 ± 0.08
Total body	1.29 ± 0.06†	1.14 ± 0.05	1.22 ± 0.08‡	1.11 ± 0.05
Left arm	0.99 ± 0.05§	0.92 ± 0.03	1.00 ± 0.09‡	0.86 ± 0.06
Right arm	1.03 ± 0.08*	0.90 ± 0.03	1.00 ± 0.07*	0.85 ± 0.06
Left leg	1.48 ± 0.09†	1.23 ± 0.04	1.32 ± 0.07‡	1.20 ± 0.07
Right leg	1.46 ± 0.08†	1.25 ± 0.04	1.35 ± 0.07‡	1.22 ± 0.06
Pelvis	1.42 ± 0.11*	1.20 ± 0.06	1.35 ± 0.14*	1.17 ± 0.09
Torso	0.94 ± 0.08‖	0.85 ± 0.05	0.87 ± 0.08‖	0.79 ± 0.04

Note: Under skeletal site, the total body includes the head, and the torso is the sum of the left and right ribs, thoracic spine, and lumbar spine from total body scan.

* $P < 0.05$; volleyball and gymnastic greater than swimming and control.

† $P < 0.05$; volleyball greater than swimming, gymnastic, and control.

‡ $P < 0.05$; gymnastic greater than swimming and control.

§ $P < 0.05$; volleyball greater than swimming and control.

‖ $P < 0.05$; volleyball and gymnastic greater than control.

Conclusions.—The type of mechanical loading activity in sports has a key effect on BMD. Women athletes in impact-loading sports—those that load the skeletal system with high-magnitude, short-duration stimuli—have greater BMD than nonathletes or athletes in sports that do not involve ground reaction forces. Thus, impact bone loading leads to site-specific increases in BMD. Menstrual irregularities in the gymnasts did not appear to have an adverse effect on BMD at any site.

► This study raises a number of interesting issues for further research. Why, for example, did year-round training with weights plus running 5–10 miles per week in the off-season have no apparent positive effect on the bone density of swimmers, compared with the controls who exercised less than 1 hour per week? Does the mechanical loading of gymnastic routines offset the negative effect of low endogenous estrogen levels on bone? If so, what is the minimum effective strain stimulus required to afford this protection? Or is it a mistake to draw conclusions about the effect of menstrual irregularities on bone when combining amenorrheic, oligomenorrheic, and eumenorrheic athletes into 1 group? Is the effect of delayed menarche on an athlete's bone density dependent on the sport? Although cross-section studies such as this one can not answer the basic questions related to cause and effect, they can—and do—raise questions that stimulate further inquiry.

B.L. Drinkwater, Ph.D.

Variations in Bone Status of Contralateral and Regional Sites in Young Athletic Women

Lee EJ, Long KA, Risser WL, Poindexter HBW, Gibbons WE, Goldzieher J (Rice Univ, Houston, Univ of Texas, Houston; Baylor College of Medicine, Houston)

Med Sci Sports Exerc 27:1354–1361, 1995 7–20

Background.—Although weight-bearing exercise is thought to have salutary effects on bone mineral density (BMD), the skeletal effects of specific athletic activities remain incompletely understood. Both cortical and trabecular bone respond to mechanical stress that loads specific sites, but trabecular bone responds more rapidly.

Objective and Methods.—Site-specific differences in regional, contralateral, and whole-body BMD were sought by examining 62 eumenorrheic athletes and controls. The athletes included 7 basketball players, 11 volleyball players, 9 soccer players, and 7 swimmers. Seventeen moderately active and 11 sedentary control women also were studied. About 40% of both groups reported oral contraceptive use. Bone mineral density was measured by dual-energy x-ray absorptiometry in the L2–L4 region of the lumbar spine, proximal femur, arms, legs, pelvis, and spine.

Findings.—Between-sport comparisons showed relatively high upper extremity BMD in basketball and volleyball players. Within-sport contralateral comparisons showed higher BMD in the right than in the left arm in all groups except swimmers. Total-body and lumbar BMD values were highest in the volleyball and basketball players (Table 3). Femoral BMD was highest in basketball players.

Discussion.—Weight-bearing activity has a favorable effect on the skeleton. Site-specific differences in BMD were demonstrated in athletes participating in different forms of sports activity. Swimmers did not differ from controls, except in the arm, which argues against the muscle pull theory for effecting positive changes in bone mass.

▶ One of the problems associated with identifying the site-specific effect of various sports on bone density is the wide use of strength training and other non–sport specific activities as an adjunct to the sport-specific training regimens. In this group of athletes, the authors report that the strength training was designed to develop "areas specific to their sport," but they do not describe these sites; the type of training; the number of sets, repetitions, weights or resistance, and so on. If we are ever going to be able to identify the effect of various sports on bone, all activities that load that site must be identified and described fully. In this study, for example, we cannot be sure whether the higher arm bone density of volleyball and basketball players was caused by the sport or caused because they trained with weights and the soccer players did not.

B.L. Drinkwater, Ph.D.

TABLE 3.—Total Body, Lumbar, Femur, Regional, and Contralateral Arm and Leg Bone Mineral Density Measurements of Athletes and Nonathletes

Variable	VB (n = 11)	BB (n = 7)	SO (n = 9)	SW (n = 7)	MOD (n = 17)	SED (n = 11)
Total body	1.23 ± 0.02§*†	1.24 ± 0.03§*†	1.20 ± 0.02	1.13 ± 0.02**‡	1.13 ± 0.02**‡	1.15 ± 0.02**‡
Lumbar	1.38 ± 0.04¶§*†	1.33 ± 0.05§*†	1.24 ± 0.04**	1.20 ± 0.05**‡	1.18 ± 0.03**‡	1.17 ± 0.04**‡
Femur neck	1.17 ± 0.04§*	1.26 ± 0.04¶§*†	1.16 ± 0.04‡§*	0.99 ± 0.04**‡¶	1.01 ± 0.03**‡¶	1.05 ± 0.04‡
Femur trochanter	0.97 ± 0.04§*	1.03 ± 0.04§*†	0.96 ± 0.04*	0.83 ± 0.04**‡	0.79 ± 0.02**‡¶	0.83 ± 0.03‡
Femur Ward's	1.08 ± 0.06	1.23 ± 0.06§*†	1.16 ± 0.05	1.00 ± 0.06‡	1.00 ± 0.04‡	1.04 ± 0.05‡
Spine	1.22 ± 0.04†	1.25 ± 0.04*†	1.21 ± 0.04	1.17 ± 0.04	1.17 ± 0.03**‡	1.15 ± 0.04**‡
Pelvis	1.25 ± 0.03§*†	1.27 ± 0.03§*†	1.22 ± 0.03*	1.10 ± 0.03**‡	1.09 ± 0.02**‡¶	1.14 ± 0.03**‡
Left arm	1.02 ± 0.02¶*†	1.02 ± 0.03¶*†	0.92 ± 0.03**‡	0.95 ± 0.03	0.89 ± 0.02**‡	0.91 ± 0.02**‡
Right arm	1.06 ± 0.03¶§*†	1.06 ± 0.03¶§*†	0.97 ± 0.03**†	0.96 ± 0.03**‡	0.93 ± 0.02**‡	0.94 ± 0.03**‡
Left leg	1.44 ± 0.03§*†	1.42 ± 0.04§*†	1.36 ± 0.03§*†	1.22 ± 0.05**‡¶	1.24 ± 0.03**‡¶	1.23 ± 0.03**‡¶
Right leg	1.41 ± 0.03§*†	1.44 ± 0.04§*†	1.37 ± 0.03§*†	1.20 ± 0.04**‡¶	1.22 ± 0.02**‡¶	1.23 ± 0.03**‡¶

Note: All values are reported as mean ± standard error in the units of g/cm^2.
** Volleyball.
‡ Basketball.
¶ Soccer.
§ Swimming.
* Moderately active control.
† Sedentary control.
**,‡,¶,§,*,† Significant difference at $P \leq 0.05$.
(Courtesy of Lee EJ, Long KA, Risser WL, et al: Variations in bone status of contralateral and regional sites in young athletic women. *Med Sci Sports Exerc* 27:1354–1361, 1995.)

Refractory Pelvic Stress Fracture in a Female Long-distance Runner
O'Brien T, Wilcox N, Kersch T (Naval Hosp, Pensacola, Fla)
Am J Orthop 10:710–713, 1995 7–21

Purpose.—No more than 2% of stress fractures occur in the pelvis. These fractures are most common in female long-distance runners and generally heal within 6 to 12 weeks of activity restriction. A case of pelvic stress fracture occurred in a female runner with amenorrhea and osteoporosis.

Case Report.—Woman, 42, sought attention for pain in her left hip after running. She jogged 35–40 miles per week and had exercise-associated amenorrhea. Dual-energy x-ray absorptiometry detected osteoporosis, which was treated with estrogen replacement therapy and calcium. An initial bone scan was normal; however, a repeat scan made after 5 more weeks of running showed increased uptake in the superior ramus and ischium.

The patient stopped running for 2 months. She required crutches and restricted weight bearing because of pain on walking. Six-month follow-up radiographs revealed sclerosis and cystic changes in the ischial stress fracture. An electrical bone growth stimulator was applied for this delayed union. After 3 months of stimulation, the patient was able to resume running up to 1 mile without symptoms. Her radiographic picture improved, and she was weaned from the electrical stimulator by wearing it at night only for 4 weeks. Thereafter she was able to run 25 miles per week without symptoms.

Discussion.—Female runners with exercise amenorrhea may be at risk of having osteoporosis develop and thus of pelvic stress fracture. This diagnosis should be considered in any runner with hip or groin pain while running. Symptoms resolve in most patients with activity restriction; the literature provides little guidance in the rare instance of delayed union. In this situation, electrical stimulation may be tried before resorting to bone grafting.

► A number of investigators have examined the incidence of stress fractures in amenorrheic and eumenorrheic athletes. Some report a higher incidence in amenorrheic athletes; others find no difference. As we know, a stress fracture is basically an overuse injury. However, the 35–40 miles per week this women averaged would not be considered excessive by most runners unless it were a sudden increase in mileage.

An interesting question is whether threshold for overuse is lowered in amenorrheic women because of a decrease in bone density. More information should be gathered about the rate of recovery in this population. It may be that delayed healing of stress fractures and irreversible bone loss share the same underlying mechanism.

B.L. Drinkwater, Ph.D.

Is Running Associated With Osteoarthritis? An Eight-year Follow-up Study

Panush RS, Hanson CS, Caldwell JR, Longley S, Stork J, Thoburn R (Saint Barnabas Med Ctr, Livingston, NJ; Univ of Medicine and Dentistry of New Jersey, Newark; Univ of Florida, Gainesville; et al)

J Clin Rheumatol 1:35–39, 1995 7–22

Background.—The long-term consequences, if any, of recreational exercise on the musculoskeletal system are only recently being examined. Eight-year follow-up observations regarding the association of recreational running and osteoarthritis were reviewed.

Methods.—Attempts were made to contact all 35 research subjects in the authors' 1984 study; 22 were located and agreed to participate. A detailed medical, family, and running history questionnaire was completed by all participants—12 runners and 10 nonrunners. Each underwent a physical examination of the lower extremities by a rheumatologist, a lower extremity joint range-of-motion evaluation by an occupational therapist, and radiographic examinations of the hips, knees, and feet.

Results.—Range-of-motion and clinical findings for lower extremity joints were not significantly different for runners and nonrunners. Similarly, x-ray scans showed no significant difference between runners and nonrunners in cartilage thickness or grades of osteoarthritis in the lower extremity joints at either original or follow-up evaluations. The numbers of osteophytes were similar in both runners and nonrunners.

Conclusions.—Reasonable recreational exercise does not predispose individuals to joint injury.

► Whether running contributes to osteoarthritis is a time-honored and never-ending debate; we review it frequently. Some studies basically agree with the 1986 report by Panush et al.[1] that reasonable long-term, high-mileage running is not associated with premature osteoarthritis of the lower extremity. Concurring with this view, for example, is a cross-section study of 30 runners (vs. controls) who had run for 40 years[2] and a 5-year longitudinal study of the Stanford 50-Plus Runners Association, which found that running did not accelerate osteoarthritis of the knee.[3] Other studies, however, do find a link between certain sports and osteoarthritis. An early study, for example, noted osteoarthritis of the hip in retired soccer players.[4] A case-control study from Sweden tied high exposure to sports of all kinds to risk of developing osteoarthritis of the hip.[5] Recent epidemiologic studies from Switzerland and from Sweden tie running and track-and-field activities to osteoarthritis of the hip.[6, 7] Now, in the current report, comes a follow-up from Panush et al. that supports their original conclusion. Eight years later, the runners, now in their seventh decade, still show no more osteoarthritis than the controls. This is a small group of research subjects, but Panush et al. still conclude that running need not be associated with a predisposition to osteoarthritis of the lower extremities. No study yet is definitive; the beat goes on.

E.R. Eichner, M.D.

References

1. Panush RS, Edward NL, Longley S, et al: The relation of running to bone and joint disease. *JAMA* 256:716, 1986.
2. 1991 Year Book of Sports Medicine, pp 354–355.
3. 1994 Year Book of Sports Medicine, pp 317–318.
4. Klunder KB, Rud B, Hansen J: Osteoarthritis of the hip and knee joint in retired football players. *Acta Orthop Scand* 51:925, 1980.
5. 1994 Year Book of Sports Medicine, pp 4–5.
6. Marti B, Knoblach M, Tschopp A, et al: Is excessive running predictive of degenerative hip disease? Controlled study of former elite athletes. *BMJ* 229:91–93, 1989.
7. Vingard E, Sandmark H, Alfredsson L, et al: Muskuloskeletal disorders in former athletes: A cohort study in 114 track and field champions. *Acta Orthop Scand* 66:289–291, 1995.

8 Gender, Age, Disability, Infections

Effects of Long-term Moderate Exercise on Iron Status in Young Women

Rajaram S, Weaver CM, Lyle RM, Sedlock DA, Martin B, Templin TJ, Beard JL, Percival SS (Purdue Univ, West Lafayette, Ind; Pennsylvania State Univ, State College; Univ of Florida, Gainesville)

Med Sci Sports Exerc 27:1105–1110, 1995 8–1

Introduction.—Women athletes commonly have problems with iron deficiency, ranging from depletion of body iron stores to more severe forms resulting in anemia. Compared with male athletes, women are at increased risk as a result of blood loss associated with menstruation and an inadequate iron intake. There is increasing attention to the possibility of similar changes in iron status among previously sedentary women who start exercise programs.

Objectives.—The effects of long-term aerobic exercise on iron status in previously sedentary young women were assessed. Causes were sought for any changes observed, and the effects of iron supplementation were assessed.

Methods.—Sixty-two previously sedentary college women were studied. After a hemoglobin screening test, the women were randomized into 4 groups. Group 1 received a 50 mg/d iron supplement and a low-iron diet; group 2 received placebo and a free-choice diet; group 3 received lean meat supplements plus a high-iron diet to achieve an iron intake of 15 mg/d; and group 4 received no supplement and followed a free-choice diet. Groups 1 to 3 participated in a 6-month aerobic exercise program in which they exercised 3 days a week at 60% to 75% of heart rate reserve. Blood was drawn for assessment of iron status at baseline and every 4 weeks thereafter for 24 weeks. Aerobic fitness and body composition were measured at baseline and 24 weeks.

Results.—None of the groups had a change in hematocrit during the study. Hemoglobin varied considerably from weeks 8 to 24, by which time groups 1 and 4 had a significant increase in hemoglobin and group 3 had a positive trend. Only group 1 had a difference in prestudy and poststudy values for serum iron. Group 1 also had a significant increase in transferrin saturation, whereas all other groups had a decline (Fig 1). Serum ferritin

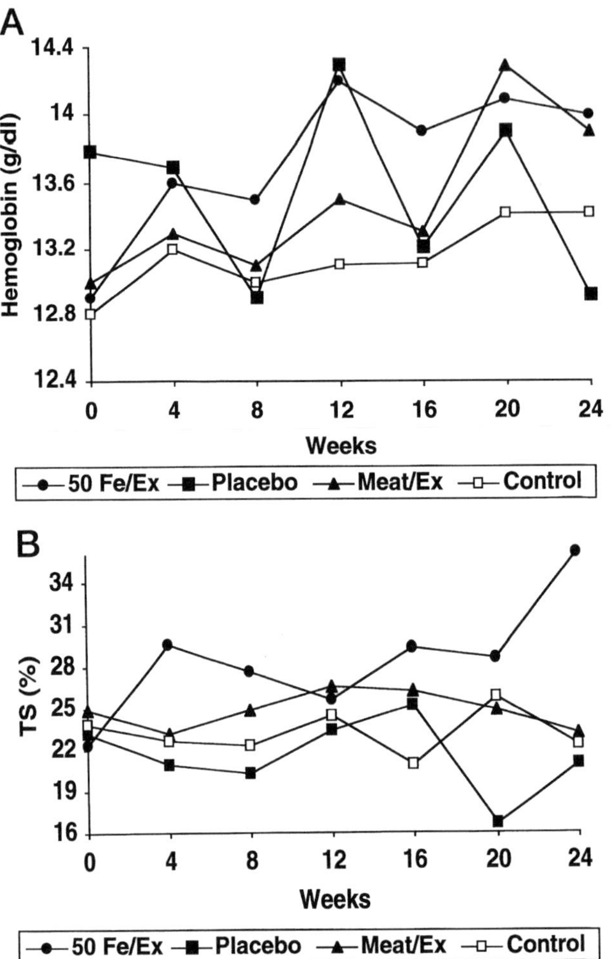

FIGURE 1.—**A:** Hemoglobin (grams per deciliter) from baseline to 24 weeks in the experimental groups. **B:** Percentage transferrin saturation from baseline to 24 weeks in the experimental groups. (Courtesy of Rajaram S, Weaver CM, Lyle RM, et al: Effects of long-term moderate exercise on iron status in young women. *Med Sci Sports Exerc* 27:1105–1110, 1995.)

value remained less than 15 ng/mL in all groups, indicating that the women were iron depleted. Group 3 had a significant increase in haptoglobin. There were no differences between groups in serum erythropoietin.

Conclusion.—In previously sedentary young women who begin an exercise program, hemoglobin levels may be compromised if dietary iron intake is inadequate. Iron supplementation improves iron status in such women. Lean meat supplementation may improve only hemoglobin levels, while failing to increase iron stores. It cannot be concluded that exercise causes decreased hemoglobin; rather, the impact of exercise most likely depends on various factors, including initial iron status, the nature and intensity of exercise, and the dietary iron level. The public should be advised to maintain normal iron status when starting an exercise program.

► Perhaps the most sobering result of this study was finding that ferritin levels in all 4 groups of sedentary college women indicated that they were iron depleted when the study began and remained so during the course of the study. After returning from a 2-week break, their iron status had improved, leading the investigators to speculate that dietary iron intake had increased and/or exercise compliance had decreased while they were on break. Although wholesale iron supplementation for college-age women is not the answer, young women—especially those involved in strenuous exercise programs—do need to be aware that low dietary iron intake does place them at risk for iron depletion.

B.L. Drinkwater, Ph.D.

Effects of Menstrual Cycle Phase on Athletic Performance

Lebrun CM, McKenzie DC, Prior JC, Taunton JE (Univ of British Columbia, Vancouver, Canada)

Med Sci Sports Exerc 27:437–444, 1995 8–2

Background.—Most past studies on how exercise performance is affected by menstrual function have involved moderately trained women. Relatively few have dealt with highly trained athletes—those most likely to be affected by subtle decrements in performance. Conceivably, the metabolic actions of female steroid hormones influence different components of performance variables in the course of an ovulatory cycle.

Objective.—Sixteen women 18–40 years of age with regular menstrual cycles participated in a study relating performance to aerobic capacity, anaerobic capacity, high-intensity endurance (at 90% of peak oxygen uptake), and isokinetic strength. The participants had not used oral contraception for at least 6 months. All regularly performed some type of intensive aerobic activity and had an initial peak oxygen uptake of at least 50 mL/kg per minute.

Methods.—Physiologic testing was performed in the early follicular phase (days 3–8) of a normal cycle and also in the midluteal phase (4–9 days after ovulation), as determined by a sustained rise in basal body temperature and confirmed by serum estrogen and progesterone estimates. Subjects performed continuous treadmill exercise at a level grade (starting at 2.2 m/sec) and increasing by 0.22 m/sec each minute to the point of fatigue. The anaerobic speed test used time to fatigue as the performance index. Endurance capacity was the running time to fatigue at about 90% of maximal oxygen uptake. Knee flexion and extension isokinetic strength was measured at 30°/sec.

Results.—Body composition did not change appreciably in the course of the menstrual cycle, nor did hemoglobin or hematocrit levels differ. Absolute peak oxygen uptake was slightly higher in the follicular than in the

TABLE 3.—Effect of Menstrual Cycle Phase on Performance Variables

Variable	Phase of Cycle Follicular	Luteal	Paired *t*-Test (df= 15)	Mean Difference
$\dot{V}O_{2max}$ ($l \cdot min^{-1}$)	3.19 ± 0.09	3.13 ± 0.08	P = 0.04	+0.06 ± 0.03*
$\dot{V}O_{2max}$ ($ml \cdot kg^{-1} \cdot min^{-1}$)	53.7 ± 0.9	52.8 ± 0.8	P = 0.06	+0.93 ± 0.46†
HR(max) (bpm)	189.4 ± 2.3	189.5 ± 2.6	P = 0.92	−0.13 ± 1.28
RER(max)	1.17 ± 0.01	1.15 ± 0.01	P = 0.56	+0.01 ± 0.01
$\dot{V}_E$(max) ($l \cdot min^{-1}$(BTPS))	105.4 ± 2.3	106.3 ± 2.4	P = 0.32	−0.89 ± 0.88
AST (s)	28.5 ± 2.2	28.4 ± 2.3	P = 0.92	+0.13 ± 1.21
Endurance (s)	753.8 ± 58.8	769.3 ± 64.1	P = 0.72	−15.50 ± 44.44
R Quadriceps (N · m)	143.9 ± 7.9	142.5 ± 6.2	P = 0.78	+1.44 ± 5.09
R Hamstrings (N · m)	80.6 ± 4.4	83.3 ± 4.9	P = 0.27	−2.69 ± 2.37
L Quadriceps (N · m)	141.9 ± 8.4	141.8 ± 7.2	P = 0.98	+0.13 ± 5.94
L Hamstrings (N · m)	82.5 ± 5.6	83.6 ± 4.4	P = 0.66	−1.19 ± 2.62

Note: Values are means ± standard deviation (N = 16).
* $P < 0.05$.
† $P < 0.10$.
Abbreviations: Vo_{2max}, maximum oxygen consumption; $\dot{V}_{E(max)}$, maximum recorded minute ventilation; *HR(max)*, maximum heart rate; *RER(max)*, maximum respiratory exchange ratio; *AST*, anaerobic speed test; *Endurance*, at 90% Vo_{2max}; *R*, right and *L*, left (measurements of muscle strength are peak torque, measured at 30°/sec, best of 3 trials).
(Courtesy of Lebrun CM, McKenzie DC, Prior JC, et al: Effects of menstrual cycle phase on athletic performance. *Med Sci Sports Exerc* 27:437–444, 1995.)

luteal phase of the cycle, but relative values did not differ (Table 3). There were no significant changes in peak minute ventilation, maximal heart rate, or maximum respiratory exchange ratio in different menstrual cycle phases. There also were no differences in anaerobic speed test results, endurance performance, or isokinetic leg muscle strength.

Conclusion.—With the possible exception of aerobic capacity, indices of performance are not substantially influenced by the phase of the menstrual cycle in highly trained women.

▶ The effect of hormonal fluctuations on athletic performance throughout the menstrual cycle has been the subject of numerous investigations over the years. Results have varied depending on the performance and physiologic variables studied, the protocol and design of the study, the sport involved, and even the power of the statistical tests as determined by the size of the sample. As we all know, the performance variables important for success vary from sport to sport. The slight change in aerobic power noted in this study would be of little consequence to the golfer, whereas small changes in eye-hand coordination could be significant. Overall, the literature suggests that the effect of the cycle on those variables that have been studied is minimal. However, the authors do make the important point that the effect may be important for individual athletes, even when mean differences are not significant.

B.L. Drinkwater, Ph.D.

Effects of Oral Contraceptives on Fibrinolytic Response to Exercise

de Paz JA, Villa JG, Vilades E, Martin-Nuño MA, Lasierra J, Gonzalez-Gallego J (San Millán Hosp, Logroño, Spain; Inst of Physical Education, León, Spain; Univ of León, Spain)

Med Sci Sports Exerc 27:961–966, 1995 8–3

Background.—Many studies have shown that blood coagulation and fibrinolysis are modified in women using oral contraceptives. Some researchers have claimed that patients in whom thrombosis develops while they are taking oral contraceptives have an increased risk of thromboembolic events and a defective fibrinolytic system. Because an increasing number of women are participating in regular endurance exercise, it is important to know whether oral contraceptive use affects the exercise-induced changes of the fibrinolytic system.

Methods.—Eighteen moderately active women were enrolled in a study to determine the effects of low-dose oral contraceptives on the different components of the fibrinolytic system before and immediately after maximal exercise. Nine women used oral contraceptives and 9 did not. All underwent a maximal effort treadmill protocol.

Findings.—The oral contraceptive group had higher plasma fibrin degradation product (FbDP), plasminogen, α2-antiplasmin, and protein C levels and lower plasminogen activator inhibitor (PAI) activity. Plasma levels of tissue plasminogen activator (t-PA) antigen, t-PA activity, PAI antigen, antithrombin III, and protein S did not differ between groups. Acute maximal exercise significantly increased t-PA antigen, t-PA activity, t-PA/PAI complexes, and FbDP in both groups. Plasminogen activator inhibitor activity was reduced in both groups after acute maximal exercise. There were no significant between-group differences in changes in those parameters. Exercise did not induce any variations in either group for PAI antigen, α2-antiplasmin, plasminogen, protein C, or protein S.

Conclusion.—Increased t-PA release is an important mediator in exercise-induced hyperfibrinolysis. A lower PAI activity and a stimulated extrinsic fibrinolysis were documented among oral contraceptive users in this study. However, oral contraceptives apparently do not affect the changes in the fibrinolytic system induced by physical exercise.

▶ Many physicians are prescribing oral contraceptives for oligomenorrheic and amenorrheic athletes to prevent a decrease in bone mineral density. There is relatively little information regarding the effectiveness of this strategy in preserving bone or—even more importantly—in the effect of oral contraceptives on other physiologic systems. This is an area that should be explored, particularly because many of these athletes are adolescents. In the specific area addressed by these authors, oral contraceptives do not affect the fibrinolytic response to exercise, although oral contraceptive use per se increased fibrinolysis.

B.L. Drinkwater, Ph.D.

Physical Activity and the Menopause Experience: A Cross-sectional Study

Guthrie JR, Smith AMA, Dennerstein L, Morse C (Univ of Melbourne, Australia; Univ of Wollongong, Australia)

Maturitas 20:71–80, 1995 8–4

Objective.—It has been suggested that exercise in midlife women may reduce the frequency of vasomotor symptoms. This study hypothesized that these and other symptoms associated with menopause may be less of a problem for women with higher levels of physical activity. Benefits in terms of well-being, self-rated health, and body mass index (BMI) are also possible. These issues were examined in a cross-sectional study of Australian women in midlife.

Methods.—A telephone interview was conducted with 2,000 Australian-born women between the ages of 45 and 55 years. A physical activity questionnaire was then sent to 1,181 women who agreed to participate and were classified as premenopausal, perimenopausal, or naturally menopausal. Women with surgical menopause were excluded; naturally menopausal women who were taking hormone replacement therapy were included as a separate sample within menopausal status. The questionnaire asked about the women's physical activity during the past 12 months. The average hours and average total energy expended per week in all leisure physical activities, and in all leisure physical activities excluding those related to outdoor labor (i.e., gardening and yard work) were calculated.

Results.—The response rate to the physical activity questionnaire was 62%. Of the 728 respondents, more than 70% participated in walking and gardening activities. Swimming, home exercise, and dancing were also popular. Missing data reduced the final analysis to 555 women. Significant relationships were noted between all 4 physical activity categories and self-rated health, past vascular and neurologic surgery, worries about the respondent's partner in the previous 12 months, the death of a friend or co-worker, and the amount of alcohol consumed in the past week. Inverse associations were noted between BMI and hours of nongardening leisure time activity and energy expenditure. Women whose BMI exceeded 25 were less physically active, and older women spent more time and expended more energy in leisure-time physical activity than younger women. The physical activity level had no apparent effect on the extent to which the women were bothered by symptoms during the menopause transition.

Conclusion.—Women with higher levels of physical activity have better self-rated health and lower BMI, as well as other indicators of better health. Better self-rated health may itself be considered a benefit of exercise. The physical activity level is not significantly related to psychological well-being or menopausal symptoms, however. An in-progress longitudinal study of women who are currently premenopausal and perimenopausal will yield more information on the contribution of exercise to midlife symptoms and well-being.

► Concern about the possible side effects of hormone replacement therapy has led many women to look to exercise and nutrition as a means of attenuating bone loss and other menopausal symptoms in the years after the menopause. This study looked specifically at the effect of physical activity on the occurrence of vasomotor symptoms as well as perceived health and health-related behaviors. Women who were active reported better health, but, as is usual in cross-sectional studies, the question is whether healthier women exercise more. The most interesting conclusion—that physical activity had no effect on menopausal symptoms—is not supported by data presented in this paper. There was no mention of what symptoms were considered, the method of quantifying those symptoms, or the actual data supporting this conclusion.

B.L. Drinkwater, Ph.D.

Strenuous Exercise With Caloric Restriction: Effect on Luteinizing Hormone Secretion

Williams NI, Young JC, McArthur JW, Bullen B, Skrinar GS, Turnbull B
(Boston Univ; Univ of Nevada, Las Vagas; Hybridon, Worcester, Mass)
Med Sci Sports Exerc 27:1390–1398, 1995 8–5

Introduction.—How strenuous exercise training suppresses gonadotropin-releasing hormone and luteinizing hormone (LH) secretion remains unclear. There is increasing evidence that abnormal hormone secretion may result not directly from the physical effects of exercise, but rather from the energy deficit that is incurred when energy expenditure exceeds energy intake.

Objective and Methods.—Whether decreased LH secretion in exercising women is caused by an energy deficit was determined by monitoring LH pulses in moderately trained subjects who, without altering their caloric intake, abruptly increased their training volume. The effects of caloric restriction were also studied. Four moderately trained, regular-cycling women had blood sampled 5 hours before, during, and for 5 hours after running for 90 minutes at 74% of peak oxygen uptake. In control studies, the subjects remained eucaloric for 7 days. In test studies, they completed 90-minute runs on days 5 through 7, taking either the same diet or 60% of the calories needed to maintain weight during days 1 through 7.

Results.—Plasma estradiol levels were well within the normal range for ovulatory cycles. The participants lost an average of 2.3 kg of body weight under conditions of caloric restriction. Luteinizing hormone pulse frequency was reduced by nearly one fourth in these tests, compared with the control condition or eucaloric exercise (Fig 2). Peak LH pulse amplitudes did not differ significantly, and overall average serum LH levels were comparable under all conditions.

Implications.—Short-term changes in energy supply may alter neuroendocrine control of reproductive function. Strenuous training may disrupt

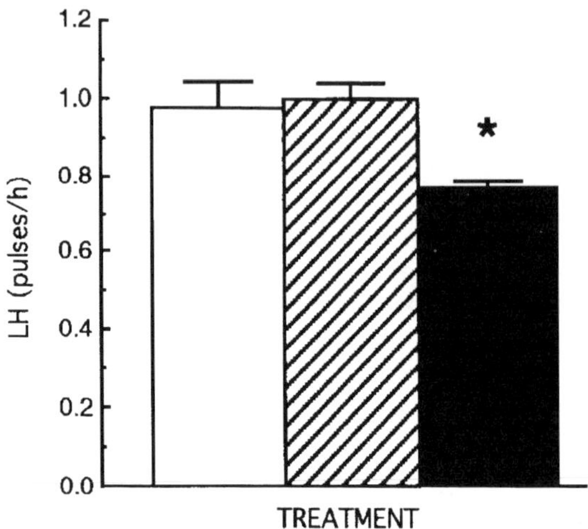

FIGURE 2.—Overall (0700 h–1830 h) luteinizing hormone pulse frequency during all treatment periods. *White bar* indicates controls; *striped bar,* short-term increase in training volume (*STTI*); and *black bar,* caloric restriction (*DIET*)/STTI. Values are expressed as mean ± standard error of the mean. Pulse frequency was significantly lower during DIET/STTI vs. control and STTI ($P < 0.05$). (Courtesy of Williams NI, Young JC, McArthur JW, et al: Strenuous exercise with caloric restriction: Effect on luteinizing hormone secretion. *Med Sci Sports Exerc* 27:1390–1398, 1995.)

the secretion of reproductive hormones and restrict gonadotropic support of the ovaries only if the caloric intake is not appropriately increased.

► More and more evidence is accumulating to suggest, with some confidence, that menstrual irregularities are related to an "energy deficit." This is an important concept that should be described when the suggestion is made that "exercise" per se causes amenorrhea or oligomenorrhea. Although this study has a small number of subjects, the results are consistent with those of other investigators who have also reported changes in LH pulse frequency when energy expenditure exceeds energy availability. If a deficit threshold that induces changes in LH pulsatility can be identified, it may be possible to plan a weight-loss program for athletes that will not adversely affect the reproductive cycle.

B.L. Drinkwater, Ph.D.

Validation of a Cycle Ergometry Equation for Predicting Steady-rate $\dot{V}O_2$ in Obese Women

Andersen RE, Wadden TA (Univ of Pennsylvania, Philadelphia)

Med Sci Sports Exerc 27:1457–1460, 1995 8–6

Background.—The metabolic equations outlined by the American College of Sports Medicine (ACSM) are frequently used for fitness assessments, such as the oxygen cost of cycle ergometry. A new equation for predicting the oxygen cost of cycle ergometry has been developed by Latin et al., and they have found that this equation provides more accurate estimates of oxygen consumption. The accuracy of the ACSM and the Latin et al. equations in predicting oxygen cost of cycling was evaluated in a group of obese, deconditioned women.

Participants and Methods.—Fifty-one obese women were studied. Average age, weight, and height were 39 years, 97 kg, and 164 cm, respectively. The mean body mass index was 36. All women were tested on an electrically braked ergometer. Steady state oxygen consumption was measured as participants pedaled at 3 different loads: 0, 50, and 100 W. Each testing phase lasted 3 minutes.

Results.—Oxygen consumption was significantly underestimated when the ACSM equation was used, with differences of 478, 235, and 151 mL/min noted at 0, 50, and 100 W, respectively. Similarly, oxygen consumption was also significantly underestimated at the 0 load when using the Latin equation; however, no significant differences were observed at 50 or 100 W. A mean bias of 287.6 mL/min was observed for all 3 workloads with the ACSM equation, vs. 58.3 mL/min for the Latin equation. When evaluating hypothesized differences between measured and predicted caloric expenditure that would have occurred if the workload were extended to 25 minutes, both the ACSM and Latin equations would have predicted significantly smaller caloric expenditures than were actually expended at 0 load. At 50 and 100 W, the ACSM equation also would have underestimated energy output by 29 and 19 kcal, respectively. In contrast, no differences were found between actual and predicted energy expenditure at 50 and 100 W when using the Latin equation (Fig 3).

Conclusion.—When compared with the ACSM equation, the Latin equation appears to provide more accurate estimates of oxygen consump-

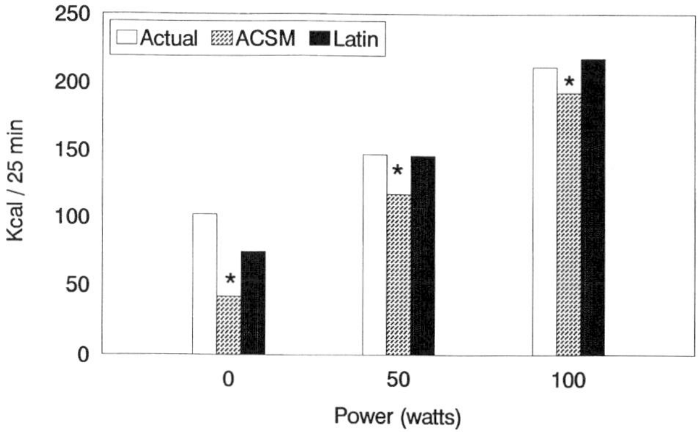

FIGURE 3.—Measured vs. predicted energy expenditure using the American College of Sports Medicine (*ACSM*) and the Latin et al. equations extended to a 25-minute exercise session at each workload. (From Andersen RE, Wadden TA: Validation of a cycle ergometry equation for predicting steady-rate $\dot{V}O_2$ in obese women. *Med Sci Sports Exerc* 27:1457–1460, 1995. Courtesy of the ACSM *Guidelines for Graded Exercise Testing and Training*, 4th ed., Philadelphia, Lea & Febiger, 1991, and Latin RW, Berg K, Smith P, et al: Validation of a cycle ergometry equation for predicting steady-rate $\dot{V}O_2$. *Med Sci Sports Exerc* 25:970–974, 1993.)

tion during loaded cycling in obese women. However, caution is advised when using the Latin equation to predict the caloric cost of unloaded cycling.

► Although it is not good news that the ACSM equation for estimating oxygen consumption significantly underestimates the actual oxygen uptake of obese women, the data do confirm the importance of validating a prediction equation for the specific groups to which it may be applied. Once again, we are reminded that error is always present when attempting to predict performance and that the magnitude of the error increases when the prediction equation is used for a group other than the one for which it was validated.

B.L. Drinkwater, Ph.D.

Military Body Fat Standards and Equations Applied to Middle-aged Women

Bathalon GP, Hughes VA, Campbell WW, Fiatarone MA, Evans WJ (Tufts Univ, Boston; Harvard Med School Boston; Pennsylvania State Univ, University Park)

Med Sci Sports Exerc 27:1079–1085, 1995 8–7

Background.—The military services have developed sex-specific body fat standards and prediction equations for estimating body fat. The body fat standards of the various military services vary considerably. The standards increase with age in the Army and Air Force but not in the Marine Corps and Navy. However, the underrepresentation of women older than 40 years of age in developing the prediction equations for the military services has brought the reliability of the prediction equations into questions for this population. The predictive ability of the equations used in the Army, Marine Corps, and Navy to estimate body fat was analyzed in middle-aged women, using underwater weighing as the reference for determining body fat.

Methods.—Sixty-two healthy women, between the ages of 40 and 60 years and within 25 pounds of the Army weight for height standards, were studied. Anthropometric measurements were obtained including height; weight; and circumferences of the neck, biceps, forearm, wrist, 2 abdomen sites, hips, and thighs. These measurements were used to estimate body fat percentage and were compared against body density as determined by underwater weighing.

Results.—Prediction of the percent body fat with the Navy equation was not significantly different from body density values obtained with underwater weighing. However, the Army and Marine Corps equations resulted in significantly lower body fat estimates, compared with underwater weighing findings, particularly in fatter subjects. The military equations had sensitivities ranging from 20% to 74% and specificities ranging from 80% to 98%.

Conclusion.—Among women between the ages of 40 and 60 years, the Navy equation can adequately assess mean percent body fat, whereas the Army and Marine Corps equations significantly underestimate body fat. (The low sensitivity indicates that women who exceed the body fat standard are unlikely to be identified.) It is recommended that the accuracy of the military equations be re-examined in both men and women of various ages, races, and body compositions. In addition, the ability of the equations to discriminate small changes in body fat during a weight loss program should be examined.

▶ For those of us who have used the different techniques of estimating percent body fat in a research setting, the decision of groups such as the military, police, fire departments, and even airlines to make personnel decisions based on estimates of percent body fat is indefensible. The amount of measurement error in using even the "gold standard"—hydrostatic weighing—when the assumption of a constant value for lean tissue is violated can be considerable. To disregard the changes that occur in lean tissue with aging by using a single prediction equation for all ages will result in an overestimation of body fat in older individuals. In effect, this can result in an unintentional form of age discrimination if it results in dismissal from the service or other employment.

As the authors point out, the mean values for prediction equations and underwater weighing may not differ significantly, but the agreement at the individual level is poor. Because the estimated percent body fat is used in making decisions that affect individual careers, the use of inaccurate prediction equations cannot be justified.

B.L. Drinkwater, Ph.D.

Maternal and Fetal Responses to Low-impact Aerobic Dance

McMurray RG, Katz VL, Poe MP, Hackney AC (Univ of North Carolina, Chapel Hill)

Am J Perinatol 12:282–285, 1995 8–8

Introduction.—Aerobic dance, compared with aerobic walking, has been shown to produce a higher heart rate without a proportional increase in oxygenation and higher blood pressures. The effects of these changes on pregnant women and their fetuses have not been established. Therefore, the effects on pregnant women and their fetuses of low-impact aerobic dance and of treadmill walking at a similar intensity were compared.

Methods.—Ten women with singleton pregnancies at 21–28 weeks' gestation completed both a 40-minute aerobic dance program and a 40-minute treadmill walk, which produced the same maternal heart rate responses. Each trial consisted of 10 minutes of warm-up of increasing intensity, 20 minutes of moderate to high intensity, and 10 minutes of decreasing intensity and cool-down. Maternal oxygen uptake (VO_2) and fetal heart rate (with ultrasound evaluation) were measured at 10-minute intervals, and maternal heart rate was measured at 5-minute intervals throughout the exercise period. During the 20 minutes of recovery after the trials, maternal heart rate and fetal heart rate and movement were assessed at 5-minute intervals.

Results.—The average maternal heart rate was similar in the 2 trials. However, the average VO_2 values were 4 mL/kg per minute lower during aerobic dance than during walking. Fetal heart rates averaged 172 beats/min during aerobic dance and 149 beats/min during walking. The significant differences in fetal heart rates were gradually reduced during the recovery period. There were no instances of fetal bradycardia or uterine contractions during any trial.

Conclusion.—Pregnant women can perform 40 minutes of either aerobic dance or walking with fairly high intensity. However, a walking program will produce a higher maternal metabolic rate and induce less of the transient fetal heart rate responses than will aerobic dance. The clinical significance of the fetal response requires further study.

Anaerobic Threshold and Respiratory Compensation in Pregnant Women

Lotgering FK, Struijk PC, van Doorn MB, Spinnewijn WEM, Wallenburg HCS (Erasmus Univ, Rotterdam, The Netherlands)

J Appl Physiol 78:1772–1777, 1995 8–9

Background.—Carbon dioxide output ($\dot{V}CO_2$) at peak exercise is lower during pregnancy compared with post partum, even though changes in the peak oxygen uptake ($\dot{V}O_2$) are minor. This finding may likely reflect a reduction in the buffering of lactic acid above the anaerobic threshold (AT) during gestation. To explore this further, the relationship between $\dot{V}CO_2$ and $\dot{V}O_2$ was evaluated during rapidly incremental exercise, and the AT and respiratory compensation (RC) point were determined in a group of women during pregnancy and after delivery.

Participants and Methods.—Thirty-three women underwent testing at 16-, 25-, and 35-weeks' gestation and again after delivery. Heart rate, $\dot{V}O_2$, $\dot{V}CO_2$, and minute ventilation ($\dot{V}E$) were measured at rest and during cycle exercise tests, with rapidly increasing exercise intensities until maximal effort was achieved. Modification of the V-slope method permitted estimates of the AT and RC point to be made for each test by nonlinear regression analysis in a 3-dimensional space (defined by $\dot{V}E$, $\dot{V}O_2$, and $\dot{V}CO_2$) for a line presumed to have 2 breakpoints.

Results.—The mean age at delivery was 31 years. The mean gestational age was 40 weeks, and the mean birth weight was 3.43 kg. Clearly distinguishable AT and RC points were found in 125 of 132 tests. Two breakpoints were also found in at least 3 of the 4 tests in all 33 participants. The AT and RC points were identified at exercise intensities of approximately 50% and 80% peak $\dot{V}O_2$, respectively. No significant differences were noted between test periods. A significantly higher $\dot{V}E$ was observed during pregnancy than after delivery, both at rest and during incremental exercise.

Conclusion.—Compared with the postpartum period, lower peak $\dot{V}CO_2$ relative to $\dot{V}O_2$ was noted during pregnancy, as demonstrated by a more shallow slope of $\dot{V}CO_2$ vs. $\dot{V}O_2$ above the AT point. This finding indicates that the buffering of lactic acid is reduced during pregnancy.

A Comparison of Cardiopulmonary Adaptations to Exercise in Pregnancy at Sea Level and Altitude

Artal R, Fortunato V, Welton A, Constantino N, Khodiguian N, Villalobos L, Wiswell R (Univ of Southern California, Los Angeles)

Am J Obstet Gynecol 172:1170–1180, 1995 8–10

Introduction.—Physical activity during pregnancy has increased significantly in recent years. Many different groups of women—including recreational athletes, travelers, and flight attendants—need information on the effects of short-term exposure to altitude and physical exertion during pregnancy. Among lowlanders, the physiologic adaptations to exercise at altitude may be restricted, thus exposing placental reserves and eliciting compromising fetal responses. Lowlander pregnant women were studied to determine their cardiopulmonary and fetal responses to bicycle ergometer exercise at sea level and at altitude.

Methods.—The study included 10 sedentary women in their third trimester of pregnancy with no medical or obstetric complications. On 2 occasions, the women performed a symptom-limited maximal exercise test and underwent cardiac output assessments at rest and at workloads of 25 and 50 W. This was done first at sea level and, 2 to 4 days later, at an altitude of 6,000 feet. The women's blood pressure was measured as soon as they reached maximal exercise levels. For at least 30 minutes after the exercise test, the maternal ECG, fetal heart rate, and uterine activity were monitored. Blood specimens were obtained for testing before, during, and after exercise.

Results.—Seven women completed the study protocol. The women's maximal work levels and peak oxygen uptake ($\dot{V}O_2$) were lower at altitude than at sea level, although their maximal heart rates were not significantly different. There were no significant differences between tests in maximal levels of ventilation, tidal volumes, respiratory rates at peak $\dot{V}O_2$, or respiratory exchange ratio. Expired carbon dioxide at peak $\dot{V}O_2$ was significantly lower at altitude. There were no altitude-related differences in maternal heart rate or oxygen consumption at rest or during exercise. Ventilation was significantly higher at altitude at 75 W but not at rest or at 25 or 50 W. Ventilation was no different between sea level and altitude at maximal exercise levels.

The brief exercise test performed in this study had no significant effect on glucose level, and there were no altitude-related differences in plasma lactate, norepinephrine, or epinephrine concentrations. Fetal heart rates were not significantly affected by altitude, either before or after exercise.

Conclusion.—For sedentary pregnant women, altitude appears to have no significant physiologic effects. They may be somewhat limited in their ability to perform high-intensity tasks. No dangerous fetal responses are apparent when women in the third trimester of pregnancy engage in brief periods of exercise at moderate altitude.

▶ Interest in the response of the pregnant woman and her fetus to exercise continues to generate a variety of research protocols. To date, it appears that healthy women with uncomplicated pregnancies can exercise at moderate intensities and even perform a maximal stress test without harm to themselves or their fetus. The danger is that some readers may interpret these results as an indication that women can exercise safely during pregnancy without noting the careful selection of subjects, the limits imposed by the protocol, and the caveats enumerated by the authors.

B.L. Drinkwater, Ph.D.

Degenerative Joint Disease in Female Ballet Dancers

van Dijk CN, Lim LSL, Poortman A, Strübbe EH, Marti RK (Academic Med Centre, Amsterdam)

Am J Sports Med 23:295–300, 1995 8–11

Background.—Studies have found a correlation between very strenuous physical activity and arthrosis, whereas others report no increased risk of degenerative arthritis in athletes or heavy manual laborers. The effects of endurance activities have not been prospectively evaluated in long-term follow-up studies. Hip, ankle, subtalar, and first metatarsophalangeal joints were evaluated in a group of retired female ballet dancers with long careers, and findings were compared with pair-matched controls.

Participants and Methods.—Nineteen retired professional dancers, aged 50–70 years, and 19 controls matched for age, height, and body weight were included in the study. The mean length of the dancers' professional careers was 37 years, and the mean dance time per week was 45 hours. All of the professional women had danced "on pointe." None of the controls had participated in contact sports. Medical histories were obtained, and standard clinical and roentgenographic evaluations were performed by the same examiner. Roentgenographs were independently reviewed by 2 radiologists for the presence of osteophytes, subchondral sclerosis, cysts, or bone destruction, and classified using a modified grade 0 through III scale of Hermodsson.

Results.—None of the 38 women had evidence of malalignment, genetic diseases, or arthritis. In addition, none of the professional dancers had experienced macrotrauma during their careers. Roentgenologic arthrosis of the ankle, subtalar, and first metatarsophalangeal joints was significantly greater in the dancers compared with controls. No significant differences in degenerative changes of the hip were noted. None of the dancers with roentgenographic evidence of degenerative changes offered any clinical complaints. Significant increases in hallux valgus deformities were noted in the dancers. Flexion, external rotation, and abduction of the hip joint; dorsal flexion of the first metatarsophalangeal joint; and inversion and eversion of the subtalar joint also were significantly increased in the dancers, although plantar flexion of the first metatarsophalangeal joint was decreased when compared with controls.

Conclusion.—The risk of arthrosis was increased among long-term ballet dancers in all examined joints. With the exception of the hip, the differences between controls and dancers for all other joints were significant. Arthrosis in professional dancers most likely results from an accumulation of microtraumas, given the fact that malalignment, genetic disease, macrotrauma, and arthritis—the most important causes of secondary arthrosis—were notably absent.

► The object of this study—to compare a group of retired ballet dancers' hip, ankle, subtalar, and first metatarsophalangeal joints for evidence of arthrosis with a matched pair of controls—has been accomplished. However, none of the dancers had complaints referable to the investigated joints. Essentially, the report consisted of an analysis of roentgenographic findings without clinical relevance.

J.S. Torg, M.D.

Lifetime Occupational Physical Activity and Risk of Hip Fracture in Women

Jaglal SB, Kreiger N, Darlington, GA (Univ of Toronto)

Ann Epidemiol 5:321–324, 1995 8–12

Objective.—Countries differ in their incidence of hip fracture, and cultural differences in physical activity patterns are one suggested explanation. In the Western world, occupational activity may still have a major impact on people's total physical activity. The influence of women's occupational activity on their risk of hip fracture was evaluated in a case-control study.

Methods.—The cases were 331 women 55–84 years of age in the Toronto metropolitan area who had a hip fracture diagnosed during 1989. The controls were a population-based random sample of 1,002 women without hip fracture, frequency-matched for age. All women in both groups had been employed full-time or part-time for longer than 6 months and for more than 15 hr/week since they were 16 years of age. Lifetime occupational physical activity was estimated, along with other factors, and associations with hip fracture were sought.

Results.—Compared with women who worked for more than 20 years in a sedentary occupation, those who worked 20 years or less in any type of job had no decrease in their risk of hip fracture (odds ratio, [OR] 0.96).

TABLE 2.—Distribution of Cases and Controls by Occupational Physical Activity Level

Occupational Activity Level	No. of Cases	No. of Controls	Adjusted OR (95% CI)
> 20 y in sedentary to light-activity jobs	133	452	1.00
1–20 y in any type activity job	109	352	0.96 (0.70–1.32)
> 20 y in a moderate- to heavy-activity job	19	104	0.53 (0.30–0.95)

Note: Odds ratios are adjusted for age, recent leisure-time activity, past leisure-time activity, estrogen, epilepsy, previous fracture, obesity, and education. Because of missing data, the total numbers for cases and controls in the logistic model are less than the available study population.

Abbreviations: OR, odds ratio; *CI*, confidence interval.

(Reprinted by permission of the publisher from Jaglal SB, Kreiger N, Darlington GA: Lifetime occupational physical activity and risk of hip fracture in women. *Ann Epidemiol* 5:321–324, Copyright 1995 by Elsevier Science Inc.)

In contrast, working for more than 20 years in jobs entailing moderate-to-heavy activity conferred significant protection against hip fracture (OR, 0.53) (Table 2). Risk factors for hip fracture included past and present leisure activities, estrogen use, obesity, epilepsy, and a history of previous fracture. Women with a very high level of leisure activity had a significantly reduced risk of hip fracture (OR, 0.41). Occupational and leisure activity were not significantly correlated with each other.

Conclusion.—A woman's history of occupational physical activity may influence her risk of hip fracture. For postmenopausal women, working for more than 20 years in a job requiring heavy activity may reduce the risk of hip fracture by half. Occupational and leisure physical activity appear to have independent effects on hip fracture risk. It is likely that fewer women today are working in heavy-activity occupations, so the incidence of hip fracture may increase in the future.

▶ Many investigators have concluded that there is little to learn from occupational studies of physical activity, as the energy demands of supposed "heavy" work have now fallen to extremely low levels. It is, thus, interesting that there is still sufficient stimulus in the heavy work of North American women to increase their bone density and, thus, reduce the risk of hip fracture.

A part of the explanation may lie in gender; the heavy work of female employees (for example, the operation of cleaning machines) is much less susceptible to automation than the traditional heavy work of male employees. It is also possible that the older woman who has had a career of heavy work has had a harder domestic life than her sedentary peers. The authors attempted to allow statistically for extraneous factors—such as current and past leisure activity, estrogen use, epilepsy, previous fractures, obesity, and education—but they did not control for either the number of children or the need to care for elderly relatives, both of which demand a significant volume of work from many women.

R.J. Shephard, M.D., Ph.D., D.P.E.

Lifetime Leisure Exercise and Osteoporosis: The Rancho Bernardo Study

Greendale GA, Barrett-Connor E, Edelstein S, Ingles S, Haile R (Univ of California, Los Angeles; Univ of California, San Diego, La Jolla)

Am J Epidemiol 141:951–959, 1995 8–13

Introduction.—Modest gains in bone density have been reported as a result of physical activity. However, it is not clear whether the increase in bone density can be attributed to current activity or former activity. The effect of self-reported current and previous leisure-time physical activity on axial and appendicular bone mineral density (BMD) and osteoporotic fracture were evaluated in a population-based sample of older adults.

Methods.—The relationship between leisure time, physical activity, BMD, and osteoporotic fracture was evaluated in 1,014 women and 689 men with a mean age of 73 years. A self-administered, standardized questionnaire was used to determine the history of alcohol consumption, cigarette use, thiazide use, estrogen use (women only), and occurrence of bone fracture. Dietary intake and exercise history were also assessed. Height, weight, and body mass index were calculated.

Results.—For men and women combined, 24% exercised moderately as teenagers and this proportion remained stable with age. The proportion of heavy exercisers diminished with age: 50% during teenage years, 18.7% at age 30, and 12.7% at age 50; only 3% reported current strenuous activity. Men reported 2–3 times more strenuous leisure activity than women, at all ages. Bone mineral density at the total hip was significantly associated with increasing intensity of current exercise for men and women combined. Lifetime exercise was positively associated with BMD of the total hip in males and females combined. Current and past exercise was not associated with BMD at the ultradistal radius, midradius, or lumbar spine. A borderline significant beneficial effect was found for lifelong exercisers at the lumbar spine. Current exercise was unrelated to BMD of the ultradistal radius, midradius, or lumbar spine. No relationship between osteoporotic fracture and exercise was detected (Table 2).

Conclusion.—A substantial protective effect of current and lifelong exercise on BMD of the hip was observed in older men and women. No protective effect of BMD or current or lifelong exercise was detected for osteoporotic fracture.

► Although BMD at some sites was higher in the more active men and women, it seems curious to speak of a "protective effect of exercise" when the risk for osteoporotic fracture was unrelated to either current or lifetime exercise habits. Physical activity has many health benefits, but no study to date has shown that exercise alone can prevent bone loss as one ages. The mean BMD for the femoral neck may be related to current exercise habits, but the absolute values would place about half the group in an "at risk" area for osteoporotic fractures. We should be careful that in our enthusiasm for exercise, we do not encourage women to dismiss the well-documented

TABLE 2.—Relative Odds of Experiencing Any Osteoporotic Fracture, by Exercise Level at Various Ages and by Sex

Age and level of exercise	Age-adjusted relative odds						Multiply adjusted* relative odds†‡			
	Both sexes		Women		Men		Women		Men	
	RO	95% CI	RO	95% CI	RO	95% CI	RO	95% CI	RO	95% CI
Teenage years										
Moderate	1.03	0.69–1.06	1.04	1.02–1.07	0.93	0.34–2.52	1.08	0.65–1.81	0.72	0.24–2.16
Strenuous	0.86	0.59–1.24	1.35	0.88–2.08	0.80	0.33–1.93	1.37	0.84–2.26	0.86	0.32–2.32
30 years										
Moderate	0.76	0.35–1.60	0.81	0.52–1.25	1.33	0.64–2.76	0.63	0.36–1.11	1.51	0.60–3.76
Strenuous	0.79	0.27–2.26	1.56	0.83–2.94	0.54	0.22–1.33	1.12	0.48–2.55	0.52	0.19–1.43
50 years										
Moderate	1.23	0.50–3.00	1.12	0.74–1.69	1.36	0.68–2.75	1.34	0.80–2.22	1.50	0.64–3.52
Strenuous	0.76	0.15–3.77	1.36	0.71–2.61	0.68	0.25–1.87	1.31	0.58–2.93	0.68	0.21–2.15
Lifetime to age 50§										
Medium	0.97	0.69–1.36	1.30	0.89–1.91	0.72	0.33–1.56	1.38	0.91–2.09	0.58	0.25–1.31
High	0.87	0.59–1.29	1.39	0.85–2.28	0.91	0.41–1.99	1.43	0.84–2.43	0.86	0.38–1.94

Note: First fractures totalled 160 among women and 45 among men.
* Models were adjusted for age, body mass index, alcohol, cigarettes, thiazide, estrogen use (women only), and dietary calcium intake.
† n = 868 women and 624 men because of the cumulative effect of missing data.
‡ The referent category for the teenage years, age 30 years, and age 50 years was composed of those who reported engaging in mild exercise or less during each of the time periods. The referent category for lifetime to age 50 years was the lowest tertile.
§ Lifetime to age 50 was lifetime exercise score up to age 50 years (excluding current age). Medium and high refer to population tertiles.
Abbreviations: RO, relative odds; *CI*, confidence interval.
(Courtesy of Greendale GA, Barrett-Connor E, Edelstein S, et al: Lifetime leisure exercise and osteoporosis: The Rancho Bernardo Study. *Am J Epidemiol* 141:951–959, 1995.)

effect of hormone replacement therapy in the prevention of bone loss and to rely instead on exercise to protect their bones.

B.L. Drinkwater, Ph.D.

Additive Effects of Weight-bearing Exercise and Estrogen on Bone Mineral Density in Older Women

Kohrt WM, Snead DB, Slatopolsky E, Birge SJ Jr (Washington Univ, St Louis)

J Bone Miner Res 10:1303–1311, 1995 8–14

Objective.—Exercise and female sex hormones appear to have independent effects on the skeleton. However, the possible interactive effects of exercise and hormone replacement therapy (HRT) remain unclear; their independent and combined effects have never been studied simultaneously. The effects of weight-bearing exercise and HRT, alone and together, on bone mineral density (BMD) were studied in postmenopausal women.

Methods.—Thirty-two healthy women 60–72 years of age participated in the study. None exercised regularly; all were at least 10 years past menopause and had not taken estrogen for at least 6 years. The women were assigned to 4 groups matched for body weight: control, exercise, HRT, and exercise plus HRT. The HRT regimen used was continuous conjugated estrogens, 0.625 mg/day, and medroxyprogesterone acetate, 5 mg/day for 13 consecutive days every third month for 11 months. Women in the exercise groups received 2 months of flexibility training followed by 9 months of relatively vigorous weight-bearing exercise consisting of walking, jogging, and/or stair climbing. The women exercised at least 3 days a week. Outcome measures included maximal aerobic power and quadriceps and hamstring muscle strength. Dual-energy x-ray absorptiometry was performed to measure BMD of the proximal femur, lumbar spine, wrist, and total body before and after flexibility training and 3 times during weight-bearing exercise. Bone turnover was assessed by measurement of serum osteocalcin.

Results.—Women who exercised had significant reductions in weight and body fat content and significant increases in maximal aerobic power and peak torque. Throughout the study, the groups were similar in total energy intake and dietary macronutrients. Women who received HRT showed a progressive decline in serum osteocalcin level, whereas the control and exercise-only groups showed no change. The HRT groups also had a significant reduction in serum insulin-like growth factor 1 levels.

Compared with controls, women in the exercise-only group had significant increases in BMD at the lumbar spine, femoral neck, trochanter, and Ward's triangle. Women in the HRT-only group had significant increases in total body, lumbar spine, femoral neck, trochanter, and Ward's triangle BMD. At most sites, the greatest gains in BMD occurred with exercise plus HRT (Figs 2 and 3). The 2 interventions together seemed to have additive effects at the lumbar spine and Ward's triangle and synergistic effects for the total body.

Conclusion.—In postmenopausal women, a relatively vigorous program of weight-bearing exercise significantly increases BMD in the proximal femur. Furthermore, weight-bearing exercise and HRT have independent positive effects on BMD, which are additive at the lumbar spine and Ward's triangle and synergistic in the total body. On its own, HRT significantly increases BMD at the proximal femur, lumbar spine, and total body. The efficacy of estrogen in preventing osteoporosis could be enhanced by combining it with weight-bearing exercise. Not only do the 2 interventions have additive effects on BMD, the improved strength and functional capacity gained through exercise probably would help reduce the risk of falls.

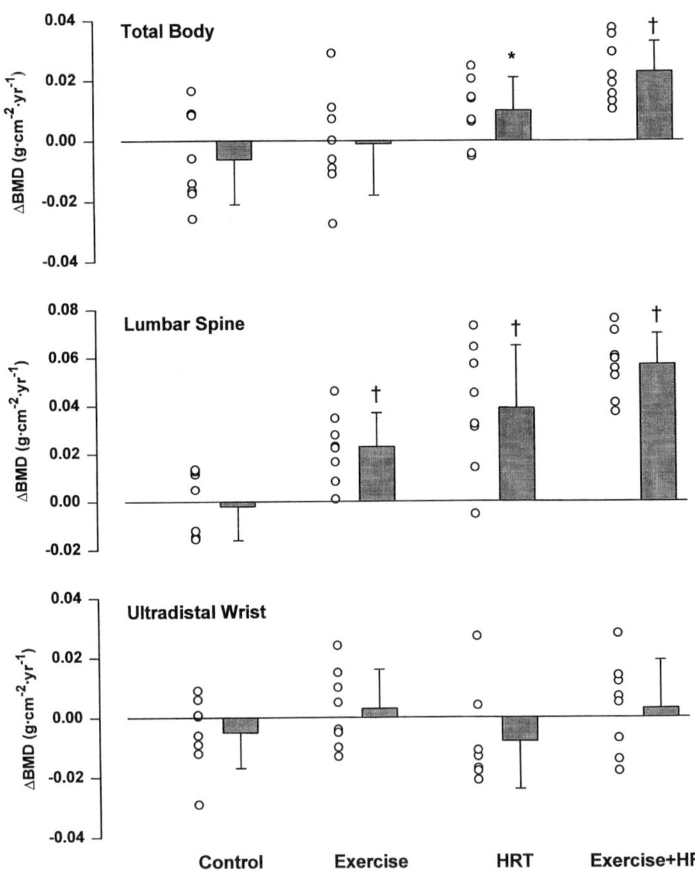

FIGURE 2.—The individual (*circles*) and mean ± standard deviation (*bars*) changes in bone mineral density (*BMD*), in grams per square centimeter per year, of the total body (**top panel**), lumbar spine (**middle panel**), and ultradistal wrist (**bottom panel**) that occurred in controls and in response to exercise and/or hormone replacement therapy over 1 year. *Asterisk* indicates significantly different from 0, $P < 0.05$; *single dagger* indicates significantly different from 0, $P < 0.01$. (Courtesy of Kohrt WM, Snead DB, Slatopolsky E, et al: Additive effects of weight-bearing exercise and estrogen on bone mineral density in older women. *J Bone Miner Res* 10:1303–1311, 1995.)

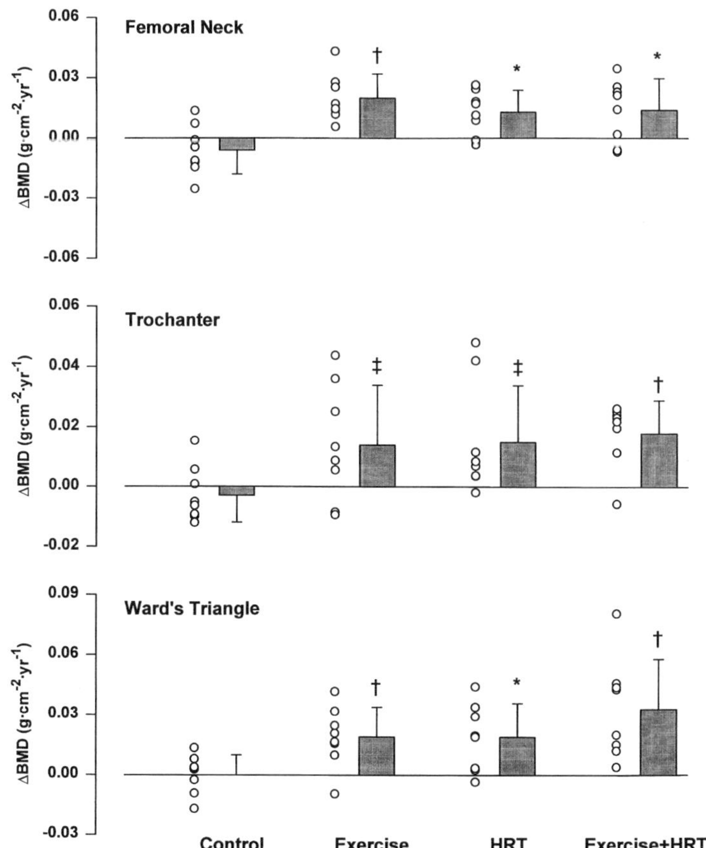

FIGURE 3.—The individual (*circles*) and mean ± standard deviation (*bars*) changes in bone mineral density (*BMD*), in grams per square centimeter per year, of the femoral neck (**top panel**), trochanter (**middle panel**), and Ward's triangle (**bottom panel**) that occurred in controls and in response to exercise and/or hormone replacement therapy over 1 year. *Asterisk* indicates significantly different from 0, $P < 0.05$; *single dagger* indicates significantly different from 0, $P < 0.01$; *double dagger* indicates significantly different from 0, $P < 0.10$. (Courtesy of Kohrt WM, Snead DB , Slatopolsky E, et al: Additive effects of weight-bearing exercise and estrogen on bone mineral density in older women. *J Bone Miner Res* 10:1303–1311, 1995.)

▶ Most women who have reason to be concerned about their risk of osteoporosis want to know what steps they can take to minimize that risk. Many of them have concerns about the use of estrogen and would prefer to rely on nonpharmacologic means to protect their bones. Although exercise alone did increase BMD significantly at some sites, the increase of approximately 0.02 g/cm^2 is unlikely to protect against fracture if a woman already has a bone density in the osteoporotic region (more than 2.5 SD below young adults). Keep in mind, too, that these were sedentary women, those most likely to benefit from the program, and the least likely to continue it. Increases in bone density gained through physical activity are lost when that activity stops. Although women who elect HRT plus exercise have the most to gain, they would benefit even more by initiating the program at the time of menopause, not 10 years later.

B.L. Drinkwater, Ph.D.

Dynamic Muscle Strength as a Predictor of Bone Mineral Density in Elderly Women

Taaffee DR, Pruitt L, Lewis B, Marcus R (Veterans Affairs Med Ctr, Palo Alto, Calif; Stanford Univ, Calif)

J Sports Med Phys Fitness 35:136–142, 1995 8–15

Background.—Several studies have shown that muscle strength can predict bone mineral density (BMD) among older individuals, although the variance explained by isometric and isokinetic testing has generally been less than 20% and confined to a limited number of exercises and muscle groups. Dynamic muscle strength and BMD, therefore, were examined in a group of older women to clarify their relationship at multiple sites and to identify the best predictor of BMD, using isotonic strength testing equipment.

Participants and Methods.—Forty healthy women aged 62–82 years were included in the study. Eighteen of the women were receiving exogenous estrogen. Dual x-ray absorptiometry was used to evaluate BMD of the spine (L2–4), proximal femur (neck, trochanter, Ward's triangle), midradius of the forearm, and whole body. Dynamic muscle strength was measured for 10 exercises involving the major upper and lower body muscle groups using 1-repetition maximum (1RM).

Results.—The average age of the women was 68.5 years. No significant differences in age or measured body composition variables were noted between women taking and not taking exogenous estrogen, although a significantly higher spine, midradius, and whole body BMD were observed among estrogen-treated women. No estrogen-related effects were noted for proximal femur BMD or muscle strength for any exercise. Significant correlations between leg press and all skeletal sites were observed (Table 4). Leg press was identified as the only independent predictor of spine, neck and trochanter, forearm, and whole body BMD, whereas bench press was found to be an independent predictor of Ward's BMD in stepwise multiple regression analyses. Leg press also was identified as the best predictor of regional and whole body BMD using isotonic equipment. This finding may be indicative of the overall skeletal health in this population.

Conclusion.—Isotonically determined dynamic muscle strength independently predicts BMD in elderly women and accounts for up to 21% of the variance at various skeletal sites. A considerable portion of the variance is not, however, explained by knowledge of muscle strength. Nutritional habits, physical activity, heredity, lifestyle, and mechanical factors also have an effect on bone mineral, and, therefore, should be considered when predicting bone mineral status.

TABLE 4.—Correlations of Muscle Strength on Bone Mineral Density

Exercises	Spine (L2–4)	Femoral neck	Femoral trochanter	Ward's triangle	Midradius	Whole body
Bench press	0.23	0.28	0.41†	0.34*	0.28	0.27
Military press	0.15	0.16	0.26	0.16	0.13	0.19
Pull down	0.14	0.13	0.24	0.08	0.21	0.12
Biceps curl	0.30	0.39†	0.41†	0.23	0.03	0.25
Back extension	0.06	0.06	0.21	0.04	0.22	0.08
Leg press	0.33*	0.46‡	0.43†	0.32*	0.46‡	0.44‡
Leg extension	0.17	0.20	0.24	0.08	0.28	0.19
Leg curl	0.10	0.29	0.07	0.16	0.12	0.07
Hip adduction	0.11	0.06	0.17	0.05	0.10	0.04
Hip abduction	0.21	0.18	0.22	0.05	0.03	0.07

* $P < 0.05$.
† $P < 0.01$.
‡ $P < 0.005$.
(Courtesy of Taaffee DR, Pruitt L, Lewis B, et al: Dynamic muscle strength as a predictor of bone mineral density in elderly women. *J Sports Med Phys Fitness* 35:136–142, 1995.)

▶ Study after study has shown a moderate relationship between muscle strength and BMD. However, the amount of variance explained by measures of strength has consistently averaged about 20% or less and may reflect overall physical activity rather than a cause and effect relationship between strength and BMD. Although the lack of agreement betweeen studies may, indeed, reflect differences in protocol and testing equipment, there still remains the nagging question of why prospective strength training studies demonstrate so little effect on BMD.

B.L. Drinkwater, Ph.D.

Physiological Determinants of 10-km Performance in Highly Trained Female Runners of Different Ages

Evans SL, Davy KP, Stevenson ET, Seals DR (Univ of Colorado, Boulder)
J Appl Physiol 78:1931–1941, 1995 8–16

Objective.—Starting at about age 35, the ability to perform endurance exercise deteriorates progressively with advancing age in both men and women. The physiologic basis of this change remains uncertain, particularly in women. An attempt was made to learn whether and to what degree this age-related decline in performance is caused by changes in peak oxygen consumption, running economy (RE), and the blood lactate threshold (LT).

Methods.—Thirty-one highly trained elite female distance runners 23–56 years of age participated in the study by running at the pace they used to complete a 10-km race. There were 10 women aged 23–35 years (group I), 11 aged 37–47 years (group II), and 10 aged 49–56 years (group III). The LT was estimated using a 7-stage discontinuous treadmill exercise protocol. Running economy was calculated as the average of four 30-second oxygen consumption estimates taken after 6–7 minutes of running.

TABLE 5.—Physiologic Responses at 10-km Race Pace

	Velocity, m/min	$\dot{V}O_2$, ml · kg^{-1} · min^{-1}	% $\dot{V}O_{2max}$	$\dot{V}O_2$, %LT	HR, beats/min	%HR_{max}	RER	RPE	Lactate, mM
Group I	265 ± 3	52.3 ± 1.2	91 ± 2	110 ± 2	173 ± 4	94 ± 2	1.01 ± 0.01	17 ± 1	3.5 ± 0.4
(*n* = 10)	(244 – 285)	(45.5 – 57.7)	(81 – 97)	(99 – 126)	(151 – 190)	(86 – 100)	(0.96 – 1.06)	(14 – 19)	(2.1 – 5.5)
Group II	244 ± 3*	49.2 ± 0.7	91 ± 1	109 ± 1	170 ± 1	96 ± 1	1.01 ± 0.01	15 ± 1	4.1 ± 0.3
(*n* = 11)	(234 – 263)	(45.1 – 53.1)	(89 – 97)	(105 – 115)	(166 – 181)	(90 – 100)	(0.98 – 1.10)	(13 – 18)	(2.5 – 6.0)
Group III	210 ± 4*†	42.1 ± 1.4*†	93 ± 2	108 ± 2	158 ± 4*†	96 ± 2	1.01 ± 0.01	16 ± 1	4.2 ± 0.5
(*n* = 10)	(185 – 230)	(36.4 – 48.5)	(82 – 100)	(101 – 116)	(138 – 174)	(84 – 100)	(0.97 – 1.08)	(11 – 20)	(1.9 – 6.2)

Note: Values are means ± standard error. Numbers in parentheses are range.
* $P < 0.05$ vs. group I.
† $P < 0.05$ vs. group II.
Abbreviations: $\dot{V}O_2$, oxygen uptake; *FFW*, estimated fat-free weight; V_E, minute ventilation; *HR*, heart rate; *RER*, respiratory exchange ratio; *RPE*, rating of perceived exertion.
(Courtesy of Evans SL, Davy KP, Stevenson ET, et al: Physiological determinants of 10-km performance in highly trained female runners of different ages. *J Appl Physiol* 78:1931–1941, 1995.)

Results.—Nearly 80% of the variance in 10-km performance was explained by the running velocity at the point of the LT. Together with aerobic power, it accounted for 85% of variance. Race performance correlated strongly and inversely with age. Age was closely associated with the LT and with peak oxygen uptake, but not with RE. The age groups did not differ significantly in body size or percent body fat. At the 10-km pace, the oldest runners had significantly lower heart rates and oxygen uptake levels (Table 5).

Conclusion.—The age-related decrement in endurance exercise ability is most closely related with a reduced peak oxygen consumption and a decline in the running velocity at the LT.

▶ It is difficult to say whether the decrease in aerobic power and the LT are an inevitable consequence of aging or reflect the less intense training program of the older women in this study. The 2 older groups had been training fewer years, which means they had started training later in life. They trained fewer days per week and ran fewer miles per week. The authors suggest that the reduction in training level may, itself, be an effect of aging. If so, the decrease in aerobic power and LT would still be related to aging. It would be interesting to compare group I with runners of their age but with a training regimen similar to group III to see if the results differed from those reported in this study.

B.L. Drinkwater, Ph.D.

Aging, Physical Activity and Sports Injuries: An Overview of Common Sports Injuries in the Elderly

Kallinen M, Markku A (Peurunka-Med Rehabilitation and Physical Exercise Centre, Laukaa, Finland)

Sports Med 20:41–52, 1995 8–17

Benefits.—Because immobilization and inactivity are especially problematic for elderly individuals, many older persons engage in regular physical activity. Physical capacity is clearly augmented as a result. Strength may be retained up to an advanced age. Lifelong activity may enhance neurophysiologic function in the later years, although this has not been established. Vigorous activity helps preserve bone structure.

Risks.—Aging is accompanied by elevated blood pressure, increasing the load on the heart and making the cardiovascular system susceptible to atherosclerotic disease. Atherosclerosis may lead to musculoskeletal symptoms. Muscle damage is repaired less rapidly in older animals. Aerobic capacity declines by an estimated 10% per decade and may decrease more rapidly after age 65.

Injuries.—Whether physical activity reduces the risk of falling remains uncertain. Sudden cardiovascular deaths are rare in the elderly. Varying proportions of the elderly (more than half in some studies) incur injuries related to walking and jogging. Most injuries occurring in the active elderly are related to speed of movement, even when merely walking. Little is known of factors related to sports injuries in the elderly. Inflammatory injuries related to overuse may be relatively frequent in older individuals, especially those who play golf. Some studies have found that muscle strain is the most typical injury incurred by older athletes.

Conclusion.—Especially in the elderly, the best "treatment" for sports injuries is to prevent them, which entails using carefully titrated physical loading to retard the aging process. Injuries that do occur should be expeditiously treated.

► Importantly, this article emphasizes the fact that immobilization and inactivity have a more deleterious effect in the elderly than in younger adults. Also, the functional capacity and rate of aging vary greatly between individuals. Thus, in the elderly, it is necessary to try doses of exercises on an individual basis.

J.S. Torg, M.D.

Antecedents and Consequences of Physical Activity and Exercise Among Older Adults

Wolinsky FD, Stump TE, Clark DO (Regenstrief Inst for Health Care, Indianapolis, Ind)

Gerontologist 35:451–462, 1995 8–18

Background.—Previous research on the health benefits of physical activity and exercise in elderly persons is limited methodologically. To ad-

TABLE 3.—Adjusted Odds Ratios, Partial *r* Statistics, and *P* Values Obtained From Using Logistic Regression to Model Mortality and Nursing Home Placement Among 6,668 Self-Respondents

Independent Variable	Mortality	Nursing Home Placement
More active than peers	.8126 (−.0343) [.0010]	.6023 (−.0791) [.0001]
Gets enough exercise	.8850 (−.0161) [.0467]	
Has a regular exercise routine	.8597 (−.0213) [.0199]	
Walks a mile at least once a week	.8017 (−.0327) [.0015]	.7931 (−.0226) [.0426]

Notes: Adjusted odds ratios (*AORs*) not significantly different from one at the $P \leq 0.05$ level, as well as the AORs associated with the predisposing, enabling, need, and health services utilization characteristics are omitted for clarity (although those variables were included in each of the 8 equations represented by the above cells. Partial *r* statistics appear in parentheses and *P* values in brackets.

dress these limitations, the antecedents to and consequences of physical activity and exercise were investigated among a large group of older adults.

Methods.—The subjects were 6,780 self-respondents in the Longitudinal Study on Aging. Four dichotomous baseline perceptions of physical activity and exercise were included: subjects' level of physical activity compared with their peers; whether subjects got as much exercise as they needed; whether they had a regular exercise routine; and the frequency with which they walked 1.6 kilometers (1 mile) or more.

Findings.—Responses indicated that 45.8% of the subjects perceived their level of physical activity as greater than their peers, 58.9% got as much exercise as they needed, 28.4% had a regular exercise routine, and 29.9% walked 1.6 km or more at least once a week. Engaging in these behaviors was primarily associated with having fewer bodily limitations, better perceived health, more sources of social support other than relatives, not worrying about ones health, and having a sense of control over ones health.

Conclusion.—When added to traditional models that predict 6- to 8-year mortality, nursing home placement, hospital resource use, and functional status changes, these 4 markers of activity have many significant correlations, all involving better health outcomes (Table 3). Encouraging physical activity among elderly individuals should be an important goal of federal health care policy.

► A growing volume of prospective data is now accumulating, suggesting that regular physical activity has positive long-term consequences for health and the quality of life. The importance of prospective data is that they largely overcome the main criticism of cross-sectional analyses, namely, that disability and disease impair physical activity, rather than the converse. Nevertheless, given the fairly short time frame of the prospective observations (2–6 years), it remains possible that those who had low levels of activity at entry to the study were already beginning to sense some disability. Because humans cannot be allocated to long-term exercise programs on a random basis, it is difficult to circumvent this experimental difficulty.

R.J. Shephard, M.D., Ph.D., D.P.E.

Lesser Vagal Withdrawal During Isometric Exercise With Age

Taylor JA, Hayano J, Seals DR (Hebrew Rehabilitation Ctr for the Aged, Boston; Harvard Med School, Boston; Nagoya City Univ, Japan; et al)

J Appl Physiol 79:805–811, 1995 8–19

Background.—The initial tachycardiac response to isometric exercise reflects the withdrawal of cardiac vagal effects on the sinoatrial node. Increased cardiac sympathetic outflow contributes to the subsequent increase in heart rate. For reasons that are not clear, tachycardia during sustained isometric exercise is attenuated in healthy older men.

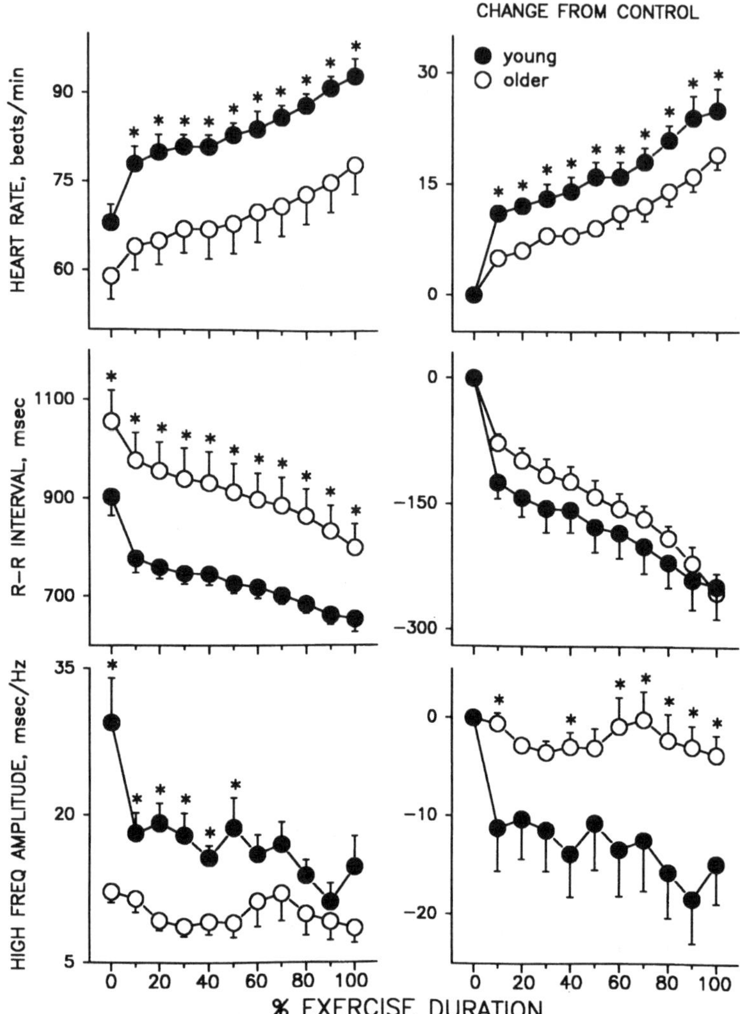

FIGURE 3.—Absolute values and changes from control value for heart rate, R-R interval, and high-frequency (*Freq*) amplitude in young and older subjects at each 10% of isometric exercise duration. Values are means ± standard error. *Asterisk* indicates $P < 0.05$ young vs. older subjects. (Courtesy of Taylor JA, Hayano J, Seals DR: Lesser vagal withdrawal during isometric exercise with age. *J Appl Physiol* 79:805–811, 1995.)

Objective and Methods.—To determine whether the age-related decline in the tachycardiac response to isometric exercise reflects less cardiac vagal withdrawal, variability of the high-frequency R-R interval (an index of cardiac vagal tone) was examined before and during handgrip exercise to exhaustion in 12 healthy men 21–29 years of age and 11 men aged 61–72 years.

Results.—The heart rate increased with exercise in both age groups, but both the absolute rate and the increase over baseline were significantly less marked in older men (Fig 3). The absolute R-R interval was significantly greater in older men at all intervals, but the decrease in R-R interval from baseline was similar in the 2 age groups. A smaller decrease in high-frequency amplitude, related to lower baseline amplitude, corresponded to a smaller increase in heart rate throughout isometric exercise.

Conclusion.—The attenuated tachycardiac response to isometric exercise in older persons is associated with the inability to reduce cardiac vagal tone below an already decreased baseline level.

▶ Various mathematical analyses of R-R intervals are used increasingly to detect the activity of sympathetic and parasympathetic nerves. The high-frequency component provides an index of parasympathetic (vagal) activity. Vagal activity is initially substantially less in the older subjects, although the curves for the young and elderly adults converge as the isometric contraction is sustained. The most reasonable explanation might seem that the older group has a lower level of fitness and, thus, a lower resting vagal activity.

Unfortunately, no details are given of aerobic fitness in the 2 samples, other than the bald statement that they are normal for age, but, somewhat surprisingly the subjects aged 61–72 years have a handgrip strength that matches or even exceeds that of those aged 21–29 years. The sustained isometric contraction also elicits no greater rise of blood pressure in the older subjects than in the young adults. Finally, it is a little puzzling that the resting heart rates do not differ significantly but the R-R intervals do! These experiments should plainly be repeated on individuals who have shown the normal, age-related decrease in fitness, with loss of muscle strength.

R.J. Shephard, M.D., Ph.D., D.P.E.

Personal Health Benefits of Masters Athletics Competition

Shephard RJ, Kavanagh T, Mertens DJ, Qureshi S, Clark M (Univ of Toronto)
Br J Sports Med 29:35–40, 1995 8–20

Introduction.—Regular physical activity confers substantial health dividends on the middle-aged adult, but the type and intensity of activity needed to realize these benefits are not clearly defined. Competitors in the Toronto Masters Games are a select group of middle-aged and older individuals who practice substantial and well-documented types and amounts of physical activity. A prospective study was conducted among Masters athletes to examine the long-term health value of endurance exercise training in this select group.

Methods.—Of the 1,689 Masters athletes recruited in 1985, 750 responded to questionnaires sent in 1992, for a response rate of 44.4%. The questions examined health status, injury, and health behavior during the 7-year period. Current ages ranged from 40 to 81 years. The participants were divided into endurance competitors (endurance running, orienteering, swimming, rowing, and cycling) and those involved in social, recreational sports such as racquet sports. The majority had initially completed maximal exercise tests. The weekly time devoted to training, competition, and exercise-related travel ranged from 10 to 30 hours, and the annual expenditure on clothing, equipment, and entrance fees ranged from Canadian $500–C$1,500.

Results.—Only 1.4% of Masters athletes experienced a nonfatal heart attack and 0.6% underwent bypass surgery. Slightly more than half (56.7%) experienced some injury which had limited their training for 1 or more weeks. Most respondents (76%) considered themselves as less vulnerable to viral illnesses, and 68% regarded their quality of life as much better than that of their sedentary colleagues. The majority (90%) were very interested in good health, 85.7% had stopped smoking before they began training, and 37% indicated that exercise had helped them in smoking withdrawal. More than half (59%) had regular medical check-ups, and 86% always used a seat belt when driving. In contrast to other older persons, 88% slept well or very well.

Conclusion.—Participation in Masters competition is apparently associated with favorable prospects in terms of quality of life and health benefits. It appears that older individuals can sustain activity levels substantially higher than those in some recent public health recommendations without adversely affecting their resistance to infectious diseases. The threat of physical injury with intensive endurance training appears to be an acceptable risk from an active lifestyle. In part, the favorable health experience of the Masters athletes may reflect an overall healthy lifestyle.

▶ This 7-year questionnaire follow-up of Masters athletes suggests that their general health is well above average, although, as the authors note, the fairly low response rate of 45% may create a reporting bias (perhaps healthier athletes were more apt to respond). Also, Masters athletes are largely a self-selected group, and this study involved some self-rating. Given these limitations in interpretation, these Masters athletes sustained physical activity levels well above some public health guidelines, yet they seemed broadly to benefit from their lifestyle and had a low injury rate and no increase in infections.

An intriguing tip for physicians who counsel patients is that the endurance athletes (compared to the social, recreational athletes, mainly racket-sport players) were more likely to quit smoking after they became involved in sport. In light of reports that some runners are at fault when struck by vehicles,[1, 2] it may be alarming that 11% of the runners in this study claimed to develop enough of a "runner's high" to tempt them to take risks with traffic.

E.R. Eichner, M.D.

References

1. Williams AF: *US Publ Health Rep* 96:448, 1981.

2. Shephard RJ: Vehicle injuries to joggers: Case report and review. *J Sports Med Phys Fitness* 32:321–331, 1992.

Associations of Physical Activity With Performance-based and Self-reported Physical Functioning in Older Men: The Honolulu Heart Program

Young DR, Masaki KH, Curb JD (Univ of Hawaii at Manoa, Honolulu)

J Am Geriatr Soc 43:845–854, 1995 8–21

Background.—Individuals who lead physically active lives may not experience the typical age-related declines in psychomotor and physical functioning that are generally seen in sedentary persons. The greater functional reserve associated with regular aerobic exercise may allow elderly people to perform activities of daily living with less fatigue and may prolong independence. However, more epidemiologic evidence is needed to support such claims. The relationships between self-reported physical activity and performance-based and self-reported physical functioning 3–5 years later were assessed.

Methods.—A longitudinal study, conducted on the island of Oahu, Hawaii, included 3,640 Japanese-American men older than 70 years of age. The estimated daily energy expenditure was determined from self-reported engagement in a variety of activities which had been reported in a mail survey in 1988. Three to 5 years later, physical functioning status was ascertained from self-report and performance-based measures.

Findings.—Among healthy persons, highly active individuals in 1988 were more likely to be functioning optimally in the basic activities of daily living, home management skills, and physical endurance–type tasks than subjects initially classified as "low active." Time to walk 3 meters (10 feet) was significantly and linearly associated with grip strength across physical activity levels. Although results were similar for subjects with chronic diseases, most of the benefit of physical activity in this subgroup occurred among subjects who were at least moderately physically active (Table 3).

Conclusion.—Being physically active predicts a high level of physical functioning in older men with and without chronic diseases. Even moderate physical activity may be sufficient to maintain optimal functioning in those with chronic diseases.

► There has been increasing recognition in recent years that many of the gains in both health and quality of life in older individuals can be achieved through quite modest increases in physical activity; indeed, these activities are sometimes insufficient to produce an increase in aerobic power. This paper provides further data substantiating this viewpoint in terms of prospective comparisons of the continuing ability to undertake the activities of daily living among a population of older men.

R.J. Shephard, M.D., Ph.D., D.P.E.

TABLE 3.—Age- and Chronic Disease–Adjusted Prevalence of Physical Functioning Variables by Physical Activity Level in 3,587 Men

	Physical Activity Level									
	Low		Medium				High			
	No.*	%*	No.	%	OR†	95% CI	No.	%	OR	95% CI
Physical performance score (n = 3108)	764	80.4	885	82.9	1.2	0.9–1.5	904	82.9	1.2	0.9–1.5
Basic activities of daily living score (n = 3428)	1002	89.0	1069	93.1	1.7	1.2–2.3§	1081	93.7	2.0	1.4–2.8§
Home management skills score (n = 3328)	698	64.6	779	69.2	1.2	1.0–1.5‡	795	70.9	1.4	1.1–1.7§
Physical endurance-type tasks score (n = 3394)	677	61.3	789	69.3	1.5	1.2–1.8§	823	71.6	1.7	1.4–2.0§
Strength-related tasks score (n = 3453)	961	85.1	1035	89.1	1.4	1.1–1.9§	1037	89.2	1.5	1.1–2.0§

* Number of subjects and percentage of subjects who scored optimally.
† Probability of optimal score compared with low physical activity level.
‡ $P < 0.05$.
§ $P < 0.01$ for the comparison with the low physical activity level.
Abbreviations: OR, odds ratio; *CI*, confidence interval.
(Courtesy of Young DR, Masaki KH, Curb JD: Associations of physical activity with performance-based and self-reported physical functioning in older men: The Honolulu Heart Program. *J Am Geriatr Soc* 43:845–854, 1995.)

The Natural History of Exercise: A 10-Yr Follow-up of a Cohort of Runners

Koplan JP, Rothenberg RB, Jones EL (Natl Ctr for Chronic Disease, Prevention and Health Promotion, Atlanta, Ga; DynCorp, Reston, Va)

Med Sci Sports Exerc 27:1180–1184, 1995 8–22

Background.—Despite recommendations on and strong interest in physical activity, little is known about patterns of exercise behavior over time, rates of perseverance, changes in types of exercise, reasons for quitting, and the frequency of various adverse events. The 10-year pattern of exercise and its associated risks were investigated in a cohort of runners.

Methods.—Participants in the 1980 Peachtree Road Race Study were sent a survey questionnaire. Five hundred thirty-five participants responded, including 326 men and 209 women. The response rate was 72% of the original cohort for whom addresses were known.

Findings.—In 1990, only 56% of the respondents said they were still running. However, 81% were still exercising regularly. The cumulative probabilities for continuing running were 0.71 and 0.56 for men and women, respectively. The main reason men quit running permanently was injury, reported by 31%. Twenty-eight percent of women quit to change to a different form of exercise. During the 10-year interval, 53% of the respondents had at least 1 injury. The probability of injury was related to greater weekly mileage. The most frequent site of injury was the knee. Verbal assaults while running were reported by 39% of the women and 35% of the men. About 10% were hit by objects thrown or were bitten by a dog.

Conclusion.—In this cohort of recreational runners, nearly half had quit running after 10 years. However, more than 80% were still physically active. Injury and other hazards were reported by many of them.

Physical Disability in Older Runners: Prevalence, Risk Factors, and Progression With Age

Ward MM, Hubert HB, Shi H, Bloch DA (Veterans Affairs Med Ctr, Palo Alto, Calif; Stanford Univ, Calif)

J Gerontol 50A:M70–M77, 1995 8–23

Objective.—The benefits of exercise have been shown to extend to elderly people, leading to recommendations that individuals in older age groups increase their level of physical activity. However, there is concern that some types of exercise—especially vigorous activity—could increase physical disability in older people. Although many different factors associated with physical disability have been identified, the role of exercise remains uncertain. Risk factors for disability were examined in older adult runners, together with the factors contributing to age-related progression of physical disability.

Methods.—The study included 454 runners aged 50 years or older, most from an association of older adult runners. The subjects' levels of physical disability were prospectively assessed by the Health Assessment Questionnaire Disability Index, which was mailed to the subjects annually over 5–7 years. The subjects' baseline sociodemographic, clinical, and lifestyle characteristics were assessed to identify factors associated with the development of disability over the course of the study. The results were compared with those of 292 older adult nonrunners with similar follow-up.

Results.—Forty-nine percent of the runners reported some type of physical disability during the study. The most important risk factor for disability was arthritis symptoms at baseline. Other significant risk factors were older age, greater body mass index, strenuous work-related physical disability, and use of more medications. The incidence of physical disability was greater (77%) among the nonrunners. Again, the presence of arthritis symptoms was the most important risk factor for disability. Both groups showed significant age-related changes in physical disability between subjects with and without arthritis symptoms at baseline. Once it had occurred, physical disability tended to persist in runners and nonrunners alike. A history of strenuous work activity was a significant risk factor only for the runners.

Conclusion.—Arthritis symptoms are an important risk factor for physical disability among older people, regardless of their level of physical activity. The identification of risk factors for disability could permit preventive strategies to decrease the burden of disability or delay its onset. Treatment of arthritis symptoms, for example, might not only restore the patient to full activity sooner but also prevent further disability. People who remain physically active throughout adulthood and maintain a lean body weight could be less likely to become disabled.

► Regarding risk factors and the inevitable development of degenerative joint disease, it is clear that the substantial benefits of exercise outweigh any untoward complications. However, stated by Koplan et al. (Abstract 8–22), "Obtaining prospective information on a population with a wide range of levels of physical activity should be a priority for future investigation."

J.S. Torg, M.D.

Effects of Strength and Endurance Training on Thigh and Leg Muscle Mass and Composition in Elderly Women

Sipilä S, Suominen H (Univ of Jyväskylä, Finland)

J Appl Physiol 78:334–340, 1995 8–24

Background.—One of the main reasons for impaired muscle performance in elderly individuals is age-related muscle atrophy. The effects of progressive, intensive strength and endurance training on the quadriceps, hamstrings, knee flexor compartment, and lower leg muscle mass and composition were studied by CT in elderly women.

Methods.—Forty-two women aged 76–78 years with no contraindications to intensive physical exercise were randomly assigned to groups performing strength, endurance, or no training. Twelve women in the strength training group, 12 in the endurance group, and 11 in the control group completed the study. Intensive training was performed for 18 weeks. Computed tomography was used to assess muscle cross-sectional area (CSA), lean tissue CSA, and relative proportion of fat.

Findings.—Compared with the control group, women undergoing strength training increased their total muscle lean tissue CSA of the thigh, quadriceps CSA, quadriceps lean tissue CSA, and mean Hounsfield unit of the lower leg muscles. The strength training group's change in quadriceps lean tissue CSA was also significant compared with that in the endurance group. The relative proportion of fat in the quadriceps muscle declined with strength training compared with endurance training.

Conclusion.—Intensive strength training can induce skeletal muscle hypertrophy in elderly women, thereby decreasing the relative amount of intramuscular fat. The effects of endurance training are negligible.

► Part of the increase in strength from baseline values in strength training studies has been ascribed to learning or neural adaptation. This could be an important confounding factor in studies involving older individuals who lack experience in strength training and has led to a number of studies in men examining changes in the CSA of the muscles involved. The use of CT in this study to quantify changes in the CSA of the trained muscles confirms the belief that muscle hypertrophy occurs in older women who participate in a well-planned program of strength training.

B.L. Drinkwater, Ph.D.

Strength Improvements With 1 Yr of Progressive Resistance Training in Older Women

Morganti CM, Nelson ME, Fiatarone MA, Dallal GE, Economos CD, Crawford BM, Evans WJ (Tufts Univ, Boston; Harvard Med School, Boston; Pennsylvania State Univ, State College)

Med Sci Sports Exerc 27:906–912, 1995 8–25

Background.—Resistance training is known to improve strength in individuals of all ages. Several recent studies have also suggested that high-intensity strength training stimulates muscle hypertrophy among older people, although long-term effects of strength training in older individuals are not yet known. There have been no randomized, controlled, prospective, long-term studies investigating the effects of high-intensity progressive resistance training in older women. This study examined the association between progressive resistance training and strength gains over an extended period among postmenopausal women.

Participants and Methods.—Thirty-nine healthy women (mean age, 59.5 years) completed this 1-year, controlled clinical study. All women had been postmenopausal for 5 years or longer, were not older than 70 years of age, did not participate in any routine exercise program, weighed less than 120% of ideal body weight, were nonsmokers, and had not taken estrogen for at least 1 year. Twenty women were randomly assigned to a progressive resistance training group, and 19 served as controls. Participants in the strength training group engaged in supervised high-intensity resistance training 2 d/wk for 52 weeks. Sessions lasted approximately 45 minutes and were separated by at least 1 day of rest. Training intensity was set at 80% of the most recently measured 1 repetition maximum (1RM) for each muscle group for double leg press, knee extension, and lateral pull-down exercises. Three sets of 8 repetitions were performed on each machine during each training session, with repetitions lasting 6–9 seconds. There was a 3-second rest between repetitions and a 1.5–2 minute rest between sets. Women assigned to the control group maintained their current activity levels during the 1-year period and were instructed not to begin any strength training programs.

Both groups underwent testing at baseline, with the 1RM serving as the measure of dynamic concentric muscle strength for the double leg press, knee extension, and lateral pull-down exercises. Testing was repeated at 6 and 12 months for controls and monthly for women in the intervention group.

Results.—The women in the training group were found to be stronger than controls in all 3 exercises at 6 and 12 months. Among women in the training group, increases of 73.7% for knee extension, 35.1% for double leg press, and 77% for lateral pull-down exercises were observed, compared with 12.7%, 3.7%, and 18.4%, respectively, among controls. The

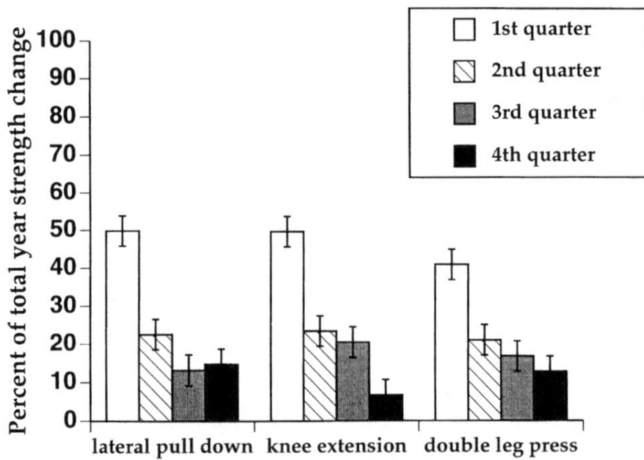

FIGURE 3.—Percentage of total strength change for the strength-training group over 1 year, divided into quarters, in the lateral pull-down, knee extension, and double leg press. (Courtesy of Morganti CM, Nelson ME, Fiatarone MA, et al: Strength improvements with 1 year of progressive resistance training in older women. *Med Sci Sports Exerc* 27:906–912, 1995.)

greatest gains were noted during the first 3 months of the study, although strength continued to increase during the 1-year period in the women undergoing training (Fig 3).

Conclusion.—High-intensity strength training leads to considerable, progressive gains in strength for at least 12 months among postmenopausal women.

► This group has been one of the leaders in calling attention to the benefits of strength training for older women and men. Now they have shown that strength can continue to increase substantially over a period of 12 months. These investigators have consistently observed gains in strength throughout the course of their previous studies as well, although other studies have reported a plateau in strength gains after 8–12 weeks. As more reports of strength training of older individuals become available, it may be possible to identify the factors, such as intensity of training, that differentiate between those protocols that produce continual gains and those that result in a plateau. Regardless of whether or when a plateau occurs, the best news is that age does not negate the benefits of strength training.

B.L. Drinkwater, Ph.D.

The Effects of Strength Conditioning on Older Women's Ability to Perform Daily Tasks

Hunter GR, Treuth MS, Weinsier RL, Kekes-Szabo T, Kell SH, Roth DL, Nicholson C (Univ of Alabama, Birmingham)

J Am Geriatr Soc 43:756–760, 1995 8–26

Background.—The increased incidence of disability in older adults partially results from the decreased muscle size and strength that occurs with age. The functional capacity of older, healthy adults may also be affected by strength. Studies have shown that strength training can increase muscle size and strength in older adults. Because of the positive relationship between surface electromyographic activity and force in muscles, normalized integrated electromyographic activity may be used as an index of relative muscular stress. The effects of strength conditioning on walking speed and normalized integrated electromyographic activity were evaluated in older women performing daily activities.

Methods.—The subjects were 14 healthy, sedentary women between 60 and 77 years of age. Women receiving estrogen replacement therapy were not excluded. Subjects completed a fitness questionnaire before training and after 8 and 16 weeks of training. Before and after the 16 weeks of strength conditioning, all subjects were evaluated for (1) normalized integrated electromyographic activity of the right biceps while walking at 2 mph and carrying a box of groceries; (2) normalized integrated electromyographic activity of the right quadriceps while sitting in and rising from a chair; (3) maximal walking velocity during a 6-m walking test; and (4)

TABLE 1.—Performance Tests: Pre- and Post-strength Training

	Pre	Post	% Change
1-RM strength tests (kg)			
Elbow flexion	10.8 ± 0.6	15.2 ± 0.7*	+40.7
Latissimus pull down	23.5 ± 1.3	33.9 ± 1.4*	+44.2
Bench press	14.7 ± 0.9	24.1 ± 1.1*	+63.9
Leg press	70.4 ± 4.4	116.0 ± 8.6*	+64.8
Leg extension	20.2 ± 1.6	29.4 ± 1.3*	+45.6
Leg curl	15.6 ± 1.8	24.1 ± 1.0*	+54.5
Isometric strength (N)			
Knee extension	219 ± 20	317 ± 26*	+44.7
Knee flexion	131 ± 06	154 ± 09*	+17.5
Walking velocity (meters/sec)	1.64 ± .16	1.94 ± .17*	+18.3

Note: Figures are for mean ± standard error.
* Significantly different from pretest at 0.01 level.
Abbreviation: 1 RM, repetition maximum, the largest amount of weight that can be lifted 1 time.
(Courtesy of Hunter GR, Treuth MS, Weinsier RL, et al: The effects of strength conditioning on older women's ability to perform daily tasks. *J Am Geriatr Soc* 43:756–760, 1995.)

isometric and dynamic strength. The isometric strength, dynamic strength, weight-loaded walking, standing, and maximal walking velocity tests were described in detail.

Results.—In all subjects, strength increased significantly in the dynamic strength tests. Upper body strength increased 48.4% and lower body strength increased 60.3% (Table 1). Peak isometric force also increased significantly. The increase was 17.5% in the elbow flexion test and 44.7% in the knee extension test. Walking velocity increased significantly. Velocity of standing and sitting remained the same, but normalized integrated electromyographic activity of the rectus femoris decreased significantly at 110 degrees and 130 degrees of knee flexion; it also decreased an average of 40% while standing and an average of 47% while sitting. Normalized integrated electromyographic activity decreased significantly while holding a box of groceries before, during, and after walking. Scores from the fitness questionnaire increased throughout the training program.

Discussion.—In these subjects, increased strength was associated with improved ability to perform everyday activities. These are the first documented objective changes in relative muscle activation during a daily activity. These findings indicate that older women are as trainable as younger adults.

▶ This is another example of how strength training can enable older women to function independently in their "golden years." The beneficial effects of encouraging women to participate in some form of weight training will extend beyond the effect on the quality of life for individual women to a decrease in cost to the health care system. The challenge will be to structure inexpensive programs that will be readily available and attractive to older women. As anyone who has attempted to retain formerly sedentary women in an exercise study knows, compliance and continued participation are the 2 biggest challenges the investigator faces. There is a reason sedentary women are inactive: They prefer inactivity to activity. The expertise of psychologists and sociologists will be needed if we are to put the work of the physiologists to practical use.

B.L. Drinkwater, Ph.D.

Sports Injuries in Athletes With Disabilities: Wheelchair Racing
Taylor D, Williams T (Loughborough Univ, England)
Paraplegia 33:296–299, 1995 8–27

Background.—Individuals with physical disabilities are participating in sports activities more and more. The types of injuries they sustain may be specific to their disabilities and the athletic event. There is little research regarding the incidence, causes, and treatment of sports injuries in disabled athletes. The training activities and number and kinds of injuries sustained by wheelchair racers were examined.

Methods.—Members of the British Wheelchair Racing Association completed questionnaires that asked about the nature of their impairment, their experience in wheelchair racing, their training program, and sports-related injuries.

Results.—Of 53 respondents, 72% had sustained at least 1 injury in the previous 12 months. Training variables were not associated with injury occurrence; training variables included distance pushed per week, amount of speed training, frequency of weight training sessions, and length of time participating in wheelchair racing. The most common injuries were overuse injuries, and these recurred more often than other types of injuries. Athletes with recurring injuries were more likely to have started training again before the pain from the previous injury was gone.

Conclusion.—The incidence and type of injuries were not affected by the training activities of these wheelchair athletes. Further research is needed to investigate the relationship between overuse injuries, early return to training after injury, and the injury recurrence rate. The responses provided by these athletes indicated that they were not knowledgeable regarding sports injuries, causes of sports injuries, or treatment.

▶ Although this study is beset with many of the problems inherent in a retrospective questionnaire protocol, it is important to point out that it was not intended to be a diagnostic or injury registry. Rather, this study was an attempt to provide subjective historical information from wheelchair racers in a "first step" attempt to understanding the nature of injuries in this particular group of individuals with disabilities. The authors have, in fact, accomplished this goal.

J.S. Torg, M.D.

Peripheral Neuropathies in the Upper Extremities of Paraplegic Wheelchair Marathon Racers

Dozono K, Hachisuka K, Hatada K, Ogata H (Univ of Occupational and Environmental Health, Fukuoka, Japan; Oita Nakamura Hosp, Japan)
Paraplegia 33:208–211, 1995 8–28

Background.—Wheelchair races are becoming more competitive, and participants must train more vigorously to be successful. The wheelchair marathon race may cause nerve injury in paraplegic individuals. Nerve conduction studies were performed on the upper extremities of paraplegic wheelchair marathon racers and on sedentary paraplegic persons to determine whether the racers have peripheral neuropathy in the upper extremities.

Methods and Findings.—Nerve conduction studies were performed bilaterally on the median, ulnar, and radial ulnar nerves of 10 male wheelchair marathon racers and 10 sedentary paraplegic men. Reduced motor nerve conduction velocities and/or prolongation of motor or sensory nerve distal latencies were documented in 5 racers and 9 sedentary subjects. In the nerve conduction studies, findings were abnormal in 3.2% of the racers and in 13.6% of the sedentary paraplegics. Although the racers had fewer peripheral neuropathies in the upper extremities than the sedentary subjects, ulnar lesions from involvement of the deep motor branch and at the elbow were characteristic, most likely resulting from marathon racing.

Conclusion.—Wheelchair marathon racing is generally a safe sport. However, participants must wear gloves and handle their wheelchairs correctly during the race to prevent nerve injuries.

► The existing literature dealing with injuries incurred by paraplegic wheelchair marathon racers supports the conclusion that this is "generally a safe sport." Curtis has reported 291 "wheelchair athletic injuries" in 128 paraplegic persons.[1] These were mainly soft-tissue injuries, blisters, lacerations, and pressure ulcers. Nilson et al. also reported on complications occurring in paraplegic athletes while participating in sports, the major injuries being strains and sprains.[2]

With regard to the paper at hand, I question whether abnormal nerve conduction studies can be equated with "peripheral neuropathies." Also, all measurements were performed 1 month before a wheelchair marathon race, perhaps not the preferable time to demonstrate physically induced abnormalities.

J.S. Torg, M.D.

References

1. Curtis KA, Dillon DA: Survey of wheelchair athletic injuries: Common patterns and prevention. *Paraplegia* 23:170–175, 1985.
2. Nilsen R, Nygaard P, Bjorholt PG: Complications that may occur in those with spinal cord injuries who participate in sports. *Paraplegia* 23:152–158, 1985.

Human Immunodeficiency Virus (HIV) and Other Blood-borne Pathogens in Sports: Joint Position Statement

American Medical Society for Sports Medicine and the American Academy of Sports Medicine (American Academy of Sports Medicine, Rosemont, Ill)

Am J Sports Med 23:510–514, 1995 8–29

Background.—Transmission of HIV and hepatitis B virus (HBV) is by similar routes, namely, sexual contact, parenteral blood exposure, and perinatal exposure. However, HBV is far more readily transmitted than HIV because of the higher number of infectious viral doses in the blood of HBV patients. Because of the nature of these bloodborne illnesses, many athletes will be healthy enough to compete for several years after their infection. The American Medical Society for Sports Medicine and the American Academy of Sports Medicine have issued a joint position statement regarding the management of these patients in athletic competition.

Discussion.—Although transmission of HIV and HBV is theoretically possible, the risk is so small as to nearly defy quantitation. Even for HBV, there is only 1 documented case of sport-related transmission. No such case has been reported for HIV. The decision to continue competitive athletics is highly individual and is related more to the patient's health than to the infectious status. By itself, HIV or HBV infection is not sufficient reason to prohibit athletic activity. Education of athletes regarding these diseases is encouraged. Mandatory testing of athletes for these pathogens is not justified by the minimal degree of risk.

Specific guidelines emphasize common sense, basic hygiene, and adherence to universal precautions. They are as follows:

1. Existing wounds should be cleaned and covered before competition.
2. Supplies needed for universal precautions should be available at all times.
3. Uncontrolled bleeding during competition should be immediately controlled and the wound cleaned and dressed before the player returns to competition.
4. The athlete must understand his or her responsibility to report preexisting or on-field injuries in a timely manner.
5. All caregivers must follow universal precautions.
6. Minor cuts and abrasions can be cleaned and dressed during scheduled breaks in play.
7. Emergency care for life-threatening injuries must take place, even in the absence of protective equipment.
8. Equipment or surfaces soiled with blood should be wiped, disinfected with a fresh bleach solution, and dried before further use.
9. Postevent, wounds should be re-evaluated and dressed, and blood-soiled laundry should be collected for hot laundering.
10. Training room procedures should include universal precautions.

11. Some team health personnel may be covered by Occupational Safety and Health Administration (OSHA) regulations, including HBV immunization.

Legal considerations include the following. (1) only the athlete or the guardian of a minor may decide to whom medical information is given, except for mandatory reports; (2) team physicians may not share this information with others, including coaches; (3) there is no precedent for legal responsibility for disease transmission in athletics, although responsibility lies with the infected person in other situations; and (4) team physicians should be aware of applicable rules, including OSHA regulations.

Conclusion.—Although there is a slight risk of transmitting HIV or HBV during athletic competition, it is extremely small. Proper attention to basic hygiene and routine use of universal precautions are necessary. The presence of HIV is, in itself, not a reason to withdraw from athletics. Mandatory testing of athletes for HIV and HBV is not appropriate.

► I would like to repeat some of my comments from the 1993 YEAR BOOK OF SPORTS MEDICINE regarding HIV infection in athletes. Old habits are sometimes hard to break. Athletic trainers and team physicians must take the time to stop, put on a pair of gloves, and take whatever other precautions are necessary before treating a bleeding athlete. This is not only necessary to protect the physician or athletic trainer, but also the next athlete we may be treating. We seem to have the situation pretty much under control in the training room or doctor's office, but we need to be equally careful on the field and in the gymnasium, hockey rink, or mat-side.[1]

I continue to observe athletic trainers treating bleeding or open wounds and not adhering to universal precautions. You owe it to yourself and your athletes to use universal precautions in all situations where they are required.

F.J. George, A.T.C., P.T.

Reference

1. 1993 YEAR BOOK OF SPORTS MEDICINE, p 450.

Bleeding Injuries in Professional Football: Estimating the Risk for HIV Transmission

Brown LS Jr, Drotman DP, Chu A, Brown CL Jr, Knowlan D (Addiction Research and Treatment Corp, Brooklyn, NY; Columbia Univ, New York; Emory Univ, Atlanta, Ga; et al)

Ann Intern Med 122:271–274, 1995 8–30

Introduction.—Because bleeding injuries can occur during athletic competition, there is concern regarding the possibility of the transmission of

HIV and other bloodborne pathogens. An investigation was undertaken to quantify the risk of HIV transmission via bleeding injuries in professional football competition.

Methods.—A total of 155 regular season games of 11 National Football League teams were observed to record the number and types of bleeding injuries, and selected environmental and athletic factors. Associations between these variables were analyzed. The probability of HIV transmission from a single contact during football competition was calculated as the product of the prevalence of college men infected with HIV × the risk for percutaneous HIV transmission × the risk for laceration injury in an opponent × the risk for bleeding injury for each player per game.

Results.—There were 575 observed bleeding injuries, of which 87.5% were abrasions and 12.5% were lacerations. The frequency of bleeding injuries, particularly abrasions, increased in association with games played on artificial surfaces, in domed stadiums, and with teams that had an even or losing season record (Table 1). The probability of HIV transmission was calculated as follows: 1 infected player/200 players × 1 HIV transmission/300 exposures × 0.41 lacerated players per game/45 players per game × 3.46 bleeding players per game/45 players per game = 1 HIV transmission per 85,647,821 game contacts.

Discussion.—Using data documenting the frequency of bleeding injuries together with prevalence and transmission risk data, the risk of HIV transmission during professional football competition was calculated as

TABLE 1.—Bleeding Injuries Per Game: Environmental and Athletic Factors

Variables	Games (n = 155)	Games With at Least 1 Injury, n (%)	Mean Number of Bleeding Injuries Per Game		
			Abrasions	Lacerations	Total
Month of game					
September or October	68	61 (90)	3.25	0.50	3.74
November or December	87	81 (93)	3.24	0.44	3.68
Game location					
Home	85	75 (88)	3.13	0.41	3.53
Away	70	67 (96)	3.39	0.53	3.91
Playing surface					
Artificial	81	77 (95)	3.94*	0.49	4.42*
Grass	74	65 (88)	2.49	0.43	2.92
Stadium type					
Domed	41	39 (95)	3.93	0.63	4.54†
Open-air	114	103 (90)	3.00	0.40	3.40
Outcome of game					
Win	82	74 (90)	3.28	0.40	3.67
Loss	73	68 (93)	3.21	0.53	3.74
Margin of victory or loss					
≤10 points	76	71 (93)	3.37	0.38	3.73
>10 points	79	71 (90)	3.13	0.54	3.67
Season winning percentage					
≤0.500	69	66 (96)	3.72	0.54	4.25†
>0.500	86	76 (88)	2.68	0.41	3.27

* $P < 0.005$.

† $P < 0.05$. Student t-test to detect differences used 2-tailed univariate analyses with alpha = 0.05.

(Courtesy of Brown LS Jr, Drotman DP, Chu A, et al: Bleeding injuries in professional football: Estimating the risk for HIV transmission. *Ann Intern Med* 122:271–274, 1995.)

less than 1 in 85 million contacts. This risk is extremely low, particularly when compared with the risk of HIV transmission associated with sexual and drug-using activities. Therefore, professional athletes can most effectively reduce their risk of contracting or spreading HIV infection by modifying their nonathletic behaviors.

▶ This report, although limited by statistical assumptions and estimates, concludes that the chance of HIV transmission in professional football is extremely low or negligible. Surely this is correct. But the chance of HIV transmission in boxing or wrestling, for example, is greater. As reviewed last year,[1] in the medical literature are 2 reports of HIV transmission from bloody fistfights. In 1996, heavyweight boxer Tommy Morrison tested HIV-positive before a bout and retired. This led to calls for the mandatory HIV screening of boxers, on the premise that, in this "blood sport," public health outranks civil rights.

Five states (including New York) now screen professional boxers for HIV. California and New Jersey, which (along with New York) are major boxing states, are expected to follow suit. If national screening is mandated, at what level should it start? The Junior Olympics? The Golden Gloves? How often should boxers be screened? And who will ensure the integrity of screening in a sport sullied with scoundrels?

E.R. Eichner, M.D.

Reference

1. 1995 Year Book of Sports Medicine, pp 494–496.

Osteitis Pubis in the Active Patient

Sing R, Cordes R, Siberski D (Sports Science Ctr, Glen Mills, Pa; Geisinger Med Ctr, Danville, Pa; Chicago College of Osteopathic Medicine, Downers Grove, Ill)

Physician Sportsmed 23:67–68, 71–73, 1995 8–31

Introduction.—Persistent pain in the groin region, especially when unresponsive to conservative management, may indicate osteitis pubis. This overuse injury occurs most often in sports that require support of body weight on 1 leg and/or abrupt changes in direction. A representative case of sport-related osteitis pubis was presented.

Case Report.—Boy, 17 years, was a high school soccer player with continuous bilateral groin pain of 3 months' duration. Although straight running did not exacerbate the pain, the patient was unable to play soccer for more than 15 minutes. No symptoms of a urinary tract infection were present. The most notable finding at physical examination was significant tenderness on palpation of the symphysis pubis. A diagnosis of osteitis pubis was confirmed

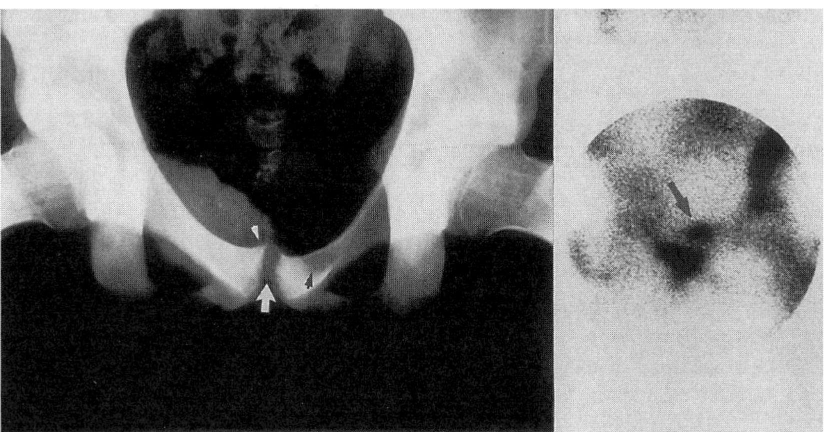

FIGURE 1.—A, plain radiograph of a 17-year-old male soccer player's pelvis exhibits findings consistent with osteitis pubis: widening of the pubic symphysis (*arrow*), osteolysis of the left pubic ramus (*large arrowhead*), and an irregularity of the superior border of the right pubic ramus (*small arrowhead*). **B,** third-phase bone scan of the patient's pelvis reveals asymmetric uptake at the public ramus (*arrow*). This finding, combined with the osteolysis on the left side, indicates bilateral osteitis pubis. (Courtesy of Sing R, Cordes R, Siberski D: Osteitis pubis in the active patient. *Physician Sportsmed* 23:67–68, 71–73, 1995, reproduced with permission of McGraw-Hill, Inc.)

with technetium pyrophosphate bone scanning which revealed increased uptake at the right symphysis pubis (Fig 1). The patient was successfully treated by 6 months of flexibility and strength training, including in-water conditioning at an aquatics rehabilitation center. He was able to resume full soccer competition.

Discussion.—Osteitis pubis occurs most often among athletes whose sports create shearing forces at the pubic symphysis. Simultaneous contraction of the adductor and abdominal muscles contributes to antagonistic pulling on the pubic anastomosis, leading to the repetitive motion disorder. The pain develops gradually and may be confused with a groin pull. All recalcitrant cases of "pulled groin" should be evaluated with x-ray studies; if radiographic findings are nondiagnostic, a triple-phase bone scan is recommended. Therapy consists of rest, oral nonsteroidal anti-inflammatory medications, and hydrotherapy. The disease appears to be self-limited, and conservative treatment is usually successful.

▶ Osteitis pubis is an overuse injury that is especially common in sports that require frequent support on 1 leg, as in a soccer kick or rapid cutting. It also occurs in distance runners and race walkers. It is thought that a repeated shearing force leads to a self-limited erosion of the pubis symphysis, followed by spontaneous healing. Osteitis pubis should be suspected when a "groin pull" shows no sign of improving after 2 weeks of conservative therapy. This article covers the classic clinical features, diagnostic measures, and management. Another recent article covers the rarer problem of pyogenic osteomyelitis of the pubis in otherwise healthy athletes. This condition is seen as extreme, acute groin pain; point tenderness; and fever.[1]

E.R. Eichner, M.D.

Reference

1. Karpos PA, Spindler KP, Pierce MA, et al: Osteomyelitis of the pubic symphysis in athletes: A case report and literature review. *Med Sci Sports Exerc* 27:473–479, 1995.

Pyomyositis in an Adolescent Female Athlete

Meehan J, Grose C, Soper RT, Kimura K (Univ of Iowa, Iowa City)

J Pediatr Surg 30:127–128, 1995 8–32

Introduction.—Historically, pyomyositis often occurs in men, especially among those who participate in strenuous physical activity. A case of pyomyositis in a healthy adolescent girl was discussed.

Case Report.—Girl, 13 years, a volleyball player, complained of left hip and gluteal pain that was exacerbated while playing volleyball, as well as fever and chills. There was no history of trauma, but she would frequently fall on that area during volleyball drills when "digging" for balls. The patient appeared toxic and lay on her right side with the left hip flexed. Psoriasis was evident in the face and extremities. Aspiration of the left hip joint failed to yield any fluid; a bone scan showed uptake in the iliac and femoral nodes but not in the bone. Magnetic resonance imaging clearly showed a left iliopsoas abscess (Fig 1). Incision and drainage was performed, revealing pus within the iliopsoas muscle surrounded by necrotic tissue. The lymph nodes and blood grew *Staphylococcus aureus*. The patient improved with IV antibiotics.

Discussion.—Competitive sports and vigorous exercise programs are becoming more widely available to young girls. Pyomyositis should be suspected in the differential diagnosis of unexplained localized muscle pain in any adolescent who has been engaged in strenuous physical activity. Magnetic resonance imaging is undoubtedly the most accurate method of defining a lesion within a muscle. In this patient, the abscess was located in muscle tissue, a common site of impact when a volleyball player dives for a ball. The bacteremia most likely developed from intercurrent staphylococcal infection of psoriatic lesions.

► This case has practical clinical importance for the sports medicine physician: Fever and chills in the face of muscle trauma or injury should suggest the rare complication of pyomyositis, and the MR image can be diagnostic. I doubt that, as the authors suggest, the iliopsoas muscle—the site of the staphylococcal abscess here—is really a "point of impact when a volleyball

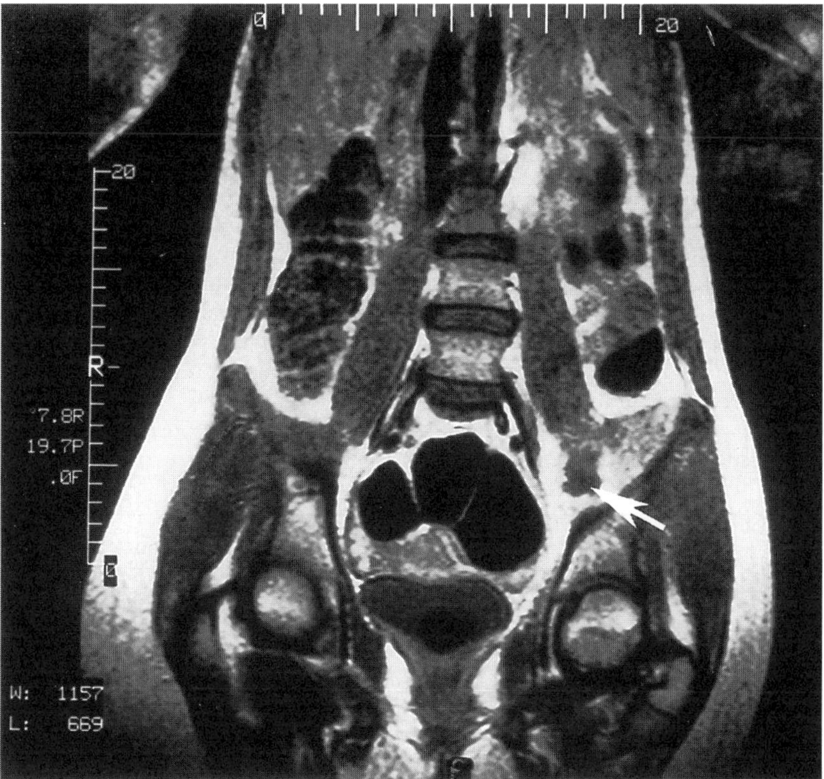

FIGURE 1.—Coronal MR image of the pelvis shows an abscess in the medial left iliacus muscle (*arrow*), adjacent to the psoas muscle (superior to the iliacus). The vertebral column is visible in the center of the image. (Courtesy of Meehan J, Grose C, Soper RT, et al: Pyomyositis in an adolescent female athlete. *J Pediatr Surg* 30:127–128, 1995.)

player dives for a ball." It is key, however, to considering the possibility of bacterial myositis in athletes like this, and to moving fast. Although fewer than 100 cases of bacterial myositis have been reported in the American literature, late diagnosis can be lethal, as in the tragic case of streptococcal myositis in a young quarterback originally given the diagnosis of a "thigh bruise."[1]

E.R. Eichner, M.D.

Reference

1. 1995 YEAR BOOK OF SPORTS MEDICINE, pp 491–493.

An Epidemic of Tinea Corporis Caused by *Trichophyton tonsurans* Among Wrestlers in Sweden

Hradil E, Hersle K, Nordin P, Faergemann J (Univ Hosp, Malmö, Sweden; Frölunda Hosp, Gothenburg, Sweden; Sahlgrenska Univ, Gothenburg, Sweden)

Acta Derm Venereol 75:305–306, 1995 8–33

Purpose.—*Trichophyton tonsurans* is commonly involved in tinea corporis outbreaks among United States wrestlers. However, *Trichophyton verrucosum*, rather than *T. tonsurans*, was the causative organism in the only documented tinea corporis outbreak among Swedish wrestlers. Two tinea corporis outbreaks caused by *T. tonsurans* were reported.

Patients.—During the summer of 1993, 2 young men belonging to the same wrestling club in Malmö were seen with discrete, slightly scaling annular skin lesions on the cheek and arm. *Trichophyton tonsurans* was cultured from the lesions of both wrestlers. Subsequent screening of the other wrestling club members revealed scaling lesions in 19, and 14 of them had laboratory-confirmed *T. tonsurans* infections. Several months later, 4 young men belonging to a wrestling club in Gothenburg were seen with tinea corporis and received a diagnosis of *T. tonsurans* infections. The wife of one of the wrestlers was also infected with this organism. Systemic oral treatment with griseofulvin, fluconazole, or terbinafine completely cured the infection in all cases.

Findings.—Investigation of the outbreaks revealed that the members of a United States wrestling team who had participated in an international competition in Sweden earlier that year were the most likely source of infection.

► In 1992, we covered a large outbreak of herpes gladiatorum at a high school wrestling camp in Minnesota.[1] In that outbreak, herpes gladiatorum developed in 60 (35%) of 175 young wrestlers. Transmission was mainly skin-to-skin. In 1993, we reported on how best to prevent herpes gladiatorum, and we reviewed other reports of skin-to-skin infections in athletes, including furunculosis, tinea corporis gladiatorum, and (via mud-wrestling) gram-negative pustular dermatitis.[2] This report covers the first skin-to-skin epidemic of tinea corporis gladiatorum in Sweden. Team physicians can help to prevent such epidemics by examining athletes for sores or rashes and by strictly applying universal precautions. Another recent article outlines the risk of plantar warts from communal showers.[3]

E.R. Eichner, M.D.

References

1. 1992 Year Book of Sports Medicine, pp 248–249.
2. 1993 Year Book of Sports Medicine, pp 447–448.
3. Johnson LW: Communal showers and the risk of plantar warts. *J Fam Pract* 40:136–138, 1995.

Immune Function in Marathon Runners Versus Sedentary Controls

Nieman DC, Buckley KS, Henson DA, Warren BJ, Suttles J, Ahle JC, Simandle S, Fagoaga OR, Nehlsen-Cannarella SL (Applachian State Univ, Boone, NC; East Tennessee State Univ, Johnson City; Loma Linda Univ, Calif)

Med Sci Sports Exerc 27:986–992, 1995 8–34

Background.—It is not known whether marathon runners who repeatedly participate in races and regular long distance training have altered immunity. One study involving a small number of individuals concluded that leukocyte phagocytosis and killing, lymphocyte proliferative response, and immunoglobulin levels were similar between runners and sedentary persons. A larger group of marathon runners was compared with sedentary control subjects in this study to test the hypothesis that long-distance running does not affect immune function.

Methods.—Twenty-two male marathon runners and 18 sedentary men were included in the study. The runners had completed at least 7 marathons and had been training for marathon races for at least 4 years. The mean ages were 38.7 years and 43.9 years in the running and sedentary groups, respectively. Height was also comparable between groups. However, the runners were significantly leaner and had a maximum oxygen consumption 60% greater than that of the control subjects (Table 1).

Findings.—Runners tended to have lower neutrophil counts than sedentary subjects. Other leukocyte and lymphocyte subsets were similar in the 2 groups. Mitogen-induced lymphocyte proliferation was also comparable. The runners had significantly higher natural killer cell cytotoxic activity (NKCA) than the sedentary men. For all subjects combined and within the group of marathon runners, percent body fat was negatively

TABLE 1.—Subject Characteristics

	Marathoners (n = 22)	Controls (n = 18)
Age (yr)	38.7 ± 1.5	43.9 ± 2.2
Height (m)	1.77 ± 0.01	1.77 ± 0.01
Weight (kg)	71.7 ± 1.8	89.6 ± 3.9*
Body fat %	11.2 ± 0.8	25.0 ± 1.3*
VO_2max ($ml \cdot kg^{-1} \cdot min^{-1}$)	57.9 ± 1.1	36.2 ± 1.2*
HRmax (bpm)	182 ± 1	179 ± 4
VEmax ($l \cdot min^{-1}$)	157 ± 5	128 ± 3*
RERmax	1.20 ± 0.02	1.23 ± 0.02
Running distance ($km \cdot wk^{-1}$)	78.6 ± 6.5	—
Running experience (yr)	12.3 ± 1.3	—
Marathon personal best (min)	175.3 ± 5.0	—
Total marathons completed	23.6 ± 5.7	—

Note: Figures are mean ± standard error.
* $P < 0.001$.
(Courtesy of Nieman DC, Buckley KS, Henson DA, et al: Immune function in marathon runners versus sedentary controls. *Med Sci Sports Exerc* 27:986–992, 1995.)

TABLE 2.—Cross-Sectional Comparison of Leukocyte Subset Counts ($10^9/l^{-1}$) Between Marathoners and Sedentary Controls

	Marathoners	Controls	*P*-Value
Total leukocytes	5.23 ± 0.27	6.05 ± 0.38	0.09
Neutrophils	2.66 ± 0.20	3.29 ± 0.27	0.06
Lymphocytes	1.80 ± 0.14	1.96 ± 0.16	0.47
$CD3^+$ (T cells)	1.42 ± 0.17	1.44 ± 0.13	0.95
$CD3^-CD16^+CD56^+$ (NK cells)	0.35 ± 0.06	0.31 ± 0.04	0.58
Monocytes	0.51 ± 0.04	0.55 ± 0.04	0.44
Eosinophils	0.23 ± 0.03	0.20 ± 0.02	0.45
Basophils	0.03 ± 0.004	0.05 ± 0.01	0.20

Abbreviation: NK, natural killer.
(Courtesy of Nieman DC, Buckley KS, Henson DA, et al: Immune function in marathon runners versus sedentary controls. *Med Sci Sports Exerc* 27:986–992, 1995.)

associated with NKCA, and age was negatively related to Con A–induced lymphocyte proliferation (Table 2; Figs 1 and 2).

Conclusion.—Compared with sedentary men, male marathon runners have higher NKCA but not mitogen-induced lymphocyte proliferation. These findings concur with others suggesting that endurance athletes do not experience chronic impaired natural killer– or T-cell function.

► This cross-sectional study set out to explore various facets of immune function in marathoners actively training and racing. (See Abstract 8–36 for background on exercise and natural killer [NK] cells). The study found no increase in NK cell *count* but a significant, 57% higher *activity* of NK cells in marathoners at rest, compared with sedentary controls. Nieman et al. have found the same trend in active elderly female athletes[1], but not in highly

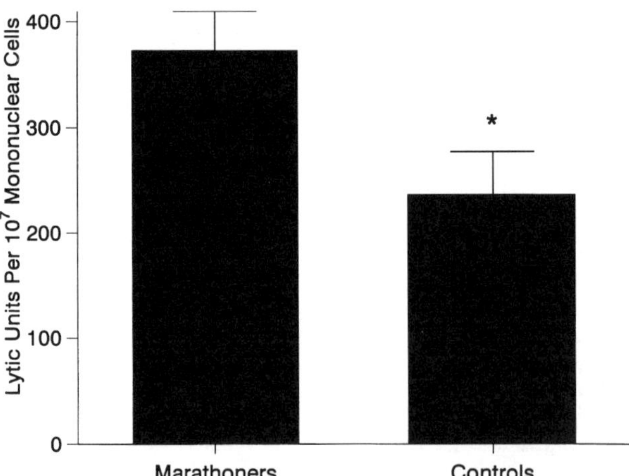

FIGURE 1.—Natural killer cell cytotoxic activity was 57% higher in the marathon runners vs. sedentary controls when expressed in lytic units per 10^7 mononuclear cells. $*P < 0.05$. (Courtesy of Nieman DC, Buckley KS, Henson DA, et al: Immune function in marathon runners versus sedentary controls. *Med Sci Sports Exerc* 27:986–992, 1995.)

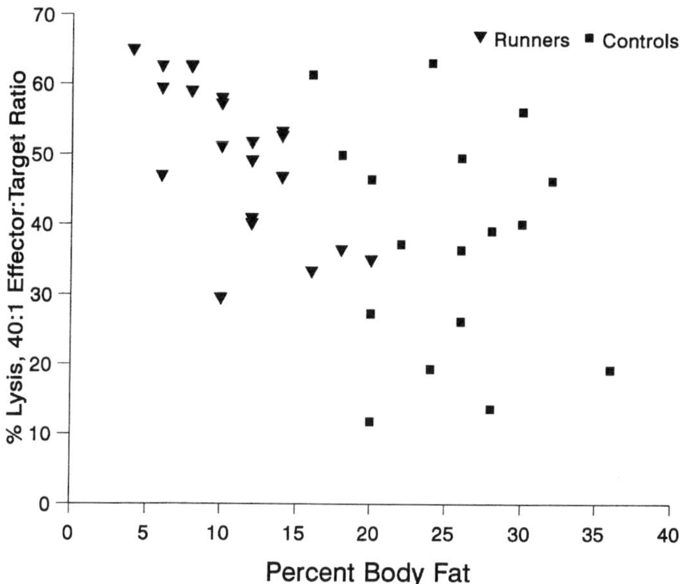

FIGURE 2.—For all subjects combined (n = 39 in this comparison), natural killer cell cytotoxic activity (percent lysis at the 40:1, effector to target ratio) was negatively correlated with percent body fat ($r = -0.52$, $P = 0.001$.) (Courtesy of Nieman DC, Buckley KS, Henson DA, et al: Immune function in marathon runners versus sedentary controls. *Med Sci Sports Exerc* 27:986–992, 1995.)

conditioned college athletes, as discussed in this report. This report at least suggests that active marathoners do not have chronic impaired NK- or T-cell function, even though it is established that various measures of immune function are suppressed for several hours during recovery from prolonged, intense bouts of endurance exercise. (See also Abstract 8–37.)

E.R. Eichner, M.D.

Reference

1. Nieman DC, Henson DA, Gusewitch G, et al: Physical activity and immune function in elderly women. *Med Sci Sports Exerc* 25:823–831, 1993.

Exercise-associated Collapse in Cyclists Is Unrelated to Endotoxemia

Moore GE, Holbein MEB, Knochel JP (Presbyterian Hosp of Dallas)

Med Sci Sports Exerc 27:1238–1242, 1995 8–35

Background.—The entrance of endotoxin into the systemic circulation triggers a cascade of cytokines involving interleukin-1 (IL-1), interleukin 6 (IL-6), and tumor necrosis factor–α (TNF-α). These cytokines probably mediate the sepsis syndrome and are involved as well in heat stroke. Systemic endotoxemia is reported in ultramarathon runners and triathletes who require medical attention after competition. To examine a potential relationship between postexertional illness and endotoxemia, researchers studied cyclists after a 100-mile ride.

Methods.—Thirty-nine of the more than 14,000 cyclists who took part in a bicycle rally in Texas volunteered for the study. Those recruited were 26 control cyclists and 13 cyclists who came to the medical tent after the ride with an aural temperature > 40°C, rigors, nausea, vomiting, diarrhea, syncope, or heat stroke. Control cyclists completed a questionnaire on the day before the rally and were examined 90 minutes before the ride and immediately after. Ill cyclists underwent a similar assessment. Blood samples were obtained from all participants for endotoxin and TNF-α assays.

Results.—Weather on the day of the August rally was somewhat milder than in previous years, with a maximum temperature of 32.9°C and a relative humidity of 78% at the beginning of the ride. The wind speed averaged 8 mph. Two of the control cyclists became ill; thus, 15 cyclists had rigors, nausea, vomiting, syncope, or diarrhea. There were no cases of hyperthermia or heat stroke. Cyclists who became ill were generally less well trained than controls. One of the ill cyclists had endotoxemia, with an endotoxin level of 330 pg/mL; 1 asymptomatic control had an endotoxin level of 150 pg/mL. Levels in all remaining participants were ≤ 64 pg/mL. Only 1 ill cyclist had a very low titer of TNF-α; controls were not measured for TNF-α. No evidence was found to support or refute an association between gastrointestinal disease and exercise-related endotoxemia.

Conclusion.—Endotoxemia does not appear to cause mild postexertional illness in cyclists. However, a similar study performed under greater thermal stress might yield different results.

► Endotoxemia mediates the septic syndrome and may play a role in heat stroke. Endotoxin, a cell-wall component of gram-negative bacteria, is abundant in the colon. For systemic endotoxemia to occur, the endotoxin must pass through the bowel wall barrier, the immune barrier of the gut-associated lymphoid tissue, and the liver filter. Pilot studies in triathletes and runners suggested that more than 80% of exhausted runners with high plasma endotoxin levels also had nausea, vomiting, or diarrhea, whereas these symptoms were present in less than 20% of runners with low endotoxin levels.[1, 2]

This study asked whether high plasma endotoxin levels played a role in the postrace illnesses of cyclists who raced 100 miles in the heat. In essence, results were "negative." Perhaps because conditions were milder than usual for this August race, most of the "ill" cyclists were only mildly ill and the generally low (or nil) endotoxin levels did not correlate with symptoms. Whether endotoxemia plays a role in postrace collapse or illness remains unclear. (See also Abstract 6–2.)

E.R. Eichner, M.D.

References

1. Bosenberg AT, Brock-Utne JG, Gaffin SL, et al: Strenuous exercise causes systemic endotoxemia. *J Appl Physiol* 65:106–108, 1988.
2. Brock-Utne JG, Gaffin SL, Wells MT, et al: Endotoxaemia in exhausted runners after a long-distance race. *S Afr Med J* 73:533–536, 1988.

Effect of Eccentric Exercise on Natural Killer Cell Activity

Palmø J, Asp S, Daugaard JR, Richter EA, Klokker M, Pedersen BK
(Rigshospitalet, Copenhagen; Univ of Copenhagen)
J Appl Physiol 78:1442–1446, 1995 8–36

Background.—Physical exercise can induce dramatic changes in the cellular immune system, including effects on natural killer (NK) cell activity and cytokine production. These effects have been noted in relation to whole body exercise, such as bicycling and running. This study examined the effect of isolated eccentric exercise on the NK cell activity.

Methods.—Eight healthy young men 20–29 years of age were studied while performing eccentric 1-legged exercise (quadriceps muscle) in 4 sessions. Blood samples were obtained from veins in the exercising leg and veins in a resting arm to distinguish between local and systemic effects, respectively. To eliminate diurnal variations, the results were compared with a control group that did not exercise.

Results.—Results of blood studies did not differ between the exercising leg and the resting arm samples. During eccentric exercise, plasma epinephrine and norepinephrine increased more than twofold (Fig 1) and plasma creatine kinase increased progressively. The percentage of CD16$^+$ NK cells increased; this was paralleled by an increase in the NK cell

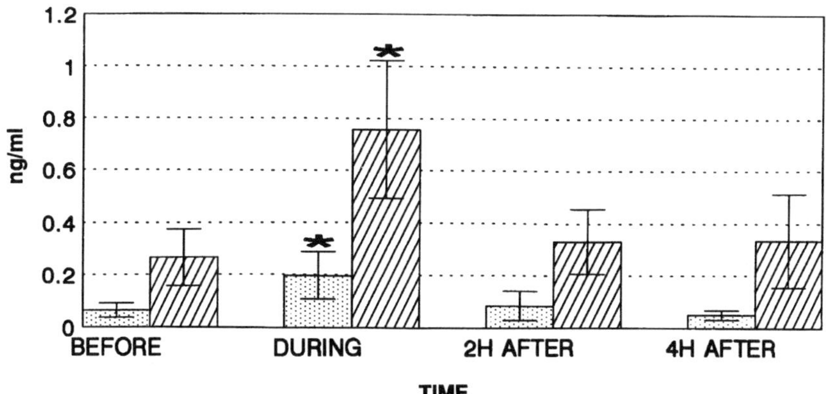

FIGURE 1.—Effects of 1-legged eccentric exercise on plasma levels of epinephrine (*stippled bars*) and norepinephrine (*hatched bars*). Values are means ± standard error; n = 8 observations. *Asterisk* indicates significant difference ($P < 0.05$) from pre=exercise value. (Courtesy of Palmø J, Asp S, Daugaard JR, et al: Effect of eccentric exercise on natural killer cell activity. *J Appl Physiol* 78:1442–1446, 1995.)

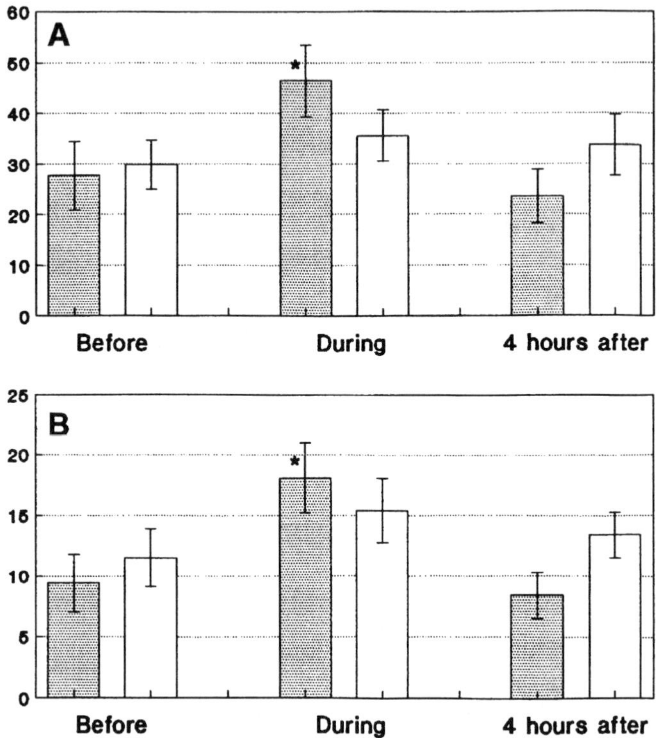

FIGURE 2.—Natural killer cell activity ([**A**] lysis per fixed number of blood mononuclear cells) and percentage of $CD16^+$ cells (**B**) in subjects performing eccentric exercise (*stippled bars*) and in a resting control group (*open bars*). Data from blood draining femoral vein of exercising leg and resting arm were obtained from the exercising group and did not differ; therefore, only data from the arm vein are shown, and the control group had blood collected only from the arm vein. Muscle biopsy specimens were obtained from the exercising group but not the control group. *Asterisk* indicates significant difference ($P < 0.05$) from pre-exercise value. (Courtesy of Palmø J, Asp S, Daugaard JR, et al: Effect of eccentric exercise on natural killer cell activity. *J Appl Physiol* 78:1442–1446, 1995.)

activity per fixed number of blood mononuclear cells (Fig 2). However, the NK cell activity per NK cell did not significantly change. There were no changes in the percentage of $CD3^+$, $CD4^+$, $CD8^+$, $CD19^+$, and $CD14^+$ cells.

Summary.—Eccentric exercise engaging only the knee extensors of 1 leg causes recruitment of $CD16^+$ cells to the blood, thereby increasing NK cell activity of blood mononuclear cells without an increased change in the function of the individual cell. The increase in plasma epinephrine during eccentric exercise may explain the increase in the percentage of $CD16^+$ cells.

▶ This report extends much recent research on exercise and NK cells. As we have extensively reviewed,[1-3] exercise can change the levels and functions of white blood cells, especially NK cells and neutrophils, and also the levels of immunoglobulins, complement, and other immune factors. In general, however, most exercise-related immune changes are mild, mixed, and brief, making their clinical import moot. This report shows that a bout of eccentric exercise using only the knee extensors of 1 leg recruits NK cells into the blood, perhaps via an increase in plasma epinephrine level.

Other studies agree that exercise lymphocytosis comprises mainly NK cells and varies in degree with the intensity of the exercise. The evidence that physical training may increase basal NK function is sparse,[4] but 1 cross-sectional study suggests that highly conditioned elderly female athletes have higher basal NK function than sedentary controls,[5] and 2 cross-sectional studies reviewed herein (see Abstracts 8–34 and 8–37) suggest that basal NK function is elevated in young and middle-aged male marathon runners but not in elderly male recreational runners.

E.R. Eichner, M.D.

References

1. 1995 YEAR BOOK OF SPORTS MEDICINE, pp 392–406.
2. 1994 YEAR BOOK OF SPORTS MEDICINE, pp 393–395.
3. 1993 YEAR BOOK OF SPORTS MEDICINE, pp 306–317.
4. Nieman DC, Nehlsen-Cannarella SL, Markoff PA, et al: The effects of moderate exercise training on natural killer cells and acute respiratory tract infections. *Int J Sports Med* 11:467–473, 1990.
5. Nieman DC, Henson DA, Gusewitch G, et al: Physical activity and immune function in elderly women. *Med Sci Sports Exerc* 25:823–831, 1993.

Physical Activity and Immune Senescence in Men

Shinkai S, Kohno H, Kimura K, Komura T, Asai H, Inai R, Oka K, Kurokawa Y, Shephard RJ (Ehime Univ, Japan; Hiroshima Univ, Japan; Suzugamine Women's College, Hiroshima, Japan; et al)

Med Sci Sports Exerc 27:1516–1526, 1995 8–37

Objective.—Immune senescence appears to be caused by shrinkage of the thyroid. It results in a decrease in the distribution and function of T cells. Because exercise changes many immune parameters, a study was conducted to compare age-related changes of immune function between young and older sedentary men and older male runners.

Methods.—Counts of immunocompetent cells; natural killer (NK) cell activity; proliferative responses to mitogens PHA and PWM; allogenic mixed lymphocyte reaction; and interleukin (IL)-1δ, IL-2, interferon (IFN)-γ, and IL-4 cytokine production were determined from the venous blood of 17 older recreational runners (average age, 63.8 years), 10 age-matched sedentary controls (average age, 65.8 years), and 16 young sedentary controls (average age, 23.6 years). Elderly runners jogged an average of 56 minutes 5 days a week for an average distance of 39 km for 17 years. Before each of 5 blood drawings, individuals did not exercise for the previous 36 hours and did not eat or drink anything but water in the previous 10 hours.

Results.—Compared with the younger group, both of the older groups had significantly lower $CD3^+$ and $CD8^+$ counts, a significantly higher percentage of CD16$^+$, a higher CD4/CD8 ratio, and higher percentages of activated T cells and "memory" helper and cytotoxic T cells. There was no change in NK cell activity or other cytokine production in older individuals. Proliferative responses to PHA and PWM were significantly reduced in older individuals, although proliferative responses of the older runners and rates of IL-2, IFN-γ, and IL-4 production were significantly higher than were those of the older sedentary group. Production of IL-2 was somewhat decreased in the older groups. There were no significant differences between the 2 older groups in numbers of immunocompetent cells.

Conclusion.—Regular endurance exercise in older men appears to slow the development of immune senescence and the decline of cytokine production.

▶ See Abstracts 8–36 and 8–34 for background on exercise and immune function. This study explores whether regular physical activity can counteract the age-related decline in T-cell function. An earlier cross-sectional study suggested that highly conditioned and active elderly women had a greater lymphocyte mitogenesis response and greater NK cell activity than sedentary peers.[1] This study, also cross-sectional, suggests that elderly male recreational runners have no increase in NK cell activity but do have a greater lymphocyte mitogenesis response than their sedentary peers. Production of IL-2 was also higher in these elderly runners. These 2 studie s, taken together, although limited by cross-sectional design and relatively few subjects, suggest that regular endurance exercise in later life may help check certain aspects of the age-related decline in T-cell function.

E.R. Eichner, M.D.

Reference

1. Nieman DC, Henson DA, Gusewitch G, et al: Physical activity and immune function in elderly women. *Med Sci Sports Exerc* 25:823–831, 1993.

9 Physical Therapy, Drugs, Doping, Environment

Pain and Pain Tolerance in Professional Ballet Dancers
Tajet-Foxell B, Rose FD (Univ of East London)
Br J Sports Med 29:31–34, 1995 9–1

Background.—Generally, individuals who play professional sports have higher pain thresholds than controls. Professional ballet dancers may be viewed as similar to sports professionals in rigorous training, self-discipline, physical fitness, competitiveness, and performance anxiety. However, ballet is associated with beauty, grace, and sensitivity and none of the "winning is all," slightly aggressive image of professional sports. This fundamental difference in culture and how this consequent difference in self-image between ballet dancers and those who play professional sports has implications for pain experience was studied.

Methods.—Using the Cold Pressor Test, pain and pain tolerance thresholds were measured in 52 professional ballet dancers (mean age, 25.3 years) and 53 age-matched control university students (mean age, 24.3 years). Pain was reported on the Short Form McGill Pain Questionnaire. All participants completed the Miller Behaviourial Style Questionnaire, which evaluated coping style, and the Eysenck Personality Inventory, which gave a measure of introversion/extroversion and neuroticism.

Results.—Professional ballet dancers had significantly higher pain thresholds and pain tolerance thresholds than controls. However, the dancers also reported a more acute experience of the sensory aspect of pain. The raised thresholds in dancers could not be explained in terms of differential coping strategies nor the higher neuroticism scores.

Discussion.—Like sports professionals, professional ballet dancers have higher pain and pain tolerance thresholds. It is likely that the raised thresholds lie in their greater exposure to physical training and their increased fitness. Both dancers and sports professionals explore boundaries and pain experience, allowing them to be familiar with the interface between physical activity and pain, and thus giving them an understanding or even perception of control over that interface. Because of their greater familiarity with pain, ballet dancers experience pain more acutely. The meaning of pain and the importance of acknowledging pain and learning how to respond to it should be targeted early in a dancer's training to minimize injuries and avoid chronic injuries.

▶ This study explores the implications of pain in sports. In the Cold Pressor Test, ballet dancers had higher pain thresholds and tolerance than nondancers (controls who were university students). Among both dancers and controls, men tended to have a higher pain tolerance than women, but female dancers had a higher pain tolerance than male controls. This type of study cannot answer why dancers have a higher pain tolerance than nondancers, but the authors speculate that it likely stems from training and fitness. The higher pain tolerance of athletes can be a double-edged sword, fostering top performance yet predisposing to overuse injuries.

E.R. Eichner, M.D.

Temperature Changes in Deep Muscles of Humans During Ice and Ultrasound Therapies: An In Vivo Study

Draper DO, Schulthies S, Sorvisto P, Hautala A-M (Brigham Young Univ, Provo, Utah; Oulu College of Health Care, Finland)

J Orthop Sports Phys Ther 21:153–157, 1995 9–2

Introduction.—Therapeutic ultrasound has been found to enhance wound healing and increase tendon extensibility, blood flow, and range of motion. Various protocols are used to prepare the treatment area before ultrasound use. Precooling the tissues is a common clinical practice based on the theory that cooling creates a thermal gradient and results in higher tissue temperatures with ultrasound treatment, although no studies have demonstrated this benefit. The effects of precooling on muscle temperature changes were studied.

Methods.—Sixteen volunteers (mean age, 26 years) were randomly assigned to 2 groups: treatment with ultrasound only or with ultrasound applied to precooled tissue. A 23-gauge thermistor needle was inserted to a 5-cm depth in the triceps surae muscle of the left leg in each participant. The precooling treatment consisted of cooling with ice for 5 minutes, with muscle temperatures recorded every 30 seconds. The ultrasound treatment was administered in a continuous mode at 1.5 W/cm^2 for 10 minutes, with muscle temperatures recorded every 30 seconds.

Results.—In the ultrasound-only treatment group, the tissue temperature increased by a mean of 4°C above the baseline temperature. In the precooled treatment group, the tissue temperature decreased by a mean of 0.5°C below the baseline temperature during icing and increased by a mean of 2.3°C during the ultrasound treatment, corresponding to a 1.8° increase over the baseline temperature.

Discussion.—Ultrasound treatment resulted in significantly higher deep muscle heating without precooling. In addition, the analgesic effect of ice may increase the patient's tolerance of the ultrasound treatment enough to mask the sensation of tissue damage. However, precooling combined with moderate doses of ultrasound may be appropriate in patients with an acute or subacute injury when pulsed ultrasound is not available.

▶ Many times, treatment protocols are established without sufficient research to support them. It appears this has been the situation with the use of precooling and ultrasound. In an effort to increase tissue density and thereby increase the effects of ultrasound, it had been theorized that precooling would bring about such a reaction. This study indicates that if the desired effect of the ultrasound treatment is to increase tissue temperature, the tissue should not be precooled. This study did not address the effect of precooling on the mechanical properties of ultrasound.

F.J. George, A.T.C., P.T.

Comparison of Various Icing Times in Decreasing Bone Metabolism and Blood Flow in the Knee

Ho SSW, Illgen RL, Meyer RW, Torok PJ, Cooper MD, Reider B (Univ of Chicago)

Am J Sports Med 23:74–76, 1995 9–3

Introduction.—Twenty minutes of topical icing decreases skeletal blood flow and metabolism at the knee by an average of nearly 20%. Although 20 minutes is the most commonly used duration, it is unknown whether 20 minutes is the most effective duration. A 30-minute maximum duration has been recommended as the safe period of icing to prevent peroneal nerve palsy. The purpose of this study was to determine the effect of shorter periods of icing on skeletal blood flow and metabolism.

Methods.—In 38 volunteers with no history of current bone or joint pathology (age range, 28 to 65 years), triple-phase bone scans with technetium-99m were used in 19 right and 19 left knees iced. Half of the participants were smokers and 6 were taking antihypertensive medication. Research subjects were grouped according to the icing duration; 5, 10, 15, 20, or 25 minutes. A standard ice wrap was applied to 1 knee and a room temperature wrap to the other knee. The ice wrap was applied for the specified duration before injection of technetium-99m. A blinded reviewer quantified the images. A percentage decrease in counts of the iced knee vs. the control knee was calculated.

Results.—A significant decrease in soft tissue and bone counts was found with increasing ice time. After 5 minutes of icing, there was an 11% decrease in soft-tissue blood flow and a 5% decrease in bone blood flow. After 25 minutes of icing, a 29.5% decrease in soft-tissue blood flow and a 21% decrease in bone blood flow was found. Knee circumference was unrelated to any data from scanning. The longer the icing time, the greater the difference in skin temperature from experimental to control leg. Temperature changes did not correlate with the changes in blood flow.

Conclusion.—As little as 5 minutes of the ice wrap resulted in a small but consistent decrease in soft-tissue and bone blood flow. The "ice effect" is time dependent in that the effect can increase threefold to fourfold by increasing the duration to 25 minutes.

▶ The authors compared the effects of icing a knee joint from times of 5–25 minutes. In as little as 5 minutes, there is an 11% reduction in soft-tissue blood flow, which decreased to 29.5% in 25 minutes. As stated, the authors did not extend the study beyond 25 minutes; therefore, a plateauing effect was not addressed after 25 minutes of icing. It appears that for safety reasons, i.e., peroneal nerve palsy and the chance of skin damage, icing of the knee should not be done for periods of longer than 25 minutes. The authors do mention a possible reflex vasodilation occurring after 10 minutes of icing, which was not present in the 5-, 15-, 20- or 25-minute groups.

F.J. George, A.T.C., P.T.

Agility Following the Application of Cold Therapy

Evans TA, Ingersoll C, Knight KL, Worrell T (Indiana State Univ, Indianapolis; Univ of Indianapolis, Ind)

J Athletic Train 30:231–234, 1995 9–4

Purpose.—Cryotherapy is commonly used for injury treatment and rehabilitation because of its hypalgesic effects. Although therapeutic cooling is known to affect physiologic activity, its effects on functional performance are uncertain. The effects of cryotherapy on agility test performance were studied.

Methods.—Twenty-four male college athletes were studied during 2 different treatment sessions in which they underwent 20 minutes of 1° C ice immersion of the dominant foot and ankle or 20 minutes of rest. After each treatment, the research subjects performed 3 trials of 3 agility tests in random order: the carioca maneuver, the co-contraction test, and the shuttle run. They were allowed 30 seconds of rest between trials and 1 minute between tests. Agility times were compared for differences between the cold and the control treatments and between the order of the treatment sessions.

Results.—The mean agility time scores were somewhat slower after cold treatment. However, the ice immersion treatment did not cause any significant difference in agility times. Treatment order also had no effect. Most of the men reported some type of altered sensation—for example, numbness, tingling, stiffness, or awkwardness—immediately after cold treatment.

Conclusions.—Ice immersion of the foot and ankle does not appear to affect performance on agility tests. Scores are slightly lower immediately after cold treatment, perhaps because of tissue stiffness, apprehension, or both on the part of the athlete. Cryotherapy can be applied to the foot and ankle before strenuous exercise without causing any reductions in agility.

▶ Is it safe to allow an athlete into competition after applying an ice pack? Will his or her performance or agility be affected? In the 1994 YEAR BOOK OF SPORTS MEDICINE, I commented on a study by Myrer et al.[1] In that study, cryotherapy was applied to the quadriceps muscles of research subjects, and significant strength decrements were recorded. I stated that "a warm-up period may be necessary before the athlete has attained full strength and that moderate exercise helps the recovery of concentric but not eccentric strength values."

As more studies are done on cryotherapy and its effects on performance, we will learn more about this subject. A number of factors must be considered after using cryotherapy, which include the body part injured, the length of the cryotherapy, the effects of the cryotherapy on the body part, and most important, the effects of the cryotherapy on the injury. K.L. Knight, Ph.D., A.T.C., commenting on the study, states, "The body apparently compensates for whatever changes short-term cold applications cause, and exercise is not contraindicated."[2]

F.J. George, A.T.C., P.T.

References

1. Ruiz DH, Myrer JW, Durrant E, et al: Cryotherapy and sequential exercise bouts following cryotherapy on concentric and eccentric strength in the quadriceps. *J Athletic Train* 28:320–323, 1993.
2. Knight KL: *Athletic Training Sports Health Care Perspectives* 2:143, 1996.

Management of Sports-induced Skin Wounds

Foster DT, Rowedder LJ, Reese SK (Univ of Iowa, Iowa City; Northwestern College, Orange City, Iowa; Waukesha Sports Medicine & Physical Therapy Ctr, Wis)

J Athletic Train 30:135–140, 1995 9–5

Introduction.—There is little detailed information about sports-induced skin wounds and their frequency. Athletic trainers are at risk of exposure to biohazards because they provide acute care for wounds in athletes. The most common skin wounds among athletes are abrasions, blisters, incisions, and lacerations. Abrasions are subdivided into partial-thickness and full-thickness wounds. Wound management techniques were reviewed in detail.

Wound Cleansing.—Hydrogen peroxide has been used for almost 50 years to reduce bacterial contamination and aid débridement and cleansing. In 1991, a study reported that partial-thickness wounds treated with hydrogen peroxide healed faster than wounds treated with acetic acid, povidone-iodine solution, or normal saline. At 3 months, all wounds had similar pigmentation and texture, regardless of treatment. Another study reported that Neosporin ointment does not delay or speed healing, but that bacitracin, one of the antimicrobial agents in Neosporin and Polysporin, stimulated healing when used alone. Various creams, lotions, and soaps also were studied.

Wound Dressing.—Research has shown that both acute and chronic wounds heal faster in a moist environment, such as that provided by occlusive dressings, vs. a dry environment. Because occlusive dressings retain moisture in the healing tissues, they may provide an easier route for epidermal migration.

Complications.—Pain and infection are among the most common wound complications. Important differentiating features of infection useful to those without access to cultures are tenderness, a wide margin of erythema, and seeping exudate on pressure. A common cause of widespread redness around a wound is seborrheic dermatitis and is often seen in athletes with a pre-existing dermatitis. The skin may appear to be infected but will not be painful. This condition is often treated with topical corticosteroids, but these have reportedly reduced the rate of healing by 60% and reduced the collagen biosynthesis capacity, which results in reduced wound strength. Caution is advised in using topical corticosteroids when treating seborrheic dermatitis near a wound. Hypertrophic scars, keloids, dysesthesias, unstable scars, excessive granulation, hypopigmentation, and telangiectasis are other wound complications.

Conclusions.—Athletic trainers should observe universal precautions when treating sport-induced wounds. Cleansing agents that stimulate epidermal migration and do not interfere with fibroplasia are recommended, as are closures and occlusive dressings.

► Some general rules should be followed when managing skin wounds. Use universal precautions, use saline as a cleansing agent, keep the wound clean and covered, use occlusive dressings because they promote healing. Be very cautious in the use of topical corticosteroids. An excellent study discusses how the proper protocol for wound care management differs from athletic trainers' perceptions.[1]

There has been much controversy over the use of Betadine and hydrogen peroxide. There may be times when Betadine should be used, especially in an open, dirty wound that may have many different pathogens. Studies are now being conducted on the use of ¼-strength Betadine in this type of wound.[2] Betadine should not be used on a clean, red, granulating wound. Some wounds would benefit at times from the mild débridement that occurs with the use of hydrogen peroxide. Every wound should be looked at differently with 3 questions in mind: "What is it? What caused it? What do I do for it?"[2]

F.J. George, A.T.C., P.T.

References

1. Goldenberg M: Wound care management: Proper protocol differs from athletic trainers' perceptions. *J Athletic Train* 31:12–16, 1996.
2. Gilbert RE: Tissue trauma and wound repair: A clinical approach. Presented at Rhode Island American Physical Therapy Association (R.I.A.P.T.A.) Continuing Education Conference, Warwick, Rhode Island, April 1996.

A Prospective Investigation of the Impact of Alcohol Consumption on Helmet Use, Injury Severity, Medical Resource Utilization, and Health Care Costs in Bicycle-related Trauma

Spaite DW, Criss EA, Weist DJ, Valenzuela TD, Judkins D, Meislin HW (Univ of Arizona, Tucson)

J Trauma 38:287–290, 1995 9–6

Background.—Bicycling is a popular sport and mode of transportation. At least 100 million bicycles are estimated to be in use in the United States. At least 600,000 individuals, and possibly as many as 2 million, seek medical care as a result of bicycling injuries each year. Almost one third of all bicycle-related injuries are head injuries, which are highly associated with the lack of helmet use. Bicyclists who do not wear helmets also sustain more injuries and more severe injuries in other areas of the body. The relationship between bicycle-related injuries, helmet use, alcohol consumption, and use of medical resources was investigated.

Methods.—Data were gathered prospectively from the medical records of adults involved in bicycle-related incidents who were seen in the emergency department of a university-based medical center during a 22-month period. The data included Injury Severity Scores and patient outcome.

Results.—Information about the use of helmets was available for 350 of 389 patients. Of the 350 patients, more than 31% were wearing a helmet at the time of the incident. Group 1 consisted of 29 patients with a blood alcohol level between 20 and 345 mg/dL; group 2 had 321 patients who had not consumed alcohol before the incident. About 7% of patients in group 1 and 34% of patients in group 2 wore a helmet. Of patients in group 1, 20.7% sustained at least 1 severe anatomical injury, compared with 4.4% of patients in group 2. Group 1 was much more likely to sustain major head injuries than group 2. For group 1, the mean hospital stay was 3.5 days and the mean stay in the ICU was 1.4 days; for group 2, the mean hospital stay was 0.5 days and the mean stay in the ICU care was 0.1 days. In group 1, 58.6% of patients were admitted to the hospital, compared with 13.1% of patients from group 2.

Conclusions.—Individuals involved in bicycling incidents who consumed alcohol beforehand were less likely to wear a helmet, required longer hospitalization and more days in the ICU, sustained more severe injuries, and incurred greater health care costs than those who did not consume alcohol before bicycling. These individuals might benefit from bicycle injury prevention programs.

▶ The observations and conclusions derived from this excellent study are in keeping with the recognized relationship between alchohol consumption and injury patterns involving motorcyclists and automobile drivers. The authors point out that "it remains unclear whether the higher injury severity in this group is the result of helmet nonuse (and loss of the direct protective effect) or from a greater likelihood of high-risk riding behavior and consequently a greater incidence of high-impact crashes." It would appear to this observer that it is all of the above.

J.S. Torg, M.D.

β-Adrenoceptor Blockade and Skeletal Muscle Energy Metabolism During Endurance Exercise

Van Baak MA, De Haan A, Saris WHM, Van Kordelaar E, Kuipers H, Van Der Vusse GJ (Univ of Limburg, Maastricht, The Netherlands; Vrije Universiteit, Amsterdam)

J Appl Physiol 78:307–313, 1995 9–7

Background.—β-Adrenoceptor blocking agents decrease endurance exercise performance, both in healthy individuals and in hypertensive patients who are receiving β-blocker therapy. The mechanism underlying this impairment is not well understood. After β-adrenergic blockade, the rate of glycogen utilization may be reduced in type I muscle fibers, with a compensatory rise in glycogenolysis in type II fibers. There also may be a greater recruitment of type II fibers. To elucidate the possible role of an imbalance between adenose triphosphate (ATP) formation and utilization after β-blockade, this study examined whether exhaustion from prolonged submaximal endurance exercise after nonselective β-blockade is accompanied by increased breakdown of adenine nucleotides and elevated inosine 5'-monophosphate (IMP).

Methods and Findings.—After administration of propranolol 80 mg or placebo, 12 healthy male volunteers cycled to exhaustion at a work-rate corresponding to 70% of maximal aerobic power. Exercise times to exhaustion were 39 minutes in the propranolol group and 86 minutes in the placebo group. After placebo, muscle IMP content was significantly elevated above resting levels at exhaustion. After propranolol, IMP was not significantly elevated and was lower than at exhaustion after placebo. No changes in ATP or total adenosine nucleotide content were found during exercise in either group. Muscle glycogen content was reduced significantly at exhaustion after either placebo or propranolol. However, glycogen levels at exhaustion were still significantly greater after propranolol than after placebo. No evidence of a shift in glycogen utilization was found among types I, IIa, and IIb fibers after propranolol administration.

Conclusions.—Muscle IMP content at exhaustion is significantly less after propranolol administration than after placebo administration, whereas the glycogen content of muscle as a whole and of the different types of muscle fiber is significantly greater at exhaustion after propranolol. Thus, neither an imbalance between ATP utilization and ATP regeneration nor premature glycogen depletion in whole muscle or specific muscle fiber types can explain the premature fatigue that occurs during endurance exercise after propranolol administration.

► It is common clinical experience that patients who are being treated with nonspecific β-blocking agents complain of muscle fatigue. Because the normal metabolic response to β-adrenoceptor stimulation is an increase of glycogenolysis,[1, 2] it is tempting to suppose that the fatigue is linked either to difficulty in mobilizing glycogen in the muscle as a whole or to a redistribution of effort between slow- and fast-twitch muscle fibers because of the slowing of glycogenolysis. If there were indeed a critical slowing of energy delivery to the muscle fibers, one would anticipate a depletion of ATP levels, with a shift from slow- to fast-twitch muscles as local fatigue developed. Broberg et al.[3] have demonstrated such responses during high-intensity effort, but this article suggests that β-blockers induce neither of these changes during prolonged activity of more moderate intensity, despite a fatigue that halves exercise endurance time. The reason for fatigue during sustained acitivity remains a mystery.

R.J. Shephard, M.D., Ph.D., D.P.E.

References

1. Greenhaff PL, Ren J-M, Söderlund K, et al: Energy metabolism in single human muscle fibers during contraction without and with epinephrine infusion. *Am J Physiol* 260:E713–E718, 1991.
2. Raz I, Katz A, Spencer MK, et al: Epinephrine inhibits insulin-mediated glycogenesis but enhances glycolysis in human skeletal muscle. *Am J Physiol* 260:E430–E435, 1991.
3. Broberg S, Katz A, Sahlin K, et al: Propranolol enhances adenine nucleotide degradation in human muscle during exercise. *J Appl Physiol* 65:2478–2483, 1988.

Exercise-induced Acute Renal Failure Associated With Ibuprofen, Hydrochlorothiazide, and Triamterene

Sanders LR (Brooke Army Med Ctr, Fort Sam Houston, Tex)
J Am Soc Nephrol 5:2020–2023, 1995 9–8

Objective.—In certain conditions associated with decreased renal blood flow (RBF)—such as old age, hypertension, chronic renal insufficiency, diuretic use, and other conditions that decrease effective circulating volume—nonsteroidal anti-inflammatory drugs (NSAIDs) can predispose to acute renal failure. Substantial reductions in RBF also occur as a result of strenuous exercise. A case of postexercise acute tubular necrosis developing without rhabdomyolysis in a patient taking NSAIDs was reviewed.

Case Report.—Man, 37, was found to have nonoliguric acute renal failure 36 hours after a bout of strenuous exercise. He had a history of mild essential hypertension and was taking ibuprofen 800 mg as needed for knee pain plus 1 combined pill with hydrochlorothiazide 50 mg and triamterene 75 mg each day. A nephritic sediment with red blood cell casts was noted on urinalysis. Renal ^{99m}Tc-DTPA scanning revealed mildly decreased parenchymal uptake and renal cortical retention. On renal biopsy, acute tubular necrosis and mild nephrosclerosis were apparent (Fig 1). The patient remained nonoliguric and was treated with isotonic saline and nifedipine. His laboratory values quickly returned to normal, with the serum creatinine level peaking 5 days after admission, and he was discharged and given nifedipine after 19 days.

Discussion.—In patients with conditions predisposing to decreased RBF, NSAID use may potentiate renal ischemia as a result of strenuous exercise. Prescribing NSAIDs to patients with such conditions should be done with

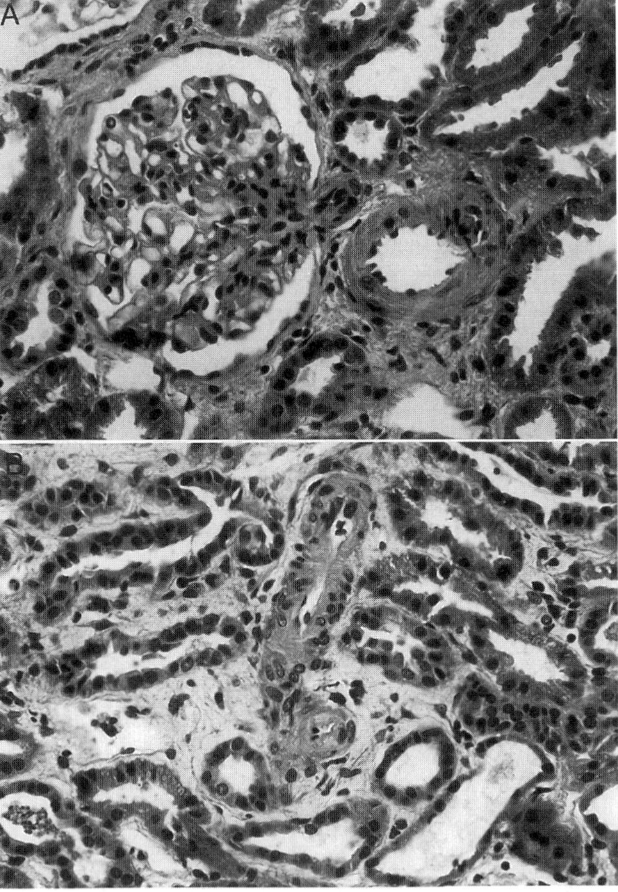

FIGURE 1.—Renal biopsy findings compatible with acute tubular necrosis, arteriolar nephrosclerosis, interstitial edema, and mild interstitial fibrosis. Two light photomicrographs with hematoxylin and eosin stain and original magnification ×400. **A**, glomerular tuft with mild segmental mesangial thickening and vascular collapse, arteriolar sclerosis of a branching interlobular artery with subintimal hyalin deposition, and thickening and hyalinization of the media. **B**, arteriolar sclerosis in a (centrally located) thickened interlobular vessel with plump endothelial-cell nuclei and a narrowed lumen, cellular and proteinaceous cast material, and interstitial edema with mild interstitial fibroses. (Courtesy of Sanders LR: Exercise-induced acute renal failure associated with ibuprofen, hydrochlorothiazide, and triamterene. *J Am Soc Nephrol* 5:2020–2023, 1995.)

caution. The patients should be warned about the risks of over-the-counter NSAIDs and advised to avoid using these drugs during exercise.

▶ In most distance runners acute renal failure does not develop, but there are sometimes warning signs of impaired renal function such as hematuria and red blood cell casts. Given the widespread self-administration of NSAIDs, particularly by athletes, it would seem important to watch for this possible complication in patients with hypertension or other potential causes of renal insufficiency.

R.J. Shepard, M.D., Ph.D., D.P.E.

Pharmacological Treatment of Soft-tissue Injuries

Buckwalter JA (Univ of Iowa, Iowa City)

J Bone Joint Surg (Am) 77–A:1902–1914, 1995 9–9

Overview.—Few individuals who do physical work or participate in recreational or sports activities escape acute musculoskeletal or soft-tissue injury. Although drugs are able to lessen the intensity and duration of inflammation and thereby relieve pain, the agents used at present—including steroids—vary substantially in their effectiveness and safety.

Nonsteroidal Drugs.—Nonsteroidal anti-inflammatory drugs have been used chiefly to treat chronic musculoskeletal disorders including rheumatoid disease, but they often are used to treat soft-tissue injuries as well. Although orally administered nonsteroidal agents are widely used in individuals incurring acute injuries, the clinical indications for such use remain to be clearly defined. Clinical observations affirm that they do limit the pain, tenderness, and stiffness consequent to acute soft-tissue injury. Topical and transdermal administration of these agents has been proposed.

Steroids.—A number of corticosteroids are used for their ability to suppress the initial events in inflammation. Orally administered steroids have a number of potential systemic side effects, and repeated intra-articular steroid injections may lead to progressive deterioration of normal joint cartilage. The effect of injected steroids on the mechanical function of normal tendons is unclear. Steroids impede and delay the healing of dense fibrous tissues. Anabolic steroids, used to augment muscle strength, frequently cause systemic complications. Like corticoids, they may have negative effects on musculoskeletal soft tissues. The value of anabolic steroids remains to be established.

Dimethyl Sulfoxide.—Topical use of dimethyl sulfoxide has been proposed for limiting pain from soft-tissue injury and hastening recovery. Experimental work has questioned the purported anti-inflammatory efficacy of dimethyl sulfoxide. Topical application has yielded inconclusive results.

▶ This article is a comprehensive current concepts review with 186 references. Interestingly, the article appears to raise as many questions as it answers. Despite the widespread use of nonsteroidal anti-inflammatory drugs, the clinical indications for their use in the treatment of acute soft-tissue injuries have not been clearly defined. Few investigators have examined the effect of corticosteroids on injured joints. Also, orally administered corticosteroids cause a number of potentially serious systemic side effects, and it is difficult to precisely define the dose as related to the wide variety of potential complications. Experimental work has raised questions regarding the reputed anti-inflammatory effect of dimethyl sulfoxide. The author concludes that pharmacologic treatments can reduce the inflammation and relieve pain after soft-tissue injury. However, the 3 classes of drugs reviewed vary considerably in their efficacy and safety.

J.S. Torg, M.D.

Effects of Local Injection of Corticosteroids on the Healing of Ligaments: A Follow-up Report

Wiggins ME, Fadale PD, Ehrlich MG, Walsh WR (Brown Univ, Providence, RI)
J Bone Joint Surg (Am) 77–A:1682–1691, 1995 9–10

Introduction.—Concerns have been raised about the use of corticosteroids to treat acutely injured ligaments and tendons, although there are only limited, conflicting data on the effects of corticosteroids on healing tendon or ligament tissue. A previous study by the authors demonstrated that corticosteroids significantly impaired the early healing process in a transected ligament. The effects of corticosteroids on the late healing process in ligaments were examined.

Methods.—A total of 101 rabbits were assigned to 4 groups. The right medial collateral ligament in the hind limb of 3 groups of rabbits were transected and a fascial pocket was constructed to receive steroid injection. Two groups of rabbits were injected with a lower and higher (human) dose of betamethasone. The third group of injured rabbits and the sham group did not receive injections. The animals were killed at 42 and 84 days, and the hind limbs were examined with biomechanical testing and histologic analysis.

Results.—The sham specimens had significantly greater biomechanical properties than the other 3 groups at both 42 and 84 days. At 42 days, the peak loads were similar in the 3 injured groups, but the peak loads were significantly lower in the 2 injected groups than in the noninjected group at 84 days. In the noninjected specimens, peak load improved significantly between 42 and 84 days, whereas peak load did not change significantly from day 42 values in the 2 injected specimens. Although all injured specimens demonstrated progressive healing, the healing tissue was significantly less mature in gross appearance in the high-dose injected specimens at 42 days. At 42 days, the noninjected specimens had significantly more type-III collagen than the other 2 injured specimen groups. The healing tissue had more histologic maturity, with well-organized, linear collagen fibers, in the noninjected specimens, as compared with the more cellular and vascular injected specimens with nonparallel collagen fiber arrangements, at both 42 and 84 days.

Conclusions.—Treatment of an acutely injured ligament with corticosteroids delays the healing process in both the early and late phases of healing, with detrimental effects extending to 84 days after the injury.

► This is an interesting study with several inconsistencies. In the concluding paragraph, the authors state that "it appears possible that corticosteroids only delay healing and do not truly inhibit healing." Then several sentences later they "conclude that acute corticosteroid treatment of an injured ligament is detrimental to the healing process in both the early and the later phase of healing." They also conclude that "intensive rehabilitation after injection of corticosteroids around injured type-I collagenous structures (ligaments and tendons) could potentially be harmful and lead to reinjury." Certainly, the data do not support this unless they are referring to mature New Zealand white rabbits.

J.S. Torg, M.D.

Treatment of Osteitis Pubis in Athletes: Results of Corticosteroid Injections

Holt MA, Keene JS, Graf BK, Helwig DC (Univ of Wisconsin, Madison)

Am J Sports Med 23:601–606, 1995 9–11

Background.—Traumatic osteitis pubis usually causes pain in the adductor muscles that is made worse by kicking, running, or pivoting on 1 leg. Athletes most often have to rest for a prolonged time for the symptoms to resolve.

Objective.—The results of treatment were reviewed in 12 intercollegiate athletes (6 football players, 3 soccer players, 2 ice hockey players, 1 diver). The 10 men and 2 women had an average age of 20 years.

Treatment.—Nine of the patients treated earlier were rested for longer than 16 weeks, during which time they received orally administered anti-inflammatory drugs and performed hip-stretching exercises. Eight of them later received steroid injections into the pubic symphysis. Three patients treated later received injections within 10 days of the onset of symptoms after noninvasive measures had proved ineffective. A 19-gauge needle was placed anteroposteriorly in the center of the pubic symphysis (Figs 1 and 2) and advanced about 1 inch, where 1 mL each of 1% lidocaine and 0.25% bupivacaine and 4 mg of dexamethasone were injected.

Results.—Conservative measures succeeded in only 1 instance. The other 8 athletes gained immediate relief of adductor pain after injection treatment, and 3 of them returned to full participation within 3 weeks. Three others returned within 4 weeks but continued to be symptomatic and received a second injection. One athlete required 3 injections. All 3 athletes who received injections early in the course returned to full activity without symptoms within 2 weeks.

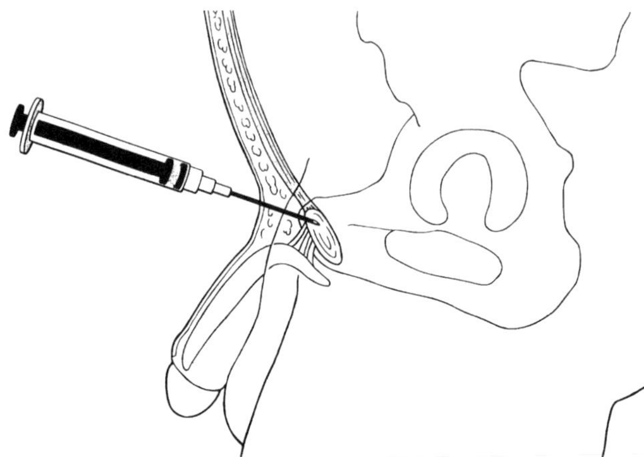

FIGURE 1.—Needle placement in the anteroposterior plane. (Courtesy of Holt MA, Keene JS, Graf BK, et al: Treatment of osteitis pubis in athletes: Results of corticosteriod injections. *Am J Sports Med* 23:601–606, 1995.)

Recommendations.—Presently, athletes with osteitis pubis are taken off activity and given anti-inflammatory medication orally for 7 to 10 days. If necessary, steroid then is injected into the pubic symphysis.

► The therapeutic response to injection of 4 mg of dexamethasone into the pubic symphysis is most impressive. It is assumed that this was in large part attributable to accurate diagnosis. As pointed out by the authors, physical

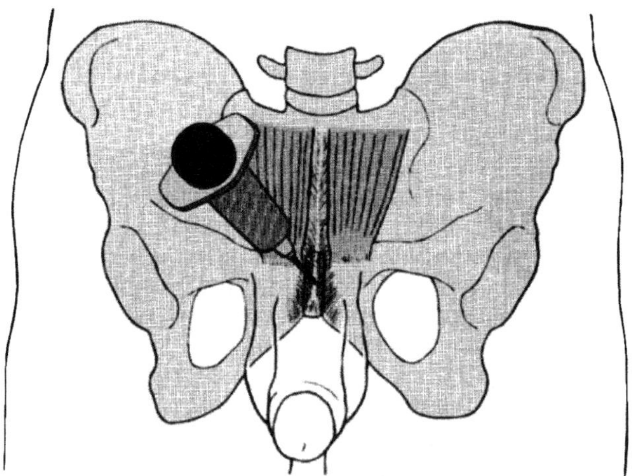

FIGURE 2.—Needle placement in the sagittal plane. (Courtesy of Holt MA, Keene JS, Graf BK, et al: Treatment of osteitis pubis in athletes: Results of corticosteroid injections. *Am J Sports Med* 23:601–606, 1995.)

examination revealed tenderness over the pubic symphysis, adductor tightness, and pain with resisted abduction of the lower extremities. Also, standard radiograph and bone scans confirmed the diagnosis. To be ruled out are other causes of growing pain such as the gracilis syndrome, stress fracture, adductor strain, inguinal hernia, prostatitis, orchitis, Reiter's syndrome, and internal abdominal oblique muscle avulsion from the superior aspect of the pubic ramus.

J.S. Torg, M.D.

Anti-inflammatory Medication After Muscle Injury: A Treatment Resulting in Short-term Improvement But Subsequent Loss of Muscle Function

Mishra DK, Fridén J, Schmitz MC, Lieber RL (Univ of California, San Diego)
J Bone Joint Surg (Am) 77–A:1510–1519, 1995 9–12

Background.—Exercise-related muscle injuries are a common cause of disability both in sports participants and at the workplace. Delayed soreness is not infrequent after sporadic exercise, and in some patients chronic symptoms develop. Nonsteroidal anti-inflammatory drugs are commonly used to relieve pain and enhance performance, but their actual effects on muscle function are not known.

Methods.—The effects of flurbiprofen, a commonly prescribed anti-inflammatory drug, were studied in rabbits subjected to an eccentric contraction injury by electrically stimulating the common peroneal nerve on a schedule mimicking intensive exercise. Contractile force and isometric dorsiflexion torque were measured, and the muscle tissue was examined ultrastructurally and immunohistochemically. In addition, fascicles near the central part of the muscle were sampled to measure the muscle fibers. Oral administration of 3 mg of flurbiprofen per kilogram was given daily for 6 days starting after muscle injury.

Results.—Functional recovery was more complete 3 and 7 days after injury in flurbiprofen-treated rabbits, but at 28 days these animals showed deficient torque and force generation. Significantly fewer muscle fibers in treated animals lacked staining for the intermediate filament protein desmin. Nevertheless, these animals remained able to mount a substantial regenerative response, as indicated by the expression of embryonic myosin. Fewer muscle fibers in treated animals expressed embryonic myosin 3 days after injury but, at 7 days, the expression of embryonic myosin exceeded that seen in muscle tissue from untreated animals. Inflammatory cells were seen within muscle fibers of untreated control animals.

Conclusions.—Although short-term administration of an anti-inflammatory agent may benefit muscle function after exercise-induced injury, muscle function may subsequently be impaired. The extent to which the muscle eventually recovers remains to be established.

▶ The authors believe that "these data suggest that the inflammatory process itself, which may occur secondary to the initial muscle injury, also results in additional delayed injury to the muscle and that the eventual functional recovery of the muscle is dependent on the inflammatory process. By suppressing the initial inflammatory reaction, the non-steroidal anti-inflammatory drug permits improved performance in early time-periods but appears to suppress the stimulus that may be needed for cellular remodeling in longer time." On the basis of this, they concluded that the results may prompt rethinking of the liberal use of nonsteroidal anti-inflammatory drugs in the treatment of muscle injury. Of course, what is required is evidence that deleterious functional changes occur in the human being and that the term "liberal use" be more specifically defined.

J.S. Torg, M.D.

Use of Capacitive Coupled Electric Fields in Stress Fractures in Athletes

Benazzo F, Mosconi M, Beccarisi G, Galli U (Universita' di Pavia, Italy)

Clin Orthop 310:145–149, 1995 9–13

Background.—Stress fractures in athletes can cause extended restriction of an athlete's activities because of delayed diagnosis and slow healing, especially of the fifth metatarsal, tarsal navicular, and tibia. It would be beneficial to accelerate the healing process because these injuries are often sustained by top-class athletes during the peak of their participation in sports. Osteogenetic electrical treatment with capacitively coupled fields can theoretically stimulate healing of these fractures. The use of this treatment for stress fractures in athletes was explored in an open study.

Methods.—In 21 athletes with 25 stress fractures, capacitively coupled electric fields were used to stimulate healing. Athletes were between 17 and 29 years of age. Treatment was administered around the clock until the fracture healed or improved or until no progress was noted. Injuries were categorized as healed, improved, or not healed.

Results.—The time between onset of symptoms, diagnosis, and start of treatment averaged 147.5 days and 223.9 days for navicular fractures alone. The average length of stimulation was 51.9 days and 60 days for navicular fractures. Of all fractures, 22 healed, 2 improved, and 1 did not heal.

Conclusions.—These injuries were primarily navicular fractures and fractures of the fifth metatarsal, which generally heal poorly and often require surgery. Capacitively coupled electric fields resulted in healing of stress fractures in a high percentage of these patients. This treatment benefits athletes because they can return to their sports activities quickly. Further research is needed before this treatment is used in nonathletes.

▶ The conclusion that capacitively coupled electric fields resulted in the healing of stress fractures in a high percentage of these patients is not supported by the data. Specifically, the design of the study is flawed because there was no controlled population treated with immobilization. It is well established that stress fractures of the tarsal navicular treated using non–weight-bearing with or without immobilization will heal within 6 weeks. Also, the case example of a Jones fracture that healed "after 85 days of stimulation" and then refractured 4 months later is classic for the natural history of this problem. Also, stress fractures of the fibula, tibia, and second metatarsal routinely heal with or without treatment. Clearly, what is needed to evaluate this modality is a prospective, randomly selected study population.

J.S. Torg, M.D.

Detection in Blood and Urine of Recombinant Erythropoietin Administered to Healthy Men

Wide L, Bengtsson C, Berglund B, Ekblom B (Univ Hosp, Uppsala, Sweden; Karolinska Hosp, Stockholm; Karolinska Inst, Stockholm)

Med Sci Sports Exerc 27:1569–1576, 1995 9–14

Background.—Erythropoietin (Epo) is the chief hormonal regulator of red blood cell differentiation in mammals. When given to patients with chronic renal disease, it markedly improves the well-being of these patients. Recombinant human Epo (rhEpo) also increases the hemoglobin in healthy individuals, enhances peak oxygen intake, and maximizes treadmill exercise performance. For these reasons, rhEpo is a potential threat to fair competition, especially in endurance sports such as skiing.

Methods.—An electrophoretic method for detecting rhEpo in the blood and urine is based on the molecule being electrically less negative than endogenous Epo. Levels of Epo were estimated in serum and urine in 15 healthy, moderately to well-trained men aged 19–40 years. The participants received subcutaneous injections of 20 IU of rhEpo per kilogram 3 times a week over 7–9 weeks. The electrical charge of Epo in blood and urine concentrate was determined by electrophoresis in 0.1% agarose suspension and expressed in terms of electrophoretic mobility. Serum and urinary Epo concentrations were determined by radioimmunoassay using ^{125}I-labeled rhEpo and a rabbit antibody against purified human urinary Epo.

Results.—All 15 participants had rhEpo detected in their sera 24 hours after injection. Seven of 9 individuals remained serum positive at 72 hours. The urine was consistently positive for rhEpo up to 24 hours after injection. Nine of 12 samples taken from 3 individuals 48 hours after injection remained positive. Elution patterns were determined (Fig 2). No rhEpo was detected in serum or urine 1–3 weeks after the last injection. The charge of both rhEpo and endogenous Epo in urine concentrates was more negative than in paired serum samples.

Conclusion.—The electrophoretic method of detecting rhEpo in serum and urine is expected to be useful in controlling doping.

► This new technique seems to have some potential in the prevention of blood doping, which has become all too prevalent among endurance com-

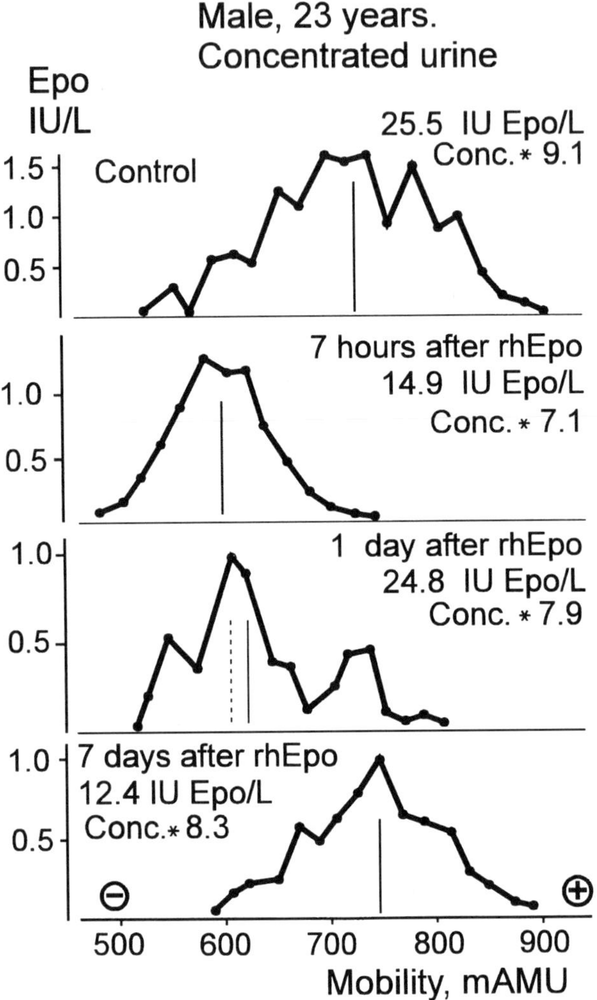

FIGURE 2.—The elution patterns of erythropoietin (*Epo*) by electrophoresis of 1 mL of concentrated urine from a man aged 23 years given 1 recombinant human *Epo* (*rhEpo*) injection (20 IU·kg^{-1} body weight) 3 times a week. The urine samples were obtained 7 hours, 1 day, and 7 days after the last (the 20th) subcutaneous injection of rhEpo. The control sample was obtained 3 weeks after the last injection. The urine samples were concentrated 7.1–9.1 times. A *vertical solid line* indicates the median mobility of all Epo isoforms and a *dashed vertical line* indicates the median mobility of isoforms in the basic peak. (Courtesy of Wide L, Bengtsson C, Berglund B, et al: Detection in blood and urine of recombinant erythropoietin administered to healthy men. *Med Sci Sports Exerc* 27:1569–1576, 1995.)

petitors. The problem is that the electrophoretic diagnosis becomes less clear-cut 48 hours after administration of Epo, whereas the competitive advantage may persist substantially longer. Random testing might help in overcoming this difficulty.

R.J. Shephard, M.D., Ph.D., D.P.E.

High-risk Behaviors Among High School Students in Massachusetts Who Use Anabolic Steroids

Middleman AB, Faulkner AH, Woods ER, Emans SJ, DuRant RH (Harvard Med School, Boston; Boston Univ)

Pediatrics 96:268–272, 1995 9–15

Background.—Adolescents' use of anabolic steroids has been associated with the use of other harmful substances, such as cigarettes, smokeless tobacco, marijuana, alcohol, cocaine, and injected drugs. However, it is unknown whether steroid use is related to other high-risk behaviors.

Methods.—A random sample of 3,054 high school students was included in the 1993 Massachusetts Youth Risk Behavior Survey. The mean age was 16 years. Fifty-one percent were female. In addition to anabolic steroid use, health risk and problem behaviors measured were sexual activity, suicidal behaviors, frequency of not wearing a passenger seatbelt, riding a motorcycle, not wearing a helmet while riding a motorcycle, driving after drinking alcohol, riding with a driver who had been drinking alcohol, fighting, and carrying a weapon.

Findings.—Frequency of anabolic steroid use was correlated with all these high-risk behaviors. In a multiple regression analysis, driving after drinking alcohol explained 12.5% of the variance. Another 9% of the variance was attributed to carrying a gun, having a number of sexual partners in the past 3 months, not using a condom during last intercourse, having an injury in a physical fight necessitating medical attention, having a history of sexually transmitted disease, not wearing a helmet on a motorcycle, not wearing a passenger safety belt, and making a suicide attempt requiring medical attention.

Conclusions.—The frequency of adolescents' anabolic steroid use is correlated with other high-risk behaviors. Thus, anabolic steroid use is part of a "risk behavior syndrome," rather than an isolated behavior. Comprehensive high-risk behavior screening and counseling is needed for adolescents using anabolic steroids.

▶ This report, which seems to be a follow-up of a groundbreaking study reviewed in 1994,[1] increases our understanding of adolescents, drugs, and behavior. The first study, of adolescents in Georgia, found that among ninth graders, about 5% of boys and 2% of girls reported using anabolic steroids, and among users, 25% shared needles and many were likely to use other drugs, including marijuana, tobacco, alcohol, and cocaine.[1] Other studies in the United States report similar trends among adolescents.[1] This study of Massachusetts high school students enlarges the concept, suggesting that drug abuse is part of a "risk behavior syndrome" that includes "problem behaviors" (drug and alcohol abuse, delinquency, sexual precocity) and "nonproblem health risk behaviors" (nonuse of safety belts, unhealthy eating, lack of exercise). Such behavior seems to reflect "the adolescent's way of being in the world" and somehow helps the adolescent affirm individuality (from parents), reach toward adulthood, and get peer acceptance. Sad but true. A recent survey of 16,000 Canadian students shows similar sad trends.[2]

E.R. Eichner, M.D.

References

1. 1994 YEAR BOOK OF SPORTS MEDICINE, pp 346–350.
2. Melia P, Pipe A, Greenberg L: The use of anabolic-androgenic steroids by Canadian students. *Clin J Sport Med* 6:9, 1996.

The Effects of Albuterol and Isokinetic Exercise on the Quadriceps Muscle Group

Caruso JF, Signorile JF, Perry AC, Leblanc B, Williams R, Clark M, Bamman MM (Univ of Miami, Coral Gables, Fla)

Med Sci Sports Exerc 27:1471–1476, 1995 9–16

Background.—β-Adrenergic agonists are able to increase muscle mass. Animals given β_2-agonists have gained significant muscle mass and strength, and these agents also enhance muscle mass and function in models of atrophy. At the same time, their cardio-acceleratory effects are minimal.

Objective.—The effects of albuterol were examined in 22 individuals 18–27 years of age who were either sedentary or engaged in recreational athletics. They performed isokinetic knee extension exercises twice a week over 9 weeks. Ten repetitions were done with the right thigh in the concentric/eccentric mode at a rate of 45 degrees/sec. Thirteen individuals received 16 mg of albuterol daily for 6 weeks, whereas 9 received a placebo.

Results.—For most eccentric strength variables, the individuals given albuterol had greater posttreatment values than controls (Table 3). Albuterol also enhanced strength when eccentric variables were expressed in relation to body mass. No significant intergroup differences in body mass were found at any interval, and there were no significant changes in pulmonary function.

Conclusion.—Albuterol may have a possible role in countering loss of muscle strength. The drug appears to be effective in therapeutic doses when given in conjunction with resistance exercise.

► Albuterol has generally been considered to have minimal effects on athletic performance. As a selective β_2-agonist, it is an effective bronchodilator for those who are troubled by asthma, yet it has little immediate influence on heart rate and thus cardiovascular function. However, a number of investigations have shown that β-agonists have long-term effects on both skeletal and cardiac muscle mass,[1-3] and such drugs have sometimes been used to increase muscle mass during the course of rehabilitation. Further, there have been suggestions that these drugs can act synergistically with other methods of training the skeletal muscles,[4] and there have been hopes

TABLE 3.—Eccentric Dependent Variable Values

Variable	*N*	Pretest	Midtest	Post-test
Eccentric peak torque (*N* · m)				
Placebo	9	255.9 ± 19.0	291.0 ± 21.2	317.6 ± 20.0
Albuterol	13	251.6 ± 18.6	327.3 ± 17.7	342.0 ± 16.5
Combined	22	253.3 ± 13.2	312.4 ± 13.8*	332.0 ± 12.7*
Eccentric total work (*N* · m)				
Placebo	9	2331.7 ± 223.7	2649.9 ± 170.8	2640.1 ± 111.2
Albuterol	13	2195.6 ± 188.9	2941.4 ± 186.4*	3190.8 ± 205.3*†
Combined	22	2251.3 ± 141.7	2822.1 ± 131.4	2965.5 ± 140.2
Eccentric average power (W)				
Placebo	9	51.1 ± 4.3	59.1 ± 3.6	59.2 ± 2.7
Albuterol	13	48.8 ± 3.7	68.0 ± 3.5*	68.9 ± 3.5*†
Combined	22	49.7 ± 2.8	64.4 ± 2.7	64.9 ± 2.5
Eccentric time to peak torque (msec)				
Placebo	9	1847 ± 87	1711 ± 65	1576 ± 95
Albuterol	13	1823 ± 115	1566 ± 75	1608 ± 39
Combined	22	1833 ± 75	1625 ± 53*	1595 ± 44*
Eccentric peak torque to bodyweight ratio [(N · m · kg^{-1}) · 100]				
Placebo	9	334.2 ± 21.9	359.5 ± 24.4	392.7 ± 24.4
Albuterol	13	353.5 ± 24.3	454.1 ± 22.4*†	473.4 ± 19.5*†
Combined	22	345.6 ± 16.7	415.4 ± 19.1	440.4 ± 17.2
Eccentric work to bodyweight ratio [(N · m · kg^{-1}) · 100]				
Placebo	9	355.9 ± 28.5	382.7 ± 21.8	384.0 ± 20.1
Albuterol	13	377.9 ± 28.3	479.3 ± 25.8*†	495.7 ± 25.8*†
Combined	22	368.9 ± 20.1	439.8 ± 20.1	450.0 ± 20.8

Note: Mean ± standard error.
* Greater than within-group pre value.
† Greater than within-time placebo value.
(Courtesy of Caruso JF, Signorile JF, Perry AC, et al: The effects of albuterol and isokinetic exercise on the quadriceps muscle group. *Med Sci Sports Exerc* 27:1471–1476, 1995.)

that β_2-agonists might facilitate hypertrophy of skeletal muscle while avoiding adverse effects on the myocardium.

The mechanism behind these long-term effects remains unclear. Possibly, mobilization of fat may allow a larger portion of dietary protein to be applied to muscle synthesis. But irrespective of the underlying mechanisms, the treatment has some interest for rehabilitation clinics, and there may be a need to rethink the permissive long-term use of β_2-agonists by athletes.

R.J. Shephard, M.D., Ph.D., D.P.E.

References

1. Alderman EL, Harrison DC: Myocardial hypertrophy resulting from low dosage isoproterenol administration in rats. *Proc Soc Exp Biol Med* 136:268–270, 1971.
2. Deshaies Y, Willemot J, Leblanc J, et al: Protein synthesis. amino acid uptake, and pools during isoproterenol-induced hypertrophy of the rat heart and tibialis muscle. *Can J Physiol Pharmacol* 59:113–121, 1981.
3. Stanton HC, Brenner G, Mayfield ED, et al: Studies on isoproterenol-induced cardiomegaly in rats. *Am Heart J* 77:72–80, 1969.
4. Signorile JF, Ferris A, Pearl A, et al: The impact of three weeks of albuterol intervention on a 13 week resistance training program. *Med Sci Sports Exerc*, in press.

Lack of Effect of Exercise Training on Dehydroepiandrosterone-sulfate

Milani RV, Lavie CJ, Barbee RW, Littman AB (Alton Ochsner Med Found, New Orleans, La; Massachusetts Gen Hosp, Boston)

Am J Med Sci 310:242–246, 1995 9–17

Background.—Previous studies have suggested an inverse association between levels of the sulfate ester of dehydroepiandrosterone (DHEA) and the risk of coronary artery disease. Levels of DHEA reportedly increase when behavioral measures are used to ameliorate stress and lessen social isolation. Enhanced physical activity may, however, be a confounding factor.

Study Plan.—The effects of exercise training alone, in the setting of cardiac rehabilitation, on plasma levels of DHEA sulfate were studied in a prospective series of 96 patients who had had myocardial infarction or had undergone angioplasty or coronary bypass surgery for acute ischemia. Participants performed aerobic and dynamic exercises 3 times a week for 12 weeks at 70% to 85% of the peak heart rate. Plasma levels of DHEA sulfate were measured by radioimmunoassay.

Observations.—Most patients studied were older, overweight men with excessive body fat. Most were fairly deconditioned at the outset. Exercise capacity (peak metabolic equivalents) improved more than 40% during the 12-week training period, but body fat decreased by only 2%. Exercise training appeared to have salutary effects on the patients' quality of life. They were less anxious and depressed and felt more energetic and generally healthier. Plasma levels of DHEA sulfate did not change significantly after exercise training, even when only patients with initially low levels were considered.

Conclusion.—Exercise training in the course of cardiac rehabilitation does not significantly alter plasma levels of DHEA sulfate.

► It is generally agreed that the difference between the sexes in the prevalence of ischemic heart disease results, at least in part, from hormonal differences between men and women; estrogens play a protective role, and male hormones have an adverse effect. It may thus be something of a surprise to find some quite early work showing an *inverse* relationship between plasma levels of DHEA and the risk of coronary disease.[1-3] Moreover, some therapeutic programs have increased DHEA levels, although it has been unclear whether psychotherapy or an associated increase in physical activity was responsible. This investigation shows that DHEA levels are unchanged by the moderate physical activity typical of most coronary rehabilitation programs (in this instance, 30–40 minutes of dynamic, aerobic exercise at 70% to 85% of maximal heart rate, 3 times per week for 12 weeks).

R.J. Shephard, M.D., Ph.D., D.P.E.

References

1. Kask E: 17-Ketosteroids and arteriosclerosis. *Angiology* 10:358–368, 1959.
2. Marmorston J, Griffith GC, Geller PJ, et al: Urinary steroids in the measurement of aging and of atherosclerosis. *J Am Geriatr Soc* 23:481–492, 1975.
3. Herrington DM, Gordon GB, Achuff SC, et al: Plasma dehydroepiandrosterone and dehydroepiandrosterone sulfate in patients undergoing diagnostic coronary angiography. *J Am Coll Cardiol* 16:862–870, 1990.

The Effects of Anabolic Steroids on Rat Tendon: An Ultrastructural, Biomechanical, and Biochemical Analysis

Inhofe PD, Grana WA, Egle D, Min K-W, Tomasek J (Univ of Oklahoma, Oklahoma City, Okla)

Am J Sports Med 23:227–232, 1995 9–18

Introduction.—Although athletes continue to abuse anabolic steroids, the underlying mechanism of action of these drugs is largely unclear. Anabolic steroids may limit the chronic catabolic state or, via specific receptors, stimulate an increase in muscle mass. Although many athletes support the effectiveness of these drugs in enhancing performance, clinical studies are equivocal. The adverse effects of anabolic steroids on many tissues are well documented, but their influence on tendons is less well understood. Studies on animals have reported some structural changes to collagen, resulting in a stiffer tendon with less ready elongation. The mechanical, ultrastructural, and biochemical changes in tendon as a result of exercise, administration of anabolic steroids, or both were studied.

Methods.—Four groups of 12 male rats were assigned a treatment: control, exercise, anabolic steroids, or exercise plus steroids. Stanozolol, 10 mg, was given intramuscularly at the beginning of the first week. After

TABLE 3.—Results of Statistical Analysis of Biomechanical Testing Using Analysis of Variance (ANOVA) and Student's *t* Tests

Parameter	ANOVA (*P* values)	
	6-Weeks	12-Weeks
Total failure		
Maximum force	0.96	0.70
Maximum elongation	0.20	0.69
Total energy	0.52	0.66
First failure		
Force	0.93	0.83
Elongation	0.01*	0.59
Energy	0.001†	0.51
Stiffness in linear region	0.002‡	0.26
Toe-limit elongation	0.051	0.21

* Student's *t* tests: group IV was 46% less than group I, group IV was 39% less than group III.

† Student's *t* tests: group II was 42% less than group I, group III was 46% less than group I, and group IV was 57% less than group I.

‡ Student's *t* tests: group II was 30% greater than group I, group IV was 46% greater than group II, and group IV was 89% greater than group I.

(Courtesy of Inhofe PD, Grana WA, Egle D, et al: The effects of anabolic steroids on rat tendon: An ultrastructural, biomechanical, and biochemical analysis. *Am J Sports Med* 23:227–232, 1995.)

5 weeks, 3 mg of nandrolone decanoate per kilogram was given once per week to mimic the "stacking" regimen practiced by many steroid users. Exercising rats ran on a treadmill 30 minutes per day, 5 days a week. At the end of the 12-week study, the rats could run at 1.8 km/hr up an 8% grade. Force-elongation curves were determined on the Achilles' tendon at 6 and 12 weeks. Cross-section and longitudinal sections of the tendon were analyzed by electron microscopy. Collagen and a variety of other proteins and enzymes were analyzed biochemically.

Results.—Biomechanical results (Table 3) indicated that steroids produced a stiffer tendon that failed with less elongation. No change in tendon strength was noted. The effects seemed reversible with cessation of drug administration. Microscopic examination showed no change in fibrils, fiber diameter, or shape, nor was there any change in type III collagen or fibronectin.

Conclusion.—Anabolic steroids adversely affect tendon mechanics. These effects seem to be reversible.

▶ This study confirms earlier work in showing that 1 of the adverse effects of the systemic administration of anabolic steroids is a weakening of tendons. However, neither the microscopy nor the biochemical tests disclosed any significant changes in the structure of the collagen fibrils. This is in contrast to 3 earlier reports that showed an association between changes in tendon mechanics and collagen dysplasia.[1–3]

R.J. Shephard, M.D., Ph.D., D.P.E.

References

1. Michna H: Tendon injuries induced by exercise and anabolic steroids in experimental mice. *Int Orthop* 11:157–162, 1987.

2. Miles JW, Grana WA, Egle D, et al: The effect of anabolic steroids on the biomechanical and histological properties of rat tendon. *J Bone Joint Surg (Am)* 74-A:411–422, 1992.
3. Wood TO, Cooke PH, Goodship AE: The effect of exercise and anabolic steroids on the mechanical properties and crimp morphology of rat tendon. *Am J Sports Med* 16:153–158, 1988.

Impotence Related to Anabolic Steroid Use in a Body Builder: Response to Clomiphene Citrate

Bickelman C, Ferries L, Eaton RP (Univ of New Mexico, Albuquerque)
West J Med 162:158–160, 1995 9–19

Purpose.—Competitive athletes and bodybuilders have become sophisticated in the use of anabolic steroids and the drugs that are used to combat their side effects. The case report of a man with recreational anabolic steroid–induced pituitary-gonadal failure was reviewed.

Case Report.—Man, 29, a college student and competitive bodybuilder, had abused anabolic steroids for 8 months, alternating between 16-week cycles of testosterone cypionate and oxymetholone. He had stopped using these drugs because of impotence and diminished libido. After completing an unsuccessful self-selected 4-week trial of human chorionic gonadotropin, he waited 9 months before seeking an endocrine consultation for continued impotence and reduced libido. He was treated with orally administered clomiphene for 2 months, which normalized his libido and potency. At follow-up 6 months later, the patient had returned to the illicit use of anabolic steroids and was considering another course of self-selected human chorionic gonadotropin therapy plus tamoxifen to prevent a worsening gynecomastia.

Conclusions.—Clomiphene can be used to reverse impotence and normalize diminished libido resulting from pituitary-gonadal failure induced by the recreational use of anabolic steroids.

► It is alarming to read that athletes are now not only abusing anabolic steroids but are also treating themselves with such drugs as human chorionic gonadotropin, clomiphene citrate, and tamoxifen citrate to counter the side effects of gynecomastia and reduced testicular volume. Although it is usually assumed that reductions of potency induced by anabolic steroids are only temporary in nature, in the case described here, pituitary function, testicular volume, and potency were still impaired 9 months after ceasing massive steroid treatment (alternating 16-week cycles of testosterone, 1,500–1,800 mg/week) and Anadrol (560 mg/week). After 2 months of medically supervised treatment with clomiphene (50 mg, increasing to 100 mg), the patient was once again capable of daily sexual intercourse. It is particularly discouraging that this successful treatment apparently encouraged a resumption of steroid abuse.

R.J. Shephard, M.D., Ph.D., D.P.E.

Cardiopulmonary Performance During Exercise in Acromegaly, and the Effects of Acute Suppression of Growth Hormone Hypersecretion With Octreotide

Giustina A, Boni E, Romanelli G, Grassi V, Giustina G (Univ of Brescia, Italy)
Am J Cardiol 75:1042–1047, 1995 9–20

Background.—Patients with acromegaly have long-term hypersecretion of growth hormone (GH), altered GH secretion dynamics, and elevated plasma levels of insulin-like growth factor-I. They also may have severe cardiovascular complications, which are a major cause of morbidity and mortality. It has been suggested that GH hypersecretion is the cause of the cardiovascular complications. The effects of acute reduction of circulating GH levels on cardiopulmonary performance during exercise were assessed in patients with acromegaly.

Methods.—Ten patients with active acromegaly were studied: 6 women and 5 men, with a mean age of 55 years and a mean body mass index of 28 kg/m^2. Blood sampling for GH measurement and 2-dimensional guided M-mode echocardiography were performed in all patients. Patients then underwent a cycloergometric exercise test on 2 occasions: once at baseline and again after treatment with octreotide in a 500-µg/24 hr subcutaneous infusion through a portable pump. The echocardiographic and exercise findings were compared with those of 10 normal age- and sex-matched controls.

Results.—Left ventricular hypertrophy was noted in all patients. The patients had abnormalities of left ventricular diastolic filling at baseline, although their systolic function indices were not significantly different from those of the controls. Work rates were significantly decreased in the patients with acromegaly vs. the controls, both at the ventilatory threshold—54 W vs. 94 W—and at maximum power output—87 vs. 152 W. Octreotide infusion produced significant reductions in heart rate and serum GH level. Improvements were also noted in systolic and diastolic functional indices at rest and in work rates and oxygen consumption at ventilatory threshold and at maximal exercise. After octreotide treatment, the exercise capacity at the ventilatory threshold in the patients with acromegaly was not significantly different from that of the controls.

Conclusions.—The GH excess that characterizes acromegaly may have important functional as well as structural effects on the hypertrophic heart. The negative functional effects may be seen both at baseline and during exercise. The functional changes are reversed by continuous octreotide infusion to produce a sustained decrease in GH levels.

► An increasing number of athletes are rumored to be treating themselves with GH preparations, and it is thus instructive to examine patients with acromegaly in whom an excess of GH has been present for a long time. Despite left ventricular hypertrophy, the end result of prolonged exposure to GH seems to be a decrease rather than an increase of aerobic power. Ventricular hypertrophy, myocardial infarction, and sudden death also are increasingly recognized as complications of the abuse of androgenic-anabolic steroids.[1]

R.J. Shephard, M.D., Ph.D., D.P.E.

Reference

1. Melchert RB, Welder AA: Cardiovascular effects of androgenic-anabolic steroids. *Med Sci Sports Exerc* 27:1252–1262, 1995.

Carbon Monoxide Poisoning Among Recreational Boaters

Silvers SM, Hampson NB (Virginia Mason Med Ctr, Seattle; Univ of Rochester, NY; Virginia Mason Clinic, Seattle)

JAMA 274:1614–1616, 1995 9–21

Introduction.—Carbon monoxide (CO) poisoning is the most common cause of death from poisoning in the United States. In many cases of CO poisoning, the source of CO is not recognized as a potential hazard. A review of cases treated at 1 institution highlights recreational boating as a source of unintentional CO poisoning.

Methods.—Records of the hyperbaric department at the study institution were reviewed for the period from July 1984 through June 1994. Thirty-nine (8%) of the 512 patients treated for acute unintentional CO poisoning during the 10-year period were affected during recreational boating activities. Patients were treated in a multiplace hyperbaric chamber, with hyperbaric oxygen administered at 2.8–3.0 atm absolute pressure for 46–92 minutes. Additional oxygen at 1.9 atm absolute pressure was required in some cases.

Results.—The 39 patients were poisoned in 27 separate incidents, all of which occurred in calm seas on a cool day and involved a boat longer than 22 feet with enclosable cabins. Most incidents took place between 10 AM and 4 PM. The boats were typically powerboats (85%) more than 10 years old (71%). Engine exhaust accounted for 21 of the 27 incidents. Patients ranged in age from 6 months to 69 years (mean, 37 years). All had exhibited signs or symptoms of CO poisoning and 65% lost consciousness, at least transiently. Other common symptoms were headache, nausea, weakness, dizziness, and dyspnea. Alcohol use was reported in 19% of incidents. Only 1 boat had an operational CO detector, but the device did not indicate the danger.

Conclusions.—Recreational boaters, particularly on larger powerboats with enclosed cabins, are at risk of CO poisoning. Some of the patients in this series did not consider CO as the cause of their symptoms. Most of the boaters were cruising with the rear cabin door open and the bow hatch closed. Accumulation of CO in the cabin appears to have been caused by exhaust drawn into the cabin, as can occur in station wagons and pickup trucks. To prevent CO poisoning on boats, educational programs and use of CO detectors are recommended.

▶ This most interesting and important article calls attention to an important problem. The authors' observations have several implications for the prevention of CO poisoning among recreational boaters. First, exhaust systems should be regularly maintained and inspected. Second, CO detectors with an audible alarm should be installed in both cabins. Third, public education programs regarding the dangers of CO poisoning should be initiated. Finally, programs should be initiated that are directed toward improving the awareness of the mechanism of CO exposure on boats and the early symptoms of CO intoxication.

J.S. Torg, M.D.

Simulated Descent *v* Dexamethasone in Treatment of Acute Mountain Sickness: A Randomised Trial

Keller H-R, Maggiorini M, Bärtsch P, Oelz O (Univ of Zurich, Switzerland; Univ Clinic of Medicine, Heidelberg, Germany; Triemli Hosp, Zurich, Switzerland)

BMJ 310:1232–1235, 1995 9–22

Background.—Recently, portable hyperbaric chambers have been advocated for emergency treatment of acute mountain sickness. Simulated descent of 1,500–2,500 m is achieved by an increase of pressure up to 220 mbar in the chamber, which also leads to increased oxygen tension. The therapeutic efficacy of a portable hyperbaric chamber for the treatment of acute mountain sickness was compared with oral dexamethasone treatment in a randomized trial during the summer mountaineering season.

Study Design.—The study was conducted in a high-altitude research laboratory at 4,559 m above sea level (Alps Valais). Thirty-one climbers with symptoms of acute mountain sickness were randomly assigned to 1-hour treatment in the hyperbaric chamber at a pressure of 193 mbar or orally administered dexamethasone 8 mg initially and 4 mg every 6 hours. Signs and symptoms of acute mountain sickness were assessed using the Lake Louise questionnaire, the AMS-C questionnaire, and clinical assessment 1 hour and about 11 hours after beginning treatment.

Outcome.—One hour of compression with 193 mbar in the hyperbaric chamber, corresponding to a descent of 2,250 m, caused a significantly greater relief of symptoms of acute mountain sickness immediately after treatment, when compared with dexamethasone; however, symptoms recurred after a mean of 11 hours (Fig 1). In contrast, treatment with dexamethasone resulted in a more gradual but longer-lasting relief of acute mountain sickness, such that patients had significantly less severe acute

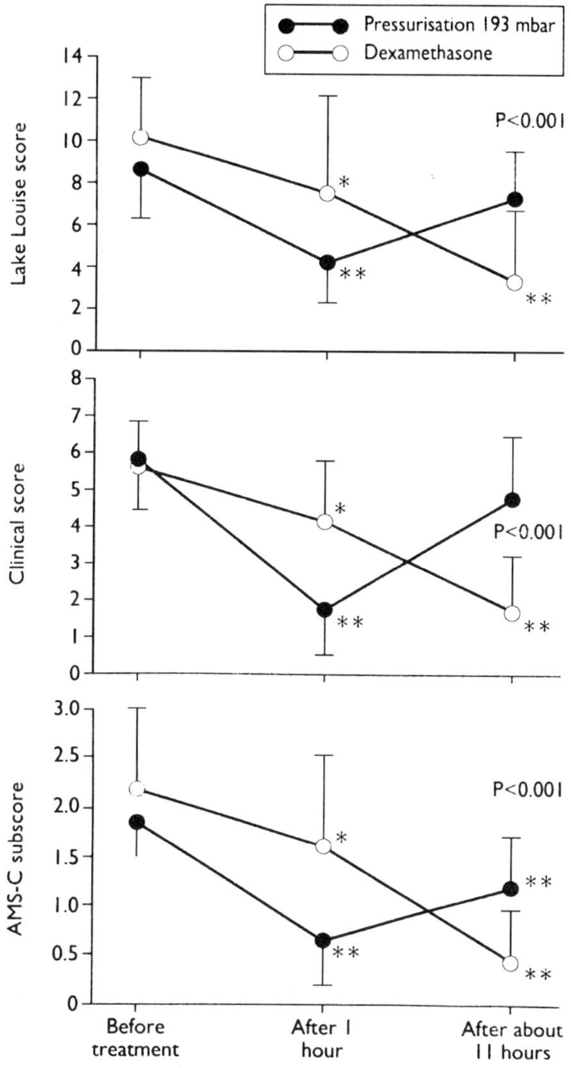

FIGURE 1.—Mean (standard deviation) score of acute mountain sickness in patients treated with simulated descent or dexamethasone. Given *P* values correspond to 2-factor analysis of variance performed with values expressed as differences from values before treatment ($*P < 0.05$, $**P < 0.01$; Scheffe F test). (Courtesy of Keller H-R, Maggiorini M, Bärtsch P, et al: Simulated descent *v* dexamethasone in treatment of acute mountain sickness: A randomised trial. *BMJ* 310:1232–1235, 1995.)

mountain sickness after a mean of 11 hours, when compared with patients treated with the hyperbaric chamber. In addition, the reduction of symptoms of acute mountain sickness with dexamethasone coincided with an increase in arterial oxygen saturation (Fig 2).

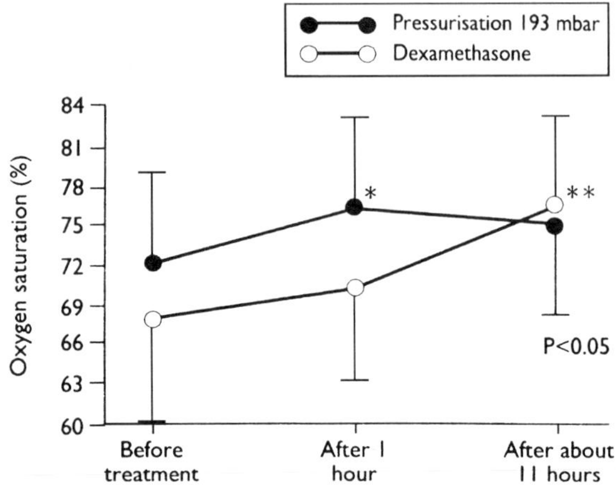

FIGURE 2.—Mean (standard deviation) oxygen saturation in patients treated with simulated descent or dexamethasone. Given *P* values correspond to 2-factor analysis of variance performed with values expressed as differences from values before treatment (*$P < 0.05$, **$P < 0.01$; Scheffe F test). (Courtesy of Keller H-R, Maggiorini M, Bärtsch P, et al: Simulated descent *v* dexamethasone in treatment of acute mountain sickness: A randomised trial. *BMJ* 310:1232–1235, 1995.)

Conclusions.—Both hyperbaric chamber and orally administered dexamethasone are effective in treating acute mountain sickness. Treatment with orally administered dexamethasone is simple and provides longer-lasting relief of symptoms: it should be the treatment of choice for the cerebral form of acute mountain sickness. The hyperbaric chamber represents an alternative to bottled oxygen in remote places and a valuable adjunct to other treatments because of its rapid action. The 2 methods can be combined for optimal efficacy if descent or evacuation is not possible.

▶ This report further erodes the case for relying on the fabric hyperbaric chamber, or Gamow Bag, as a mainstay in the treatment of patients with acute mountain sickness. Although experts in altitude medicine agree that the Gamow Bag works acutely and can help when descent is impractical and no bottled oxygen is on hand,[1] a study last year found that the benefits from the Gamow Bag were transitory and that, after 12 hours, patients treated with bed rest alone were as well off as those who had initially been treated with the Gamow Bag.[2] This report extends that research by showing that, after 11 hours, patients treated with dexamethasone were better off than those treated with the Gamow Bag.

E.R. Eichner, M.D.

References

1. 1993 Year Book of Sports Medicine, pp 412–413.
2. 1994 Year Book of Sports Medicine, pp 407–408.

Ski Sickness

Häusler R (Univ ENT Clinic, Berne, Switzerland)

Acta Otolaryngol 115:1–2, 1995 9–23

Introduction.—Downhill skiing can precipitate dizziness along with illusionary rotatory or pendular sensations that can lead to nausea and vomiting. The concept of "ski sickness" was reviewed.

Methods.—Eleven patients, 18 to 47 years of age and otherwise healthy, complained of nausea or vomiting during or shortly after downhill skiing. The symptoms were preceded by vertigo and dysequilibrium. The patients' history revealed no otologic disease. Motion sickness during car or boat rides was not uncommon in this group. Vestibular examinations were normal, and electronystagmography showed only minor abnormalities such as spontaneous nystagmus in the dark (3 patients), positional nystagmus in the dark (2 patients), and asymmetric caloric testing (4 patients). Corrective lenses were worn by 8 patients. The patients indicated that their "ski sickness" occurred on foggy days with poor visibility.

Mechanism.—Their pathophysiology seemed to be related to vestibular overstimulation resulting from winding turns or uneven ground with insufficient visual control because of the foggy conditions. The atmospheric changes caused by their descent from high to lower altitudes may have combined with psychological factors—such as fear of heights, mountains, excess speed, or falling—to further overload the sensory systems. The symptoms may be relieved by vestibular suppressants such as dimenhydrinate chewing gum, cinnarizine, or scopolamine.

Conclusions.—The nausea, vomiting, and vertigo of "ski sickness" appear to make up a distinctive form of motion sickness. Informal inquiries of many co-workers suggest that this condition is experienced by many individuals during downhill skiing.

▶ This is a newly reported syndrome of motion sickness with practical implications for skiers and their physicians. "Ski sickness" is similar to "sea sickness" and seems to result mainly from vestibular overstimulation (winding turns, uneven ground) in the face of poor visual control (fog, "white days") and poor somatosensory input (ski boots, gliding skis). The result is vertigo, nausea, and sometimes vomiting that may spoil the ski trip. In some patients, such symptoms could be compounded by alcohol use, acute mountain sickness, or both. "Ski sickness" responds best to vestibular suppressants such as dimenhydrinate chewing gum or transdermal scopolamine.

E.R. Eichner, M.D.

How Well Do Older Persons Tolerate Moderate Altitude?

Roach RC, Houston CS, Honigman B, Nicholas RA, Yaron M, Grissom CK, Alexander JK, Hultgren HN (Lovelace Inst for Basic and Applied Med Research, Albuquerque, NM; Univ of Vermont, Burlington; Colorado Altitude Research Inst, Denver; et al)

West J Med 162:32–36, 1995 9–24

Introduction.—Many older men and women are traveling more frequently to moderate-altitude resorts for vacations or business conferences; however, little research has been done on the effects of age or pre-existing disease and altitude tolerance and whether older individuals might be at greater risk of acute mountain sickness (AMS). The physiologic and clinical responses to moderate altitude were studied in a group of older visitors to a mountain resort.

Methods.—Study participants consisted of 97 men and women, 59–83 years of age, who were visiting a mountain resort at 8,200 ft. Before their visit, they completed a questionnaire that included information on hypertension, heart or lung disease, diabetes mellitus, smoking, usual exercise

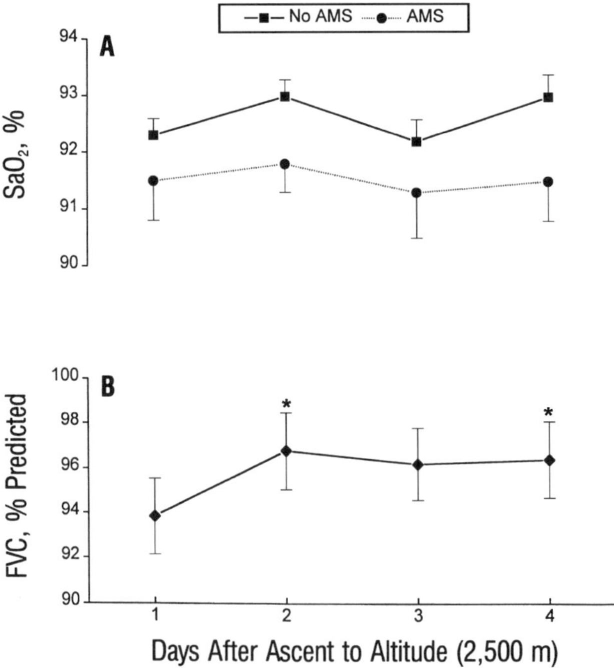

FIGURE 1.—A, the arterial oxygen saturation (*S*A_{O_2}) in elderly visitors to moderate elevations (2,500 m [8,200 ft] over a 5-day period in those with acute mountain sickness (*AMS*) is compared with SA_{O_2} values of those without AMS. Between-group differences were not statistically significant. **B,** a slight increase occurred in the forced vital capacity (*FVC*) in all patients on days 2 and 4 ($P < 0.01$.) (Courtesy of Roach RC, Houston CS, Honigman B, et al: How well do older patients tolerate moderate altitude? *West J Med* 162:32–36, 1995.)

pattern, residential altitude, and self-rated fitness. Upon arrival, each individual was given another questionnaire on activities, acute mountain sickness, AMS symptoms, and other health-related symptoms. Acute mountain sickness symptom scores were graded 0 to 3 based on self-evaluation of headache, sleeplessness, fatigue, light-headedness, and gastrointestinal problems. A score of 3 or higher defined AMS.

Results.—Of the 97 participants, 81 (84%) resided at or near sea level. Nineteen (20%) had coronary artery disease, 33 (34%) had hypertension, 9 (9%) had lung disease, and 5 (5%) had diabetes mellitus. Seventy-six

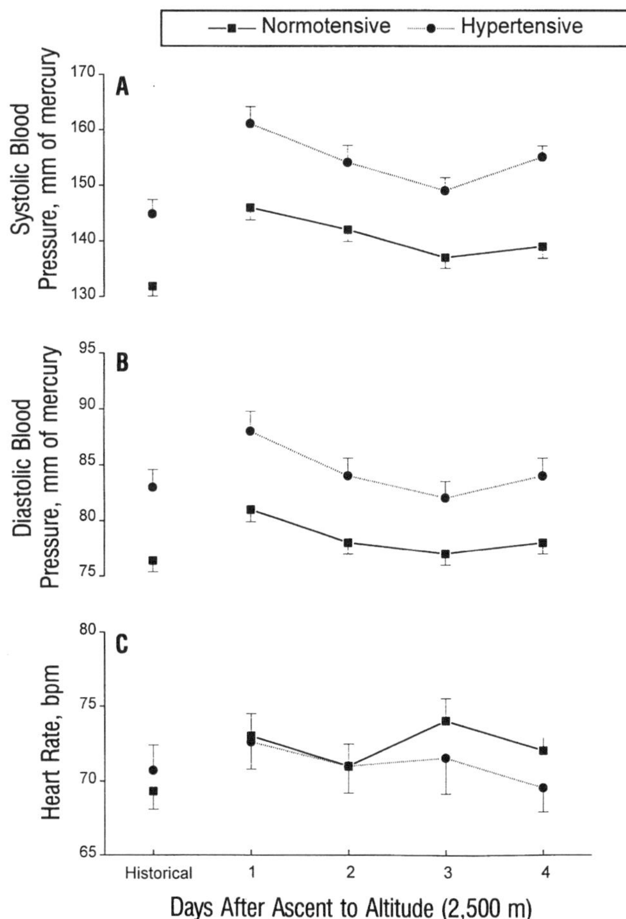

FIGURE 2.—**A**, systolic and (**B**) diastolic blood pressure and (**C**) heart rate responses are shown in hypertensive and normotensive patients on days 1 through 4 at 2,500 m (8,200 ft). Blood pressures decreased significantly on all days compared with day 1 ($P < 0.01$) in both hypertensive and normotensive patients and were significantly higher on all days in the hypertensive group compared with the normotensive group. Historical blood pressure values from each patient's physician ($n = 95$) are shown for comparison. (Courtesy of Roach RC, Houston CS, Honigman B, et al: How well do older patients tolerate moderate altitude? *West J Med* 162:32–36, 1995.)

individuals (78%) said they were in good-to-excellent physical condition, and 88 (91%) were moderately active to very active in their daily routine. The incidence of AMS in this group was 16%, slightly lower than that reported in younger individuals. Symptoms of AMS did not parallel arterial oxygen saturation or spirometric or blood pressure measurements (Figs 1 and 2). Percentages of chronic diseases were typical for the general elderly population, and despite the presence of these conditions, no adverse signs or symptoms occurred in the study group during their stay on the mountain.

Conclusions.—It is generally safe for older individuals, including those with underlying heart and lung conditions, to visit moderate altitudes. Asymptomatic coronary and pulmonary diseases, as well as hypertension, were not clinically affected by altitude. However, as a precaution, individuals with these conditions should have their blood pressure monitored if AMS symptoms occur, and they should also continue taking any medications they normally use.

► This study is the most comprehensive evaluation to date of older individuals visiting moderate altitudes. It follows a report by 1 of the authors on practical measures for safe trekking at high altitude in the face of obesity, hypertension, smoking, asthma, or coronary artery disease.[1] Only 16% of these 97 individuals, with an average age of 70 years, had AMS. This fairly low attack rate (compared with previous studies of younger individuals) may relate to these older individuals minimizing symptoms on the questionnaire, or more likely to self-selection, in that these individuals felt able, based on past experience, to go to this altitude. The proof that 20% had coronary artery disease is meager; it seems based mainly on ECG records from their personal physicians. In this study, alcohol intake was not related to AMS, but in a recent study, 1 dose of 50 g of alcohol (the alcohol in 1 L of beer) inhibited the early acute ventilatory adaptation to mild hypoxia.[2] So, alcohol use may predispose to AMS. Another study of AMS at moderate altitude (205 participants, average age, 36 years) found an attack rate of 28% and noted that habitual physical activity, as a gauge of fitness, did not correlate with development of AMS.[3]

This current study, along with 1 reviewed in 1994,[4] helps sports medicine physicians counsel their patients. It stresses that it is generally safe for older men and women, including those with hypertension or underlying heart or lung disease, to make short visits to moderate altitudes.

E.R. Eichner, M.D.

References

1. 1991 YEAR BOOK OF SPORTS MEDICINE, pp 201–203.
2. Roeggla G, Roeggla H, Roeggla M, et al: Effect of alcohol on acute ventilatory adaptation to mild hypoxia at moderate altitude. *Ann Intern Med* 122:925–927, 1995.
3. Honigman B, Read M, Lezotte D, et al: Sea-level physical activity and acute mountain sickness at moderate altitude. *West J Med* 163:117–121, 1995.
4. 1994 YEAR BOOK OF SPORTS MEDICINE, pp 408–410.

Pulmonary Barotrauma and Related Events in Divers
Raymond LW (East Carolina Univ, Greenville, NC; Baylor College of Medicine, Houston)
Chest 107:1648–1652, 1995 9–25

Introduction.—Pulmonary barotrauma (PBT) is well recognized as a complication of mechanical ventilation. It also can occur in scuba divers, in whom its recognition is sometimes delayed and its implications for future diving may be underappreciated. Diving-related PBT may occur at any significant depth and may be followed by a number of pulmonary complications, ranging from discomfort through mediastinal emphysema or pneumothorax to life-threatening gas embolization. Nine cases of PBT in divers were reviewed.

Patients.—Of the 9 cases of PBT, 4 developed when the diver was at or near the water surface. (Table 1). These cases were classified as minor, because they presented only relatively minor consequences of PBT. In these patients, PBT occurred spontaneously in the presence of increased lung volume and pressure, for example, Valsalva's maneuver with hyperinflation; with vigorous in-water activity; or as a result of equipment malfunction. The immediate sequelae, although uncomfortable, were not serious. However, 3 of the 4 divers were later found to have abnormal pulmonary function, whether as a cause or a consequence of the barotrauma.

The other 5 patients had more serious PBT, which developed while the divers were diving to depths of 5–37 m (16–20 ft). Two patients had pre-existing bullous lung disease; in both of these individuals a pyopneumothorax developed. Complications in the other 3 patients consisted of tension pneumothorax and tuberculous pleurisy, cerebral ischemia, and fatal cerebral embolism.

TABLE 1.—Pulmonary Barotrauma in Divers, Nondiving vs. Hyperbaric

Case	Age, Gender	Activity Preceding PBT	Prior Lung Disease?	Complications of PBT
Minor (Surface) Cases				
1	19, M	Drown-proofing, on surface	None	None
2	23, M	Buddy-breathing, 0 to 5 ft	None	Small airway dysfunction
3	27, M	1,000-yard swim, surface	None	Small airway dysfunction, decreased CO diffusing capacity
4	35, M	Scuba malfunction, surface	None	Pneumothorax, mild COPD
Major (Hyperbaric) Cases				
5	18, M	Hull repair, 18 ft	None	Tension pneumothorax, tuberculous pleurisy
6	23, F	Sport diving, 40 ft	Bullae	Pyopneumothorax
7	23, M	Salvage dive, 120 ft	None	Cerebral emboli, death
8	35, M	Sport diving, 40 ft	None	Cerebral ischemia
9	43, F	Sport diving, 16 ft	Bullae	Pyopneumothorax

Abbreviations: CO, carbon monoxide; *COPD,* chronic obstructive pulmonary disease.
(Courtesy of Raymond LW: Pulmonary barotrauma and related events in divers. *Chest* 107:1648–1652, 1995.)

Discussion.—Pulmonary barotrauma and associated complications may develop in divers performing a variety of in-water activities at various depths. Greater depths are associated with major PBT, probably because of the higher transpulmonary pressures, but incidents may develop in shallow water because the relative volumetric expansion for a given decrease in absolute pressure is greater at shallower depths. Patients who have sustained even minor PBT should be advised not to dive again, because these events are prone to recur and the recurrences may cause serious complications.

▶ This article makes 2 important points. If an individual has had PBT once, he is likely to have some pulmonary abnormality that predisposes to the condition. Thus, although the symptoms during a first incident may be minor, the patient should be warned against further exposure to hyperbaric conditions. Second, the relative change in breathing pressure for a given ascent is greatest as the diver nears the surface. Thus, the danger of manifest PBT is greatest during the final stages of a diving ascent.

R.J. Shephard, M.D., Ph.D., D.P.E.

Scuba Decompression Illness (DCI) and Hydrophilic Contact Lens Wear: A Case Report

Murray N (Potter & Park Optometrists, Adelaide, Australia)

Clin Exp Optom 78:14–17, 1995 9–26

Case Report.—Man, 36, with an 8-year history as an occupational abalone diver, had been fitted with hydrophilic contact lenses for better vision while diving. He was moderately myopic, with some astigmatism. His general ocular function was within normal limits. The retina and choroidal structures were intact. He wore custom-fitted toric lenses that were 38% water content. Because of the lower oxygen permeability of this type of lens, the edges were looser than normal to allow for better oxygen and gas perfusion.

An aftercare examination showed a reduction in normal acuity and contrast sensitivity. In addition, in response to coming "up a bit fast" earlier in the day, the patient had discomfort in his shoulders and elbows. The corneal surfaces showed low-degree stromal edema in both eyes and gas bubbles in the corneal epithelium of both eyes as well as the precorneal tear film. The patient's discomfort increased over the next 10 minutes, as did the number and size of corneal bubbles. Although it was expected that intraepithelial bubbles would cause some discomfort, no pain was reported by the patient. No vessel or hemodynamic irregularities occurred.

During the dive that day, the patient went deeper (26–40 m, or 125–130 ft), stayed longer (5–5.5 hours breathing compressed air from the surface), and surfaced too quickly. To make his optometric appointment, he flew in a light aircraft. He received a diagnosis of decompression illness. Hyperbaric treatment was refused by the patient.

Conclusion.—Soft hydrophilic lenses are the choice for underwater diving because of the minimal risk of loss and bubble formation. If the recommended procedures for decompression are followed, then hydrophilic lenses can still be used. If proper decompression procedures are not followed, damage to the corneal tissues can result. The damage is localized to the area of punctate erosion. These wounds should heal quickly.

▶ Reports that the eyes can have manifestations of decompression sickness date back to the 17th century British scientist, Robert Boyle, who in 1670 described the appearance of gas emboli in the anterior chamber of the eyes of snakes who were undergoing decompression. Problems can arise while a diver is at depth (particularly if goggles or rigid lenses are worn); the pressure in any trapped gas is then less than in the ocular blood vessels, and bleeding tends to occur because of the pressure differential. However, this case seems a more classic instance of decompression sickness: gas dissolved in poorly vascularized tissues (including the eyes) while at depth, and there was a failure to eliminate this gas via the bloodstream because of an overly rapid ascent. Bubble formation is always a risk if there is more than a twofold change in ambient pressure, and any problem that the diver encounters on surfacing will be enhanced by flying in a light, unpressurized aircraft.

Although no permanent damage to the eyes was incurred in this patient, decompression sickness can be a serious (and sometimes a fatal) disorder. It is thus very important to impress upon divers the need to observe diving tables carefully and to undergo early recompression if symptoms develop. Flying also should be avoided after deep diving.

R.J. Shephard, M.D., Ph.D., D.P.E.

Mask Barotrauma Leading to Sub-conjunctival Haemorrhage in a Scuba Diver

Carkeet A (Queensland Univ of Technology, Australia)

Clin Exp Optom 78:18–20, 1995 9–27

Case Report.—Woman, 27, had been recreational scuba diving. She was using a new mask. During a descent to 20 m, she felt painful negative pressure on her face. When she surfaced, she found that she had subconjunctival hemorrhages. She went to an optometry clinic 2 days later. Her unaided vision was 6/4.5 in both eyes. Her intraocular pressures were 10 and 11 mm Hg. She had discomfort with horizontal gazing but no diplopia. Externally, she had extensive subconjuctival hemorrhages and periorbital hematoma that were more prominent inferiorly. Nearly all the visible bulbar conjunctiva was affected. The patient's corneas were normal and the anterior chambers were quiet. She said her eyes had been improving over the 2 days. She received a diagnosis of mask barotrauma.

Comment.—The clinical features of "mask squeeze" include puffy edematous facial tissue, mostly under the eyelids, purpuric hemorrhages, and delayed bruising. The "squeeze" is caused by low pressure in the mask during descent. This can be prevented by breathing through the nose into the mask. The patient's new mask fitted so tightly that it was difficult for her to exhale through her nose. The pressure gradient sucks the soft tissue of the face into the mask, resulting in the trauma. Despite its dramatic appearance, mask barotrauma is a benign diving injury and resolves without specific treatment. The diver should nevertheless refrain from diving until the injury has resolved.

▶ This article illustrates a second type of problem that can affect eyes that are protected by goggles and other regions of the body that are exposed to air pockets at atmospheric pressure during diving. When a diver is underwater, the pressure within the tissues can rise to several atmospheres (depending on the depth of immersion), and this forces the tissues into the air pocket, with extravasation of fluid and rupture of small blood vessels. It is interesting that in the case described the problem was traced to a poorly fitting mask; divers should be advised to make sure they can equalize gas pressures within the mask by exhaling through the nose.

R.J. Shephard, M.D., Ph.D., D.P.E.

Doppler Assessment of Hypoxic Pulmonary Vasoconstriction and Susceptibility to High Altitude Pulmonary Oedema

Vachiéry JL, McDonagh T, Moraine JJ, Berré J, Naeije R, Dargie H, Peacock AJ (Erasme Univ Hosp, Brussels, Belgium; Western Infirmary, Glasgow, Scotland)

Thorax 50:22–27, 1995 9–28

Background.—High-altitude pulmonary edema, an uncommon but serious complication of acute mountain sickness, occurs at altitudes of more than 2,000–3,000 m in individuals who are not acclimatized to such altitudes. Although the pathogenesis of this complication is debated, it may be related to excessive hypoxic pulmonary vasoconstriction (HPV). Susceptibility to high-altitude pulmonary edema may be detectable by echo Doppler indices of HPV at sea level.

Methods.—Seven individuals with a previous episode of high-altitude pulmonary edema, 9 who had successfully climbed to altitudes of 6,000–8,842 m, and 20 healthy unselected controls were studied. Echo Doppler measures of pulmonary blood flow acceleration time (AT) and

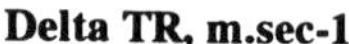

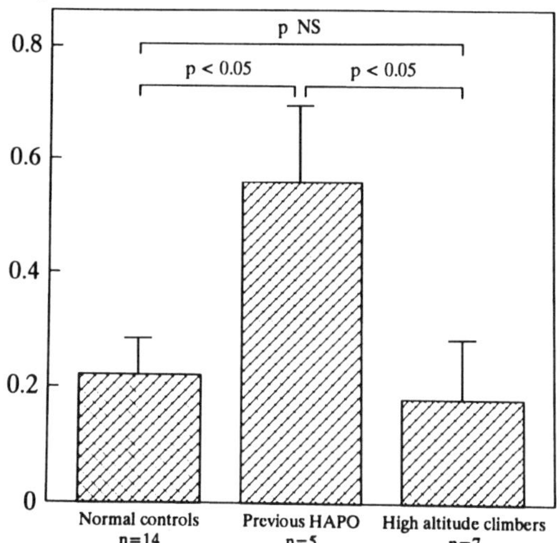

FIGURE 1.—Hypoxia-induced increases in maximum velocity of tricuspid regurgitation jets (*TR*) calculated as TR measured at a fraction of inspired oxygen (F_{IO_2}) of 0.125 minus TR measured at an F_{IO_2} of 0.21 (delta TR) in normal controls, in individuals with previous high altitude pulmonary edema (*HAPO*), and in successful high altitude climbers. Individuals with previous high altitude pulmonary edema had an increased hypoxic response compared with the other groups. (Courtesy of Vachiéry JL, McDonagh T, Moraine JJ, et al: Doppler assessment of hypoxic pulmonary vasoconstriction and susceptibility to high altitude pulmonary oedema. *Thorax* 50:22–27, 1995.)

ejection time (ET) and of the peak velocity of the tricuspid regurgitation jet (TR) were acquired under 3 conditions: normoxia, hyperoxia, and hypoxia.

Findings.—Hypoxia reduced AT/ET by a mean of 0.06 in the control group: 0.11, in the susceptible individuals, and 0.02, in the successful climbers. Hypoxia increased TR by 0.22 m/sec in the controls, 0.56 m/sec in the susceptible individuals, and 0.18 m/sec in the successful climbers. However, only 2 individuals susceptible to high-altitude pulmonary edema and 5 successful climbers had AT/ET, TR measures, or both outside the normal range (Fig 1).

Conclusions.—Individuals with previous high-altitude pulmonary edema have increased pulmonary vascular reactivity to hypoxia. Reactivity is not increased in successful high-altitude climbers. However, echo Doppler estimates of HPV at sea level do not distinguish reliably between susceptible individuals, successful climbers, and a normal control population.

► The sensitivity of the pulmonary vasculature to hypoxia has been recognized as a factor in high-altitude pulmonary edema for a number of years, but most individuals do not want to undergo cardiac catheterization to test their reactions to this stimulus. A variety of Doppler measurements show an encouraging correlation with pulmonary arterial pressures on a group basis, but like so many laboratory tests, the distinction between normal and pathologic groups is unfortunately not consistent enough to allow a reliable diagnosis of excessive susceptibility to hypoxia in the individual. Much of the problem probably relates to interindividual and interlaboratory differences in the Doppler sampling site, and it remains possible that future work may allow a better standardization of measurement variables using this equipment.

In individuals who have had repeated exposure to high altitudes, there may be anatomical changes as well as the acute physiologic spasm of the pulmonary vessels that is induced by the low oxygen pressures, and in such individuals the hypertension is not corrected by administration of oxygen.[1] The functional importance of minimizing the increase of pulmonary arterial pressure is suggested because the Tibetans, the world's best climbers, show minimal vascular reactivity to hypoxia.[2]

R.J. Shephard, M.D., Ph.D., D.P.E.

References

1. Hultgren HN, Grover RF, Hartley LH: Abnormal circulatory responses to high altitude in subjects with a previous history of high-altitude pulmonary edema. *Circulation* 44:759–770, 1971.
2. Groves BM, Droma T, Sutton JR, et al: Minimal hypoxic pulmonary hypertension in normal Tibetans at 3658 m. *J Appl Physiol* 74:312–318, 1993.

The Effect of Ambient Temperature on the Shoe-surface Interface Release Coefficient

Torg JS, Stilwell G, Rogers K (Univ of Pennsylvania, Philadelphia)
Am J Sports Med 24:79–82, 1996 9–29

Background.—Foot contact with the playing surface is known to be a possible element in the etiology of sports-related knee injuries. Past researchers have studied the correlations between shoe-surface interface and cleat length, configuration, and material composition as well as turf type and surface conditions. The effect of temperature on the rotational torsion resistance of artificial turf football shoes was investigated.

Methods.—Five models of football shoes were investigated on dry AstroTurf at 5 temperatures, ranging from 52°F to 110°F. These included a flat-soled basketball-style turf shoe, a natural grass soccer-style shoe, and 3 multistudded turf shoes. The force necessary to release a shoe from the turf surface was determined using an assay device—a prosthetic foot mounted on a loaded stainless-steel shaft. A torque wrench was used to apply a rotational force to pivot each shoe counterclockwise through an arc of 60 degrees.

Findings.—Release coefficients differed within and among the shoe models at the different turf temperatures. An increase in turf temperature combined with cleat characteristics affected shoe-surface interface friction, which could put the athlete's knee and ankle at a risk of injury.

Conclusions.—The flat-soled, basketball-style shoes are the only shoes that can be designated safe or probably safe at all 5 turf temperatures tested. Further research is needed to correlate shoe-surface interface data with the occurrence of lower extremity injuries in certain playing conditions before shoe sole parameters can be recommended definitively. Soft rubber sole shoes on warm AstroTurf may pose a risk.

▶ Torg and Quedenfeld initially reported on the effect of shoe type and cleat length on the incidence and severity of knee injuries among high school football players in 1971.[1] In a subsequent study, Torg et al. correlated the frictional relationship between football shoes and surfaces with the clinical observations.[2] Over the subsequent 25 years, even though 1,250,000 youngsters participate in tackle football in the United States, no credible effort has been made by others to either substantiate or refute the observations that shoe material and configuration contribute to knee and ankle injury risk. This more recent study emphasizes the role of environment and equipment on injury risk.

J.S. Torg, M.D.

References

1. Torg JS, Quedenfeld TC: Effect of shoe type and cleat length on incidence and severity of knee injuries among high school football players. *Res Q Exerc Sport* 42:203–211, 1971.
2. Torg JS, Quedenfeld TC, Landau S: The shoe-surface interface and its relationship to football knee injuries, *Am J Sports Med* 2:261–269, 1974.

Cystic Fibrosis Presenting as Hyponatraemic Heat Exhaustion

Smith HR, Dhatt GS, Melia WMA, Dickinson JG (Queen Elizabeth Military Hosp, London; Princess Mary Hosp, Akrotiri, Cyprus)

BMJ 310:579–580, 1995 9–30

Introduction.—Cystic fibrosis is diagnosed late in some patients, and the disease can have atypical features in such cases. One patient received a diagnosis of cystic fibrosis at age 24 years after several episodes of heat exhaustion.

Case Report.—Man, 24, an infantryman in the armed forces of the United Kingdom, was referred for evaluation. In temperate climates he was able to perform his duties, which involved strenuous physical activity, but he experienced episodes of heat exhaustion twice—in Saudi Arabia during 1991 and in Cyprus during 1993. Ten days after his arrival in Cyprus, the patient was admitted to the hospital with nausea, muscle cramps, and dizziness. He recovered within 24 hours after treatment with IV saline. Further evaluation, including assessment of sweat electrolyte concentrations, was ordered. Clinical examination was normal, as were extensive biochemical, hematologic, and endocrine investigations. The patient was azoospermic and had a family history of infertility.

Pilocarpine induced iontophoresis was carried out twice. The second time yielded a sweat sodium concentration of 103 mmol/L and a sweat chloride concentration of 143 mmol/L. Genetic testing for cystic fibrosis revealed that the patient carried the ΔF508 and R117H mutations. His lungs and pancreas were functioning normally at this time.

Discussion.—This case appears to be the first in which an adult received a diagnosis of cystic fibrosis after experiencing hyponatremic heat exhaustion. The diagnosis was confirmed by sodium and chloride concentrations in sweat and by genotyping. The genotype identified in this case is associated with older age when symptoms appeared and normally functioning lungs and pancreas. This patient has been restricted to service in temperate climates and will be followed up for signs of lung disease. A history of heat exhaustion and hyponatremia may signal an underlying diagnosis of cystic fibrosis.

▶ The sports physician usually conceives of cystic fibrosis in terms of the respiratory problems that are encountered during exercise, but this article by Smith et al. provides a useful reminder to be watchful also for hyponatremic heat exhaustion as a possible initial symptom. Because the sweat has a very high sodium content in cystic fibrosis, heat exposure can cause massive sodium loss, and if hot conditions are encountered over several weeks (as in an overseas service posting), hyponatremia becomes sufficient to cause vascular collapse. Heterozygotic forms of the disease are typically free of pulmonary problems and are thus particularly likely to be seen in this way.

R.J. Shephard, M.D., Ph.D., D.P.E.

Exercise in the Heat: Strategies to Minimize the Adverse Effects on Performance

Terrados N, Maughan RJ (Sabino Alvarez Jendin, Aviles, Spain; Univ of Aberdeen, Scotland)

J Sports Sci 13:55S–62S, 1995 9–31

Introduction.—It is widely recognized that heat adversely affects the mental and physical performance of athletes.

Objectives.—The pathophysiology of heat-induced adverse effects and their consequences on athletic performance were reviewed. Strategies to prevent, minimize, and treat these effects were investigated.

Discussion.—It is well known that heat and high humidity increase the potential for dehydration and hyperthermia during exercise. As the duration of the exercise and the exposure to these factors increase, the effects become more pronounced. Even mild dehydration will significantly impair performance, especially in endurance events, and severe dehydration may be fatal.

The development of rehydration and heat-acclimatization programs are essential in the prevention and treatment of the effects of heat and for optimal performance, especially for athletes living in a temperate climate. However, evidence shows that most athletes do not drink enough fluid during an athletic event or exercise to offset fluid losses. The thirst mechanism is relatively insensitive to fluid needs. A loss of as much as 2% of body weight may occur before a conscious awareness of the need for fluid.

Daily weight recording is valuable in monitoring intake. Increasing beverage palatability may foster fluid intake, but a conscious effort to increase fluid intake is the most effective measure and should be included in every training program. Studies have shown that rehydration is effective if sodium loss in sweat is replaced. However, salt tablets are rarely necessary, because an effective rehydration fluid will replace the sodium and thus maintain the thirst mechanism and promote retention of ingested fluid. Acclimatization is the second factor essential in combatting the effects of heat, and has been shown to reduce some of the pathophysiologic changes induced by heat. These include effects on heart rate, body temperature, blood lactate accumulation, and blood glucose concentration. The need for carbohydrate loading before an endurance event seems to be reduced by acclimatization. Numerous studies have shown that acclimatization attained by exercising in the heat will improve the thermoregulatory response during exercise. Acclimatization may actually increase fluid needs by fostering an earlier onset of sweating and a greater rate of sweating. It has been demonstrated that there is no adaptability to dehydration even by acclimatization, and if dehydration is allowed to occur, heat acclimatization will decrease and actually be lost.

Conclusions.—Rehydration and acclimatization are essential measures for preventing and correcting the pathophysiologic changes and the adverse effects on athletic performance produced by heat. Acclimatization to heat does not diminish the need for rehydration, but it actually increases fluid needs by inducing and earlier and enhanced sweat response. Strategies for rehydration and acclimatization should be incorporated into all training programs, especially those requiring endurance and those for athletes residing in temperate climates.

► This excellent article should be read with Abstract 9–32, along with the corresponding comments. The authors have narrowed the problem down to 2 major factors: rehydration and acclimatization. If an athlete is acclimated to working in high heat and humidity and is rehydrated properly, heat exhaustion should be avoided. Full acclimatization may take 14 days or more.

There are days when the heat and humidity are so high [wet bulb reading between 18°C to 23°C (65°F to 74°F)] that workout time should be decreased and adjusted or times of contests changed to earlier or later in the day, or even postponed [if the wet bulb reading is above 23°C (75°F)]. In team sports, frequently substituting athletes also can help avoid this problem.

F.J. George, A.T.C., P.T.

Heatstroke and Other Heat-related Illnesses: The Maladies of Summer
Lee-Chiong TL Jr, Stitt JT (Yale Univ, New Haven, Conn)
Postgrad Med 98:26–28,31–33,36, 1995 9–32

Background.—Heat-related illnesses, responsible for some 4,000 deaths yearly in the United States, range in severity from minor disorders, such as heat syncope, to severe, potentially life-threatening heat exhaustion and heatstroke. The various heat-related illnesses and their therapy were investigated.

Discussion.—Heat exhaustion results from plasma fluid depletion during exertion in a hot, humid environment. General symptoms, such as malaise, headache, weakness, and vomiting, occur. Neurologic symptoms are rare. The body core temperature exceeds 38°C (100.4°F) but is below 40°C (104°F). Treatment involves rest in a cool environment and repletion of fluid and electrolyte losses, with hospitalization for more severe cases.

Heatstroke is an extreme example of heat exhaustion, with body core temperature above 40°C, severe neurologic effects, such as delirium and seizures, and the potential for organ damage, cardiovascular collapse, and death. Classic heatstroke affects elderly, intoxicated, and debilitated patients, often after little exertion. Exertional heatstroke follows heavy exertion in such groups as athletes, military recruits, and unacclimatized laborers. Metabolic acidosis, myoglobinuria, acute renal tubular necrosis, and hemorrhagic diatheses may occur. Therapy involves immediate and aggressive cooling of the body with wet dressings and air convection and, in severe hyperthermia, cold water gastric or rectal irrigation, peritoneal lavage, and cardiopulmonary bypass. Antipyretics are of no benefit. Prevention involves avoidance of excessive activity and attention to oral fluid intake and ambient cooling.

Milder heat-related illnesses include heat edema, heat cramps, and heat syncope. Therapy is directed at decreasing pooling of blood and replacing fluid and electrolytes.

Conclusions.—Heat-related illnesses vary in severity, but they may be fatal. If avoidance fails, patients with heatstroke should receive aggressive cooling, fluid and electrolyte repletion, and prompt correction of any associated complications.

► With common sense, most heat-related problems in athletes could be avoided. Careful attention should be paid to the heat and humidity index, the time of day that the contest or practice will take place, the level of the athlete's hydration and rehydration, and the knowledge that thirst is a poor indicator of dehydration. The level of the athlete's acclimatization to heat and humidity is very, very important. E.R. Eichner's commentary in the 1995 YEAR BOOK OF SPORTS MEDICINE,[1] a study of heat exhaustion by Lyle et al.,[2] stated that there are 4 major risk factors of heat exhaustion: "1) History of heat exhaustion, 2) urge to improve, 3) not acclimatizing, and 4) not drinking fluids during the race." This study should be read with Abstract 9–31.

F.J. George, A.T.C., P.T.

References

1. 1995 YEAR BOOK OF SPORTS MEDICINE, pp 281–282.
2. Lyle DM, Lewis PR, Richards DA, et al: Heat exhaustion in the Sun-Herald City to Surf Fun Run. *Med J Aust* 161:361–365, 1994.

Subject Index*

A

* *All entries refer to the year and page number(s) for data appearing in this and the previous edition of the* Year Book.

B

C

D

F

G

H

L

M

O

P

T

U

X

Author Index

A

B

C

D

E

F

G

H

I

J

K

L

M

N

O

P

Q

R

S

T

U

V

W

X

Y

Z